Moderate Procedural Sedation *and* Analgesia

A QUESTION AND ANSWER APPROACH

Moderate Procedural Sedation and Analgesia

A QUESTION AND ANSWER APPROACH

Michael Kost, DNP, CRNA, CHSE

Director
Healthcare Simulation, Einstein Healthcare Network
Philadelphia, Pennsylvania

Director
Frank J. Tornetta School of Anesthesia, Einstein Medical Center
Montgomery, East Norriton, Pennsylvania

Associate Clinical Professor
La Salle University School of Nursing, Philadelphia, Pennsylvania

ELSEVIER

MODERATE PROCEDURAL SEDATION AND ANALGESIA:
A QUESTION AND ANSWER APPROACH,
FIRST EDITION

ISBN: 978-0-323-59769-2

Notice

Practitioners and researchers must always rely on their own experience and knowledge in evaluating and using any information, methods, compounds, or experiments described herein. Because of rapid advances in the medical sciences—in particular, independent verification of diagnoses and drug dosages—should be made. To the fullest extent of the law, no responsibility is assumed by Elsevier, authors, editors, or contributors for any injury and/or damage to persons or property as a matter of products liability, negligence or otherwise, or from any use or operation of any methods, products, instructions, or ideas contained in the material herein.

Library of Congress Control Number: 2019934901

Executive Content Strategist: Kellie White/Sonya Seigafuse
Content Development Manager: Lisa P. Newton
Senior Content Development Specialist: Tina Kaemmerer
Publishing Services Manager: Deepthi Unni
Senior Project Manager: Manchu Mohan
Designer: Maggie Reid

Printed in the United States of America.
Last digit is the print number: 9 8 7 6 5 4 3 2 1

3251 Riverport Lane
St. Louis, Missouri 63043

Working together
to grow libraries in
developing countries

www.elsevier.com • www.bookaid.org

To
My wonderful wife and best friend, Nancy
for her continued support, encouragement, and understanding …
and
**my mentors, Dr. Gerry Cousounis, Dr. Stu Toledano, and
Dr. Frank Tornetta**
for their profound impact and sage advice …
and
our next generation, Will, Tyler, Molly, Ella, and Emmie
for being the loving reminders of why we're really here …

Michael Kost, DNP, CRNA, CHSE, is the Director of the Frank J. Tornetta School of Anesthesia at Einstein Medical Center Montgomery/La Salle University School of Nursing and Health Sciences and Director of Healthcare Simulation for Einstein Healthcare Network, Philadelphia, Pennsylvania. He is a clinical associate professor at La Salle University School of Nursing and Health Sciences. He received his bachelor of science in nursing from Widener University, Chester, Pennsylvania, CRNA certificate from the Montgomery Hospital School of Anesthesia, and a master of science in anesthesia from Saint Joseph's University, Philadelphia, Pennsylvania. He received his master of science in nursing as a clinical specialist in gerontology from Gwynedd Mercy College, Gwynedd Valley, Pennsylvania and a post-masters certificate in nursing education from La Salle University School of Nursing and Health Sciences. His doctorate in nursing practice was completed at the University of Medicine and Dentistry of New Jersey, Newark, New Jersey. For over three decades he has presented nationally on a wide variety of sedation, ambulatory care, anesthesia, perioperative, and perianesthesia topics. In addition, he is an active member of the International Society for Simulation in Healthcare and is a certified health care simulation educator.

His first text on conscious sedation (**Manual of Conscious Sedation**) was published by W. B. Saunders Co., in 1998 and received *'Book of the Year'* honors from the American Nurses Association in both critical care and emergency nursing. His second text on moderate sedation (**Moderate Sedation/Analgesia, Core Competencies for Practice, 2nd edition**) was published by Elsevier in 2004. His latest edition (**Moderate Procedural Sedation and Analgesia: A Question and Answer Approach**) is his latest contribution to the field of moderate sedation and procedural analgesia.

Ron Eslinger, RN, CRNA, MA, APN, BCH, CMI, FNGH
Captain, USN, Retired
CEO, Healthy Visions
Clinton, Tennessee

John O'Donnell, DrPH, CRNA, CHSE, FSSH
Professor and Chair, Department of Nurse Anesthesia
Director, Nurse Anesthesia Program;
Associate Director
The Peter M. Winter Institute for Simulation Education and
    Research
University of Pittsburgh
Pittsburgh, Pennsylvania

Robert W. Simon, CRNA, DNP, MS
Staff Nurse Anesthetist
Holy Redeemer Hospital
Meadowbrook, Pennsylvania

Janice Beitz, PhD, RN, CS, CNOR, CWOCN-AP, CRNP, APNC, MAPWCA, ANEF, FAAN
Professor, School of Nursing-Camden
Director, Wound, Ostomy Continence Nursing (WOCNEP)
Rutgers University, Camden, New Jersey

John O'Donnell, DrPH, CRNA, CHSE, FSSH
Professor and Chair, Department of Nurse Anesthesia
Director, Nurse Anesthesia Program;
Associate Director, The Peter M. Winter Institute for
  Simulation Education and Research
University of Pittsburgh
Pittsburgh, Pennsylvania

PREFACE

"The error of one moment becomes the sorrow of a whole life."

Chinese proverb

The administration of moderate procedural sedation and analgesia has become common practice in a variety of clinical settings. The increased use of sedative, hypnotic, analgesic, and, in some cases, anesthetic medications in remote clinical settings has increased the demand for highly educated, clinically competent nonanesthesia sedation providers. This text focuses on the preprocedural, procedural, and postprocedural aspects of procedural sedation and analgesia patient care. Its comprehensive format is designed to function as an educational resource tool featuring best clinical practice modalities and a means for periodic self-evaluation. *Moderate Procedural Sedation and Analgesia: A Question and Answer Approach* provides a practical guide for clinicians in a wide variety of sedation settings.

This text provides a succinct question and answer format focused on patient safety in the sedation setting. The first two chapters address presedation patient care issues. Chapter 1 focuses on scope of practice and legal and regulatory issues for the sedation provider. Chapter 2 combines comprehensive presedation patient assessment strategies related to organ systems, pathophysiologic disease processes, recommended treatment strategies, and appropriate patient selection strategies.

The next nine chapters feature the comprehensive aspects related to safe sedation patient care. The administration of sedative, hypnotic, and analgesic medications requires a thorough understanding of the pharmacokinetic and pharmacodynamic effects of each medication. Chapters 3, 4, and 5 provide the reader with a review of pharmacologic concepts, medication classifications, techniques of administration, and specific sedative and analgesic medication pharmacologic profiles. Chapter 6, by Ron Eslinger, is an insightful chapter on verbal and nonverbal techniques to enhance pharmacologic sedation.

Airway and respiratory complications associated with moderate procedural sedation and analgesia are featured in Chapter 7. A comprehensive review of airway anatomy, airway evaluation, and emergency airway management strategies provides the reader with a systematic approach to crisis management in the event of respiratory depression or arrest in the sedation setting. Monitoring modalities and intravenous insertion techniques are presented and richly illustrated in Chapters 8 and 9. Sedation considerations for the geriatric patient are comprehensively presented in Chapter 10. Pediatric patient care considerations are featured in Chapter 11, by Robert Simon.

Chapter 12 encompasses the postsedation aspects of patient care, documentation, discharge planning, and recovery scoring mechanisms. The simulation strategies to enhance patient safety in the sedation setting featured in Chapter 13, by John O'Donnell, present insightful opportunities to introduce sedation simulation education and risk management strategies into all sedation patient care areas. The reader is presented with the opportunity to complete a gap analysis by completing an "Unfolding Sedation Clinical Case Study," which compares his or her performance with detailed rationales featured at the end of Chapter 14. The text appendices were carefully selected and include Answers to Chapter Review Questions and important content from the Association of Operating Room Nurses and American Society of Anesthesiologists. These complement a variety of aspects associated with sedation patient care.

Each patient care chapter features a "Patient Safety SBAR Focus" box focusing on specific clinical situations that may be encountered in the sedation setting, with appropriate sedation patient care considerations detailed. Finally, it is my hope that the information presented in this text enriches the student's fundamental knowledge of sedation patient care and ultimately enhances patient safety in all clinical settings where moderate procedural sedation and analgesia are administered.

Michael Kost, DNP, CRNA, CHSE

FOREWORD

"The man who can make hard things easy is the educator."

Ralph Waldo Emerson (1803-1882)

In his latest publication, *Moderate Procedural Sedation and Analgesia: A Question and Answer Approach,* Dr. Michael Kost continues to focus on patient safety in the sedation setting by clearly outlining the process of sedation and analgesia care for nonanesthesia health care providers. This comprehensive text is the definitive resource for all nonanesthesia practitioners working in the rapidly expanding area of moderate procedural sedation and analgesia clinical practice.

In recent years, the administration of moderate procedural sedation and analgesia sedation (procedural sedation) has grown markedly, particularly by moving outside of controlled operating room settings into diverse clinical practice sites. Physicians, nurses, and other health care providers now participate in the moderate sedation process as a primary component of their professional roles. Moderate sedation and analgesia clinical services are now a patient expectation and a valuable diagnostic or therapeutic adjunct for a wide array of tests and therapeutics. Moderate sedation offers the benefits of anxiolysis, amnesia, and analgesia. All nonanesthesia clinicians implementing moderate sedation and analgesia must recognize its associated inherent risks.

Note that the underlying theme of this text continues to focus on patient safety as the first consideration in any sedation situation, and that patient safety depends on preparation of clinicians involved. This core curriculum provides a template for the necessary educational preparation, development of resources, and understanding of the required credentialing and regulatory needs associated with the administration of sedation and analgesia. The text can be used as the cornerstone for sedation and analgesia education and credentialing programs.

Questions regarding training, resources, regulation, policy, procedure, and patient care implementation continue to arise on a daily basis. Kost originally responded to the need for a comprehensive yet practical reference by publishing the *Manual of Conscious Sedation* in 1998. His most recent edition, based on a professional standards approach, is a valuable educational resource for both daily use and as a metric for periodic evaluation. The easily understandable format targets an audience of clinicians who are actually engaged in the administration of sedation and analgesia. The text is also a resource for administrators who are developing sedation policy, procedures, and competency programs and will serve as an educational resource for experienced clinicians and a valuable guide for health care providers who are new to sedation and analgesia practice.

This first edition has several innovative chapters incorporating contemporary processes. A chapter on simulation and patient safety by John O'Donnell describes how technology and clinician practice can augment safe sedation administration. The addition of a chapter on verbal and nonverbal adjuncts by Ron Erslinger enhances clinicians' repertoire of interventions to allay patient anxiety. Pediatric and geriatric chapters offer specific sedation practice recommendations that address the substantive clinical practice challenges associated with these patient populations. These chapters also offer special insight into the specific patient care requirements for safe sedation care because they impart many of the specific skills and knowledge required for sedation secondary to the pharmacokinetic, pharmacodynamic, and developmental and physiologic variations associated with pediatric and geriatric populations. The text emphasizes critical learning outcomes by using postchapter test questions and case studies for reinforcement.

In summary, Dr. Kost has done a superlative job in compiling and writing this definitive resource in the area of sedation practice for use by nonanesthesia health care professionals. Administrators, educators, students, and clinicians will find this text to be a highly valuable resource in approaching the challenges inherent in the administration of safe moderate sedation and analgesia.

Janice M. Beitz, PhD, RN, CS, CNOR, CWOCN-AP, CRNP, APNC, MAPWCA, ANEF, FAAN
Professor, School of Nursing-Camden
Director, Wound, Ostomy Continence Nursing (WOCNEP),
Rutgers University, Camden, New Jersy

CONTENTS

Moderate Procedural Sedation *and* Analgesia:

A QUESTION AND ANSWER APPROACH

Scope of Practice and Legal and Regulatory Considerations for the Sedation Provider

At the completion of this chapter, the learner shall:

- Differentiate the contributing factors that have led to the widespread popularity of moderate procedural sedation and analgesia.
- Categorize common diagnostic, therapeutic, and surgical procedures that require moderate procedural sedation and analgesia.
- Identify the origin of the term *conscious sedation.*
- Compare and contrast the levels of consciousness within the continuum of sedation—minimal sedation, moderate sedation, deep sedation, and general anesthesia.
- Describe the goals and objectives of safe moderate procedural sedation and analgesia patient care.

- State the clinical end points of moderate procedural sedation and analgesia.
- Analyze the potential barriers that might prevent the safe administration of moderate procedural sedation and analgesia.
- Describe the impact of practice standards, practice guidelines, and position statements on the health care provider who is administering moderate procedural sedation and analgesia.
- Identify patient safety issues associated with the administration of the high-alert medication propofol in the sedation setting.

COMPETENCY STATEMENT

The health care provider administering or monitoring the patient receiving moderate procedural sedation and analgesia demonstrates knowledge of scope of practice, licensing and evidence-based policy, and procedure implementation related to sedation care.

What has led to the widespread popularity of the administration of moderate procedural sedation and analgesia?

The administration of sedation for surgical, therapeutic, and diagnostic procedures has gained widespread popularity nationally and internationally over the last several decades.[1-3] Not only has the number of procedures requiring the administration of moderate procedural sedation and analgesia increased, but also the variety of procedures in the therapeutic, diagnostic, and surgical caseload. The rationale for the proliferation of the administration of sedation is varied. Medical technology now allows physicians the ability to treat patients with minimally invasive procedures and techniques in shorter periods of time that no longer confine them to the traditional perioperative environment. In addition, as reimbursement for health care services continues to evolve, a critical review of practice patterns has ensued. As health care continues to focus on efficiency, the administration of moderate procedural sedation and analgesia by nonanesthesia personnel provides a desirable alternative for a multitude of procedures.

The clinical effects associated with moderate procedural sedation and analgesia are widely reported in the literature; these include anxiolysis, analgesia, and amnesia.[4-6] The pharmacologic effectiveness of moderate procedural sedation and analgesia has led to increased use in hospitals, ambulatory care facilities, and physician offices.[7,8] Pharmacologic advances have also contributed to the increased use of moderate procedural sedation and analgesia for specific patient populations. The introduction of intravenous (IV) medications with shorter half-lives, no active metabolites, and minimal cumulative effects has increased the margin of safety and efficacy associated with the administration of sedation.[9,10] Monitoring advances have also had a significant impact on the delivery of sedation and analgesia. The advent of pulse oximetry, which was introduced into clinical practice in the 1980s, has provided clinicians with an additional tool to aid in the diagnosis of hypoxic states. Pulse oximetry technology greatly enhanced the margin of safety associated with the administration of moderate procedural sedation and analgesia.[11] As a result, procedural sedation services continue to expand. Many registered nurses have assumed sedation subspecialty roles in gastroenterology, emergency departments, cardiac catheterization laboratories, operating rooms, fertility clinics, and interventional radiology settings.

What type of procedures would a registered nurse expect to encounter in moderate sedation practice?

The most common diagnostic, therapeutic, and surgical procedures requiring moderate procedural sedation and analgesia are identified in Table 1.1.

TABLE 1.1   Common Procedures Performed Under Moderate Procedural Sedation and Analgesia[a]

Specialty	Type of Procedure
Burns	Débridement
	Dressing changes
Cosmetic surgery	Blepharoplasty
	Breast augmentation
	Chemical peel
	Dermabrasion
	Laser skin enhancement
	Liposuction
	Otoplasty
	Rhinoplasty
	Rhytidectomy
Emergency services	Closed reduction of fracture or dislocation
	Suturing
Extremity procedures	Appliance removal (e.g., pin, screw, wire)
	Carpal tunnel release
	Closed reduction
	Trigger finger release
Gastroenterology	Colonoscopy
	Endoscopic ultrasound
	Endoscopic retrograde cholangiopancreatography (ERCP)
	Gastroscopy
	Liver biopsy
General surgery	Breast biopsy
	Chest tube insertion
	Hernia repair
	Incision and drainage
	Lipoma excision
	Superficial biopsies
Gynecology	Dilation and curettage (D&C)
	Dilation and evacuation (D&E)
	Cone biopsy
	Hysteroscopy
	Incision and drainage
	In vitro fertilization
	Lesion fulguration
Ophthalmology	Blepharoplasty
	Cataract extraction
	Lens implantation
Oral surgery	Dental caries
	Odontectomy
	Periodontal
Orthopedic	Arthroscopy
	Closed fracture reduction
	Hand surgery
	Joint manipulation
Pulmonology	Bronchoscopy
	Endotracheal intubation
	Chest tube insertion
Radiology	Arteriography
	Computed tomography scan
	Embolization
	Interventional radiology procedures
	Localization and biopsy
	Magnetic resonance imaging
Urology	Cystoscopy
	Lithotripsy

Continued

TABLE 1.1   Common Procedures Performed Under Moderate Procedural Sedation and Analgesia—cont'd

Specialty	Type of Procedure
	Vasectomy
Vascular	Angioplasty
	Cardiac catheterization
	Cardioversion
	Defibrillator insertion
	Electrophysiologic testing
	Hemodialysis access
	Invasive line insertion
	Pacemaker insertion
	Radiofrequency ablation
	Transesophageal echo
	Vascular access

[a]This is not an all-inclusive list.

Who first described conscious sedation in the literature?

In *Conscious Sedation in Dental Practice*, CR Bennett defined the term *conscious sedation*. Dr. Bennett was the first to present information related to the administration of IV sedative medications in conjunction with local anesthetics to produce a favorable operative area accompanied by intact protective airway reflexes and a minimally depressed level of consciousness.[12]

When was the term *conscious sedation* changed to *moderate sedation*?

The term *conscious sedation* was first identified in the dental literature and used for more than 2 decades. In 2002, the American Society of Anesthesiologists (ASA) published updated sedation guidelines.[13] That respective practice guideline terminology replaced the word *light sedation* with *minimal sedation* and replaced *conscious sedation* with *moderate sedation* to address differences that occur with the continuum of sedation that occurs in actual clinical practice. After the release of the 2002 ASA sedation practice guidelines, many authors and publications started to use the terms *moderate sedation, procedural sedation,* and *conscious sedation* interchangeably.[14]

Has the American Society of Anesthesiologists recently updated their sedation practice guidelines?

In October 2014, the ASA Committee on Standards and Practice Parameters recommended that new practice guidelines addressing moderate procedural sedation and analgesia be developed. In March 2018, updated guidelines were published in the journal *Anesthesiology*.[15] These new guidelines were developed by a multidisciplinary task force of physicians from several medical and dental specialty organizations and specifically address moderate procedural sedation provided by any medical specialty in any location. The updated guidelines include new recommendations that address the following:

- Patient evaluation and preparation
- Continual monitoring of ventilatory function with capnography to supplement standard monitoring by observation and pulse oximetry

- The presence of an individual in the procedure room with the knowledge and skills to recognize and treat airway complications
- Sedatives and analgesics not intended for general anesthesia (e.g., benzodiazepines, dexmedetomidine)
- Sedatives and analgesics intended for general anesthesia (e.g., propofol, ketamine, etomidate)
- Recovery care
- Creation and implementation of quality improvement processes

What is meant by the term *continuum of sedation*?

It is important for the health care practitioner providing sedation services to recognize that anxiolysis, sedation, and analgesia occur on a continuum. The continuum occurs because each patient's responses to sedative and analgesic medications vary based on the medication administered, dosage, technique of administration, and presence of concomitant disease states. The continuum of sedation and analgesia consists of four levels. Fig. 1.1 outlines the ASA's continuum of depth of Sedation and four defined levels of sedation and anesthesia, which include:

Minimal Sedation (Anxiolysis). This is a drug-induced state during which patients respond normally to verbal commands. Although cognitive function and physical coordination may be impaired, airway reflexes and ventilatory and cardiovascular functions are unaffected.

Moderate Sedation or Analgesia. This is a drug-induced depression of consciousness during which patients respond purposefully to verbal commands, either alone or accompanied by light tactile stimulation. No interventions are required to maintain a patent airway, and spontaneous ventilation is adequate. Cardiovascular function is usually maintained.

Note that reflex withdrawal from a painful stimulus is not considered a purposeful response.

Deep Sedation or Analgesia. This is a drug-induced depression of consciousness during which patients cannot be easily aroused but respond purposefully following repeated or painful stimulation. The ability to maintain ventilatory function independently may be impaired. Patients may require assistance in maintaining a patent airway, and spontaneous ventilation may be inadequate. Cardiovascular function is usually maintained.

Note that reflex withdrawal from a painful stimulus is not considered a purposeful response.

General Anesthesia. This is a drug-induced loss of consciousness during which patients are not arousable, even by painful stimulation. The ability to maintain ventilatory function independently is often impaired. Patients often require assistance in maintaining a patent airway, and positive pressure ventilation may be required because of depressed spontaneous ventilation or drug-induced depression of neuromuscular function. Cardiovascular function may be impaired.

Because sedation is a continuum, it is not always possible to predict how an individual will respond. Therefore, practitioners intending to produce a specific level of sedation must be able to rescue patients whose level of sedation becomes deeper than initially intended. Individuals administering moderate sedation/analgesia should be able to rescue patients

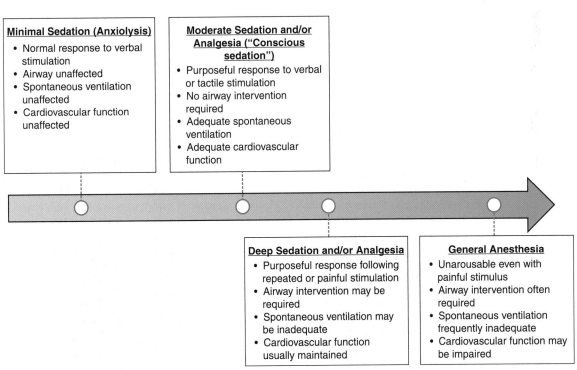

Fig. 1.1 Depth of sedation. (Adapted from the American Society of Anesthesiologists. Continuum of depth of sedation: Definition of general anesthesia and levels of sedation/analgesia. http://www.asahq.org/~/media/Sites/ASAHQ/Files/Public/Resources/standards-guidelines/continuum-of-depth-of-sedation-definition-of-general-anesthesia-and-levels-of-sedation-analgesia.pdf.)

who enter a state of deep sedation or analgesia; those administering deep sedation or analgesia should be able to rescue patients who enter a state of general anesthesia.

As noted earlier, reflex withdrawal from a painful stimulus is not considered a purposeful response.

Rescue of a patient from a deeper level of sedation than intended is an intervention by a practitioner proficient in airway management and advanced life support. The qualified practitioner corrects adverse physiologic consequences of the deeper-than-intended level of sedation (such as hypoventilation, hypoxia, and hypotension) and returns the patient to the originally intended level of sedation. It is not appropriate to continue the procedure at an unintended level of sedation.[16]

Is there a more succinct manner by which to assess the continuum of sedation?

The continuum of sedation progresses from a state of minimal sedation to general anesthesia. Changes in patient responsiveness, airway status, ventilatory status, and cardiovascular function are summarized in Table 1.2.[16]

What are the goals and objectives of moderate procedural sedation and analgesia?

The goals of moderate procedural sedation and analgesia may vary based on procedural requirements, prescribing physician preference, and the sedation technique selected. Regardless of the variables outlined above, the primary goal of moderate procedural sedation and analgesia includes administering the lowest dose of medication to achieve the following[17]:

- Maintain patient safety and welfare.
- Minimize physical pain and discomfort.
- Control anxiety, minimize psychological trauma, and maximize amnesia.
- Control behavior and movement to allow safe performance of procedures.

Patient response to the administration of sedative and analgesic medications is dependent on the total dose of medication administered, speed of injection, supplemental doses administered, patient circulatory time, and associated physiologic comorbidities. Varied patient response or the overzealous administration of sedation and analgesic medications, known as *stacking*, may result in a state of deep sedation or general anesthesia. Deep sedation or general anesthesia predisposes the patient to an increased incidence of respiratory depression, decreased response to the hypoxic drive, and the potential for cardiovascular depression. It is critically important that all moderate procedural sedation and analgesia health care practitioners recognize that unresponsiveness and unconsciousness are not the objectives of moderate sedation. Sedative techniques that prevent pharmacologic stacking are discussed in Chapter 5, "Pharmacologic Profiles: Moderate Procedural Sedation and Analgesia Medications."

What side effects are associated with moderate procedural sedation and analgesic medication administration?

Pharmacologic medications administered to achieve a sedate, amnestic, and analgesic state include the following categories and actions:

- Benzodiazepines produce amnesia and anxiolysis.
- Opioids and dissociative agents produce profound analgesia.
- Sedative-hypnotic medications produce hypnosis and sedation.

Combinations of carefully titrated sedative and analgesic medications allow the health care provider the ability to perform therapeutic, diagnostic, and minor surgical procedures with the patient in an altered level of consciousness. The combination of benzodiazepines, opioids, and

TABLE 1.2   Continuum of Depth of Sedation

Definition of General Anesthesia and Levels of Sedation and Analgesia[a]

Parameter	Minimal Sedation Anxiolysis	Moderate Sedation and Analgesia (Conscious Sedation)	Deep Sedation and Analgesia	General Anesthesia
Responsiveness	Normal response to verbal stimulation	Purposeful response[b] to verbal or tactile stimulation	Purposeful response[b] following repeated or painful stimulation	Unarousable, even with painful stimulus
Airway	Unaffected	No intervention required	Intervention may be required	Intervention often required
Spontaneous ventilation	Unaffected	Adequate	May be inadequate	Frequently inadequate
Cardiovascular function	Unaffected	Usually maintained	Usually maintained	May be impaired

[a]Monitored anesthesia care (MAC) does not describe the continuum of depth of sedation; rather, it describes "a specific anesthesia service in which an anesthesiologist has been requested to participate in the care of a patient undergoing a diagnostic or therapeutic procedure."
[b]Reflex withdrawal from a painful stimulus is not considered a purposeful response.
Adapted from American Society of Anesthesiologists. Continuum of depth of sedation: Definition of general anesthesia and levels of sedation/analgesia. http://www.asahq.org/~/media/Sites/ASAHQ/Files/Public/Resources/standards-guidelines/continuum-of-depth-of-sedation-definition-of-general-anesthesia-and-levels-of-sedation-analgesia.pdf.

sedative-hypnotic agents may produce profound synergistic effects. These synergistic effects may lead to a state of deep sedation or general anesthesia. As early as 1990, Bailey reported more than 80 deaths directly attributed to the administration of conscious sedation with benzodiazepines when combined with an opioid.[18] Decades later, adverse events associated with moderate procedural sedation and analgesia continue to be reported in the literature. Karamnov et al.[19] have reported that the most common adverse events and unplanned interventions during adult moderate procedural sedation include oversedation leading to apnea and the use of reversal agents. Oversedation, hypoxemia, reversal agent use, and prolonged bag-mask ventilation were most common in cardiology and gastroenterology suites. Miscommunication related to sedation was reported most frequently in the emergency department and on the inpatient floor.

To prevent adverse events or the development of an unconscious state during diagnostic or therapeutic procedures, it is important to understand the pharmacokinetic and pharmacodynamic profile of each sedative, hypnotic, and analgesic agent used to produce sedation. The clinician must also appreciate the potency and synergistic action of combined medications used during procedural patient care and must possess the requisite airway management competencies to support an obstructed airway and pharmacologic knowledge to reverse a patient immediately from deep sedation or general anesthetic states.

I have heard conflicting opinions from my colleagues with regard to how our procedure unit manages patients receiving moderate procedural sedation and analgesia. What are the differences among practice standards, practice guidelines, and position statements?

Scope of practice issues associated with the administration of moderate procedural sedation and analgesia include practice standards, practice guidelines, and position statements promulgated by professional organizations related to the administration of sedation. Practice standards are the highest mandate for clinical behavior. A standard represents behaviors that must be exercised by the practitioner. Standards allow for little variation in performance behavior that cannot be justified by a clear and compelling rationale. Practice standards related to sedation administration include those presented by The Joint Commission[20]; notes the following:

> The hospital plans operative or other high-risk procedures, including those that require the administration of moderate or deep sedation or anesthesia…. The standards for sedation and anesthesia care apply when patients in any setting receive, for any purpose, by any route:
> General, spinal, or other major regional anesthesia

> Moderate or deep sedation (with or without analgesia) that, in the manner used, may be expected to result in the loss of protective reflexes

Clinical Practice Guidelines. These are statements that include recommendations intended to optimize patient care that are informed by a systematic review of evidence and an assessment of the benefits and harms of alternative care options.[21] Practice guidelines are intended to reduce inappropriate variations in clinical care, minimize harm, promote cost-effective practice, and produce optimal health outcomes for patients.[22] Clinical practice guidelines promulgated by the ASA on moderate procedural sedation and analgesia patient care have been published[15]; a summary of the ASA practice guidelines is provided in Appendix B.

Position Statements. These use less forceful criteria than practice guidelines or standards. They generally represent emerging trends on a given topic, address economically driven practice modalities, or discuss procedural policies. In January 2016, the Association for Radiologic and Imaging Nursing issued a position statement endorsing the routine use of capnography for all patients receiving moderate procedural sedation and analgesia during procedures in the imaging environment. Their position statement also affirmed that the administration of moderate procedural sedation remains a critical component of the radiologic and imaging nurses' scope of practice.

In 2009, the American Society for Gastroenterological Endoscopy (ASGE) issued a position statement on nonanesthesiologist administration of propofol for gastrointestinal (GI) endoscopy. In this statement, the ASGE addressed the requirements for propofol administration by nonanesthesiologist physicians and registered nurses, focusing on specific training guidelines that included didactic training sessions, airway workshops, simulation training, and preceptorships.[23] A list of professional organizations that promulgate guidelines and position statements related to the administration of sedation is provided in Table 1.3.

TABLE 1.3 Guidelines and Position Statements on Moderate Procedural Sedation and Analgesia

Professional Organization	Website
Accreditation Association for Ambulatory Health Care, Inc.	www.aaahc.org
American Academy of Pediatrics	www.aap.org
American Academy of Pediatric Dentistry	www.aapd.org
American Association of Critical Care Nurses	www.aacn.org
American Association for Study of Liver Diseases	www.aasld.org
American Association of Moderate Sedation Nurses	www.aamsn.org

Continued

TABLE 1.3 Guidelines and Position Statements on Moderate Procedural Sedation and Analgesia—cont'd

Professional Organization	Website
American Association of Nurse Anesthetists	www.aana.com
American Association of Oral and Maxillofacial Surgeons	www.aaoms.org
American College of Cardiology	www.acc.org
American College of Emergency Physicians	www.acep.org
American College of Gastroenterology	www.gi.org
American College of Radiology	www.acr.org
American Dental Association	www.ada.org
American Gastroenterology Association	www.gastro.org
American Nurses Association	www.nursingworld.org
American Society for Gastrointestinal Endoscopy	www.asge.org
Society of Interventional Radiology	www.sirweb.org
American Society of Anesthesiologists	www.asahq.org
Association of Perioperative Registered Nurses	www.aorn.org
Association for Radiologic & Imaging Nurses	www.arinursing.org
Society for Gastroenterology Nurses and Associates	www.sgna.org
Society of Critical Care Medicine	www.sccm.org
Society for Pediatric Sedation	www.pedsedation.org
The Joint Commission	www.jointcommission.org

After reviewing multiple practice standards, practice guidelines, position statements, and consensus statements related to health care providers administering moderate procedural sedation, it becomes evident that there is significant variation among organizations, so where does this leave me legally, particularly with my state board of nursing?

Legal scope of practice issues related to nursing are delegated and administered through state boards of nursing. Individual state statutes define the practice of nursing. As registered nurses have become more involved historically in the administration of moderate procedural sedation and analgesia, scope of practice issues have been raised in many states.

In the late 1980s, the demand for registered nurses to participate in the administration of conscious sedation procedures and the monitoring of patients receiving these services increased dramatically.[24] In response, registered nurses concerned with legal scope of practice issues contacted their individual state boards of nursing to inquire about the conscious sedation practice patterns that were being developed in their institutions. At that time, responses from state boards of nursing varied in their position regarding the administration of sedation and the monitoring of patients receiving it. Some state boards adopted formal position or policy statements that specifically delineated the responsibility of professional registered nurses engaged in the administration of sedation. Many state boards of nursing have enacted formal policy statements that define and identify prescriptive responsibilities and requirements of the registered nurse participating in the administration of sedation services. However, some state boards of nursing have not taken formal action on the issue. A few select state boards of nursing do not have statutory authority to enact such legislation. Registered nurses must take the initiative to familiarize themselves with their individual state board of nursing requirements related to moderate procedural sedation and analgesia patient care (e.g., Advanced Cardiac Life Support [ACLS] course completion, patient monitoring requirements, airway management competency, appropriate credentialing for rescuing deeply sedated patients). Laws by state related to the administration of moderate procedural sedation and analgesia for registered nurses may be reviewed at the following websites: https://sedationcertification.com/resources/position-statements/position-statements-by-state/clickable-map[25] and http://www.sedationconsulting.com/laws-by-state.[26]

Box 1.1 features the North Carolina Board of Nursing position statement.[27] This example of a state board of nursing position statement related to the administration of moderate procedural sedation and analgesia by registered nurses offers clearly defined expectations of the registered nurse who is providing sedation services.

Clinical practice standards, guidelines, and position statements form the basis for hospital policy development; however, clinical staff members have continued to demonstrate confusion secondary to inconsistency in many of the

BOX 1.1 North Carolina Board of Nursing Position Statement

Procedural Sedation and Analgesia: Position Statement for RN Practice

A position statement does not carry the force and effect of law and rules but is adopted by the board as a means of providing direction to licensees who seek to engage in safe nursing practice. Board position statements address issues of concern to the board relevant to the protection of the public and are reviewed regularly for relevance and accuracy to current practice, the Nursing Practice Act, and board administrative code rules.

Issue

The administration of sedative, analgesic, and anesthetic pharmacologic agents, for the purpose of moderate or deep procedural sedation and analgesia, to nonintubated clients undergoing therapeutic, diagnostic, and surgical procedures, is within the nonanesthetist Registered Nurse (RN) scope of practice.

The administration of pharmacologic agents for moderate and/or deep procedural sedation and analgesia by an RN (who

Continued

BOX 1.1 North Carolina Board of Nursing Position Statement—cont'd

is not a licensed or certified anesthesia provider) requires all the following:

- Policies and procedures of employing agency authorize RN-administered moderate and/or deep procedural sedation and analgesia.
- The RN possesses specific knowledge and validated competencies, as described in this position statement.
- The RN responsible for sedation and analgesia administration and monitoring of a client receiving moderate or deep sedation and analgesia does not assume other responsibilities that would leave the client unattended, thereby jeopardizing the safety of the client.
- The physician, CRNA, NP, or PA ordering RN-administered moderate procedural sedation and analgesia is physically present in the procedure area and immediately available during the time that moderate procedural sedation and analgesia is administered.
- The physician, CRNA, NP, or PA ordering RN-administered deep procedural sedation and analgesia is physically present at the bedside throughout the time deep sedation and analgesia is administered.

The intended level of sedation and analgesia may quickly change to a deeper level due to the unique characteristics of the pharmacologic agents used, as well as the physical status and drug sensitivities of the individual client. The administration of these pharmacologic agents requires ongoing assessment and monitoring of the client and the ability to respond immediately to deviations from the norm.

Given the level of independent assessment, decision making, and evaluation required for safe care, nursing care of these clients exceeds the Licensed Practical Nurse (LPN) scope of practice.

Exclusions from NCBON Procedural Sedation and Analgesia Position Statement

1. Advanced Practice Registered Nurse: Certified Registered Nurse Anesthetists (APRN-CRNAs) are professional anesthesia providers qualified by education, certification, licensure, registration, and experience to administer anesthesia and all levels of procedural sedation. The CRNA scope of practice exceeds and is not limited by the constraints of this Position Statement.

    The administration of general anesthesia, including the use of inhalation anesthetics, is limited solely to anesthesia providers, including CRNAs. (Note: Nitrous oxide, used as a procedural sedative and analgesic agent, is the only agent that can be administered by nonanesthetist RNs via the inhalation route.)

2. The administration of sedation and analgesia for the purpose of intubation, including rapid-sequence intubation (RSI), is within the RN scope of practice with specific education, competence, and policies and procedures, as detailed in the North Carolina Board of Nursing (NCBON) RSI Position Statement available at www.ncbon.com.

3. The administration of medications for moderate to deep sedation and analgesia of already intubated, critically ill clients is within the RN scope of practice and is not limited by the constraints of this position statement.

4. The following are within the scope of practice for both RNs and LPNs and are not limited by the constraints of this position statement:
    - Administration of analgesia for pain control without sedatives
    - Administration of minimal sedation and analgesia (anxiolysis)
    - Administration of topical and local anesthesia and
    - Administration of sedation and analgesia solely for the purpose of managing altered mental status

Definitions: American Society of Anesthesiologists (ASA) Physical Status Classification

Class I—normally healthy client

Class II—client with mild systemic disease

Class III—client with severe systemic disease

Class IV—client with severe systemic disease that is constant threat to life

Class V—a moribund client who is not expected to survive 24 hours with or without the procedure

Anesthetic agents— medications that when administered, cause partial or complete loss of sensation, with or without loss of consciousness.

Computer-assisted personalized sedation and analgesia devices—integrated drug infusion pump and physiologic client monitoring system that administers medication (e.g., propofol) intravenously for the initiation and maintenance of minimal to moderate procedural sedation and analgesia. The device continually monitors client physiologic parameters and responsiveness, detects signs associated with oversedation and analgesia, and adjusts the medication delivery rate to limit the depth of sedation and analgesia.

Deep sedation and analgesia—drug-induced depression of consciousness during which clients cannot be easily aroused but respond purposefully following repeated or painful stimulation. The client's ability to maintain ventilatory function independently may be impaired. Clients may require assistance to maintain a patent airway, and spontaneous ventilation may be inadequate. Cardiovascular function is usually maintained.

General anesthesia—drug-induced loss of consciousness during which clients are not arousable, even by painful stimulation. The client's ability to maintain ventilatory function independently is often impaired. Clients often require assistance in maintaining a patent airway, and positive pressure ventilation may be required because of depressed spontaneous ventilation or drug-induced depression of neuromuscular function. Cardiovascular function may be impaired.

Immediately available—present on site in the unit of care and not otherwise engaged in any other uninterruptible procedure or task.

Minimal sedation and analgesia (anxiolysis)—drug-induced state during which clients respond normally to verbal commands. Although cognitive function and coordination may be impaired, ventilatory and cardiovascular functions are unaffected. The administration of medications appropriate for this purpose include benzodiazepines and opioids, but not anesthesia agents, and is within the scope of practice for both RNs and LPNs.

Continued

BOX 1.1   North Carolina Board of Nursing Position Statement—cont'd

Moderate (conscious) sedation and analgesia—drug-induced depression of consciousness during which the client responds purposefully to verbal commands, either alone or accompanied by light tactile stimulation. No interventions are required for the client to maintain a patent airway and adequate spontaneous ventilation. Cardiovascular function is usually maintained.

Monitored anesthesia care (MAC)—anesthesia care that includes the monitoring of the client by a practitioner who is qualified to administer anesthesia. Indications for MAC depend on the nature of the procedure, the client's clinical condition, and/or the potential need to convert to a general or regional anesthetic.

Procedural sedation and analgesia—technique of administering sedatives or dissociative agents, with or without analgesics, to induce a state that allows the client to tolerate unpleasant procedures while maintaining cardiovascular and respiratory function.

Rapid-sequence intubation (RSI)—airway management technique in which a potent sedative or induction agent is administered simultaneously with a paralyzing dose of a neuromuscular blocking agent to facilitate rapid tracheal intubation. The technique includes specific protection against the aspiration of gastric contents, provides excellent access to the airway for intubation, and permits pharmacologic control of adverse responses to illness, injury, and the intubation itself. (For details see NCBON RSI Position Statement at www.ncbon.com.)

Regional anesthesia—delivery of anesthetic medication at a specific level of the spinal cord and/or to peripheral nerves, including epidurals and spinals and other central neuraxial nerve blocks. It is used when loss of consciousness is not desired but sufficient analgesia and loss of voluntary and involuntary movement are required.

Rescue capacity—requires the competency to manage a compromised airway, provide adequate oxygenation and ventilation, and administer emergency medications and/or reversal agents to clients whose level of sedation becomes deeper than intended.

Sedating agent—medication that produces calmness, relaxation, reduced anxiety, and sleepiness when administered.

Topical or local anesthesia—application or injection of a medication or combination of medications to stop or prevent a painful sensation to a circumscribed area of the body where a painful procedure is to be performed. There are generally no systemic effects of these medications, which are also not anesthesia, despite the name.

RN Education and Competency Requirements for Procedural Sedation and Analgesia

Education, training, experience, and validation of initial and ongoing competencies appropriate to RN responsibilities, procedures performed, and the client or population must be documented and maintained. (**Note:** The employing agency determines the frequency with which ongoing competencies are revalidated.)

A. The RN administering moderate and/or deep procedural sedation and analgesia must possess in-depth knowledge of and validated competency to apply the following in practice:
1. Anatomy and physiology, including principles of oxygen delivery, transport, and uptake, cardiac dysrhythmia recognition and interventions, and complications related to moderate and deep procedural sedation and analgesia.
2. Pharmacology of sedation, analgesia, and anesthetic agent(s) administered singly or in combination, including appropriate administration routes, drug actions, drug interactions, side effects, contraindications, reversal agents (as applicable), and untoward effects.
3. Airway management skills required to rescue a patient from sedation and analgesia at a level deeper than intended and to manage a compromised airway or hypoventilation (i.e., establish an open airway, head-tilt, chin lift, use of bag-valve-mask, and oral and nasal airways).
4. Advanced Cardiac Life Support (ACLS) and/or Pediatric Advanced Life Support (PALS) certification, including dysrhythmia recognition, cardioversion and defibrillation, and emergency resuscitation appropriate to the status of the client or population.

B. In addition, the RN administering moderate and/or deep procedural sedation and analgesia must possess validated practice competencies needed to carry out the following:
5. Assess total client care needs before and during the administration of moderate or deep procedural sedation and analgesia and throughout the recovery phase, including implementing nursing care strategies appropriate to the client's ASA physical status classification as determined by physician, CRNA, nurse practitioner (NP), or physician's assistant (PA).
6. Perform appropriate physiologic measurements and evaluation of respiratory rate, oxygen saturation, carbon dioxide level, blood pressure, cardiac rate and rhythm, and level of consciousness.
7. Assess, identify, and differentiate the levels of sedation and analgesia and provide monitoring appropriate to the client's desired and actual level of sedation and analgesia;
8. Identify and implement appropriate nursing interventions in the event of sedation and analgesia complications, untoward outcomes, and emergencies.
9. Assess sedation and analgesia recovery, including the use of a standardized discharge scoring system.

Agency Responsibilities in Procedural Sedation and Analgesia

Based on client care needs, facility regulations, accreditation requirements, applicable standards, personnel, equipment, and other resources, each employing agency determines if the administration of moderate and/or deep procedural sedation and analgesia by nonanesthetist RNs is authorized in their setting. If the administration of moderate and/or deep procedural sedation and analgesia by nonanesthetist RNs is permitted, the Director of Nursing or lead RN in the employing agency, in collaboration with anesthesia providers and other appropriate agency personnel, is responsible for ensuring that written policies and procedures, including but not limited to the following, are in place to address the following:
1. Credentialing requirements for nonanesthesiologist physicians, NPs, and PAs approved to perform moderate and/or deep procedural sedation and analgesia
2. Required documentation of initial and ongoing RN education and competency validation in the manner and at the frequency specified by agency policy

Continued

BOX 1.1 North Carolina Board of Nursing Position Statement—cont'd

3. Physician, CRNA, NP, or PA (not the nonanesthetist RN) responsibility for preprocedure assessment of the client, including assessment and determination of the ASA physical status classification score
4. Number and qualifications of personnel to be present in the room during RN administration of moderate and/or deep procedural sedation and analgesia and requirement that designated personnel are competent to rescue the client should the airway or hemodynamic status be compromised
5. Requirement that the physician, CRNA, NP, or PA ordering RN-administered moderate procedural sedation and analgesia be physically present in the procedure area and immediately available during the time moderate procedural sedation and analgesia is administered to respond and implement emergency protocols in the event the level of sedation deepens or another emergency occurs
6. Requirement that the physician, CRNA, NP, or PA ordering RN-administered deep procedural sedation and analgesia be physically present at the bedside throughout the time deep sedation and analgesia is administered to respond in the event of an emergency
7. Requirement that the RN responsible for sedation and analgesia administration and monitoring of a client receiving moderate or deep sedation and analgesia will not assume other responsibilities that would leave the client unattended, thereby jeopardizing the safety of the client
8. Specification of nursing care responsibilities for client assessment, monitoring, medication administration, potential complications, and documentation during moderate and/or deep procedural sedation and analgesia
9. Specification of medications approved to be ordered and administered by RNs for moderate and/or deep procedural sedation and analgesia, including dosage limits as appropriate
10. Specification of emergency protocol(s), including immediate on-site availability of resuscitative equipment, medications, and personnel
11. Requirement that age and size-appropriate procedural equipment, emergency resuscitation equipment, and medications, as well as personnel qualified to provide necessary emergency measures, such as intubation and airway management, be readily available during moderate and/or deep procedural sedation and analgesia

Age and size-appropriate equipment include, but are not limited to, the following:
- Blood pressure cuff and stethoscope
- Cardiac monitor and defibrillator
- Oxygen and suction devices
- Pulse oximetry and capnography
- Positive pressure ventilation equipment
- intravenous administration devices & fluids
- Basic and advanced airway management devices
- Medications including sedatives, analgesics, reversal agents for opioids or benzodiazepines, and resuscitation drugs

NOTE: RNs retain responsibility and accountability for direct client assessment, intervention, and evaluation throughout the administration of moderate or deep procedural sedation and analgesia. Mechanical monitoring and medication administration devices (e.g., cardiac monitors, infusion pumps, and computer-assisted personalized sedation and analgesia devices) do not replace, but rather support, the RN's assessment and evaluation of client status.

NOTE: Pulse oximetry measures oxygenation, not ventilation. In the presence of supplemental oxygen, arterial oxygen desaturation as measured by pulse oximetry may represent a delayed sign of hypoventilation. For this reason, monitoring pulse oximetry is not a substitute for direct observation of the patient's ventilatory function. Capnography may be able to detect hypoventilation before pulse oximetry indicates oxygen desaturation and has been shown to be a more sensitive gauge of hypoventilation than visual observation.

RN Role in Moderate and Deep Procedural Sedation and Analgesia
1. The administration and monitoring of sedating and anesthetic agents to produce moderate or deep procedural sedation and analgesia for nonintubated adult and pediatric clients undergoing therapeutic, diagnostic, or surgical procedures is within the nonanesthetist RN scope of practice.
2. The RN must be educationally prepared; clinically competent; permitted to administer moderate and/or deep procedural sedation and analgesia by agency written policies and procedures; and not prohibited from doing so by facility-focused laws, rules, standards, and policies.
3. A qualified anesthesia provider (anesthesiologist or CRNA) or appropriately credentialed attending physician, NP, or PA must assess the client, determine the ASA physical status classification, select, and order the sedative and anesthetic agents to be administered; the intended level of sedation and analgesia must be clearly communicated.
4. The RN is accountable for ensuring that moderate and/or deep procedural sedation and analgesia orders implemented are consistent with the current standards of practice and agency policies and procedures.
5. The RN accepts the assignment to administer ordered moderate or deep procedural sedation and analgesia only if competent, and the practice setting has provided the age and size-appropriate equipment, medications, personnel, and related resources needed to ensure client safety.
6. The RN administers moderate procedural sedation and analgesia to adult and pediatric clients only if a Physician, CRNA, NP, or PA credentialed by the facility in moderate procedural sedation and analgesia, and competent in airway management, is physically present in the procedure area and immediately available to respond and implement emergency protocols in the event the level of sedation deepens or another emergency occurs.
7. The RN administers deep procedural sedation and analgesia to adult and pediatric clients only if a physician, CRNA, NP, or PA credentialed by the facility in deep procedural sedation and analgesia, and competent in intubation and airway management, is present at the bedside to respond to any emergency.
8. The RN's role in moderate and deep procedural sedation and analgesia is dedicated to the continuous and uninterrupted monitoring of the client's physiologic parameters and the administration of medications ordered.
9. The administration of all medications via any appropriate route (including nitrous oxide via inhalation) for the purpose of

Continued

BOX 1.1   North Carolina Board of Nursing Position Statement—cont'd

moderate or deep procedural sedation and analgesia is within the RN scope of practice. Medications, including etomidate, propofol, ketamine, fentanyl, and midazolam, administered for moderate and/or deep procedural sedation and analgesia purposes, if ordered by the physician, CRNA, NP, PA, or other credentialed health care practitioner, and allowed by agency policy, is not prohibited, provided the appropriate indications and precautions are in place.

LPN Role in Moderate and Deep Procedural Sedation and Analgesia

Given the level of independent nursing assessment, decision making, and evaluation required for the safe care and management of clients undergoing therapeutic, diagnostic, and surgical procedures, the administration of sedation and anesthetic agents for the purposes of moderate or deep procedural sedation and analgesia is beyond the LPN scope of practice.

RN and LPN Role in Regional Anesthesia

Regional anesthesia requires anesthetic agent delivery at a specific level of the spinal cord and/or to peripheral nerves, including epidurals, spinals, and other central neuraxial nerve blocks, when loss of consciousness is not desired but sufficient analgesia and loss of voluntary and involuntary movement are required.

In these situations, the positioning and stabilization of the client receiving regional anesthesia is sometimes challenging, and the provider performing the procedure may need mechanical assistance from the nurse (RN or LPN) to attach and/or push the medication syringe plunger while personally maintaining appropriate positioning of the medication delivery device.

In such a situation, the nurse may provide the needed manual support by functioning as the third hand of the provider.[a] When acting as the provider's third hand, the nurse is not accepting responsibility for the administration of regional anesthesia, which is beyond both RN and LPN scope of practice. Instead, the provider retains full responsibility for the appropriate medication administration and accountability for outcomes.

References

21 NCAC 36.0224 (b)(d)(e)—RN Rules
21 NCAC 36.0225 (b)(d)(e)—LPN Rules
American Association of Nurse Anesthetists (AANA). www.aana.com. The resources section provides specific policy considerations for registered nurses engaged in the administration of sedation and analgesia.
American Association of Moderate Sedation Nurses (AAMSN). www. aamsn.org . The resources section provides information on Certified Sedation Registered Nurses (CSRNs).

[a] This third-hand specification does not include the administration of anesthetic agents by the nonanesthetist nurse in any other situation. It is not permissible for the RN or LPN to function as the third hand of, or to provide only manual support or mechanical assistance to, a provider in the administration of moderate or deep procedural sedation and analgesia. To do so leaves the provider with responsibility for both performing the procedure and monitoring the patient. Moderate and/or deep procedural sedation and analgesia requires careful monitoring by a dedicated person. Therefore, the RN who administers moderate or deep sedation (this is beyond LPN scope of practice) is providing a nursing intervention and retains full accountability and responsibility for his/her actions. The RN functioning in this capacity must meet the moderate and deep procedural sedation education and competence requirements as delineated in this position statement.
It is within RN scope of practice to administer ordered additional or subsequent medication doses through a preestablished indwelling epidural or caudal device per provider order. This constitutes RN medication administration for which the RN retains full responsibility and accountability. This is not within the LPN scope of practice and is not considered manual or third-hand assistance.
Copyright North Carolina Board of Nursing (NCBON).

---

regulations created by professional organizations and licensure boards.[28] The pursuit of best sedation practice in the interest of patient safety often paves the way for individual institution sedation policy development. Ideally, a model sedation policy identifies specific standards of sedation patient care, requisite staff skill competencies, and quality improvement initiatives to be implemented throughout the inpatient or outpatient setting. A suggested structure for an evidence-based moderate sedation policy is identified in Box 1.2.[29]

How have some health care facilities implemented an effective sedation policy based on best practices and patient safety?

The safe administration of moderate procedural sedation begins with effective initial policy and procedure development. Ideally, an interprofessional committee is best suited for initiating and creating a model sedation policy, led by the Chairman of the Department of Anesthesia or the qualified anesthesia professional designee. The interdisciplinary sedation planning committee must include a wide variety of roles and expertise representing all sedation settings in the institution. The ultimate goal of the interdisciplinary sedation

committee is to produce and implement a comprehensive best practice sedation model policy. Committee members should begin with a thorough review of The Joint Commission and ASA practice guidelines and standards for sedation and analgesia by nonanesthesiologists, state board of nursing position statements, and professional organization standards, guidelines, and consensus statements.[20] The final policy should apply to all employees participating in the administration of moderate procedural sedation and analgesia, coupled with a demonstrated organization-wide commitment to sedation safety that is comparable throughout the institution.[30]

Effective moderate sedation and analgesia policy and procedure implementation also requires appointing an organizational administrative champion who demonstrates a commitment to enhanced patient safety throughout the organization. Senior personnel who are well respected by institutional managers and supervisors can use their leadership skills to ensure that the final sedation model policy adopted by the institution is uniformly applied throughout the health care facility. An effective action plan must address key questions related to specific goals in the development or revision of a sedation policy, planned initiatives, required resources,

---

BOX 1.2 Suggested Structure for a Moderate Sedation Policy

Purpose
Scope
Definitions of sedation levels
Governance
Location requirements
Equipment requirements
Personnel roles and requirements
Competency and credentialing requirements
Preprocedure evaluation
Considerations for anesthesia consultation
Periprocedure monitoring requirements
Medication administration guidelines
Postprocedure observation and discharge
Outcomes assessment
Documentation guidelines

---

processes, and ongoing outcome measures to be implemented. Key timelines must be outlined and met by all committee members to keep the project moving forward.

Facilities also look to federal agencies such as the AHRQ for resources and guidance. The mission of the AHRQ is to produce evidence to make health care safer, of higher quality, more accessible, equitable, and more affordable. In addition, they provide a number of project tools that can be implemented in the sedation setting. The Action Planning Tool for the AHRQ Surveys on Patient Safety Culture can be adapted for and used by interdisciplinary sedation team committees charged with the task of creating a model moderate procedural sedation and analgesia policy. The AHRQ Action Planning Tool can be found online at https://www.ahrq.gov/sites/default/files/wysiwyg/professionals/quality-patient-safety/patientsafetyculture/planningtool.pdf.[31]

Are there any additional barriers to implementing a model moderate sedation policy effectively in the clinical setting?

A variety of barriers may challenge the successful implementation of a moderate sedation program in any health care facility. One of the foremost obstacles encountered in many institutions is what has been termed *production pressure*. Production pressure makes speed and output, not safety, the primary objective of personnel in a system. Production pressure has been identified as a factor in important catastrophic events in nonmedical industries, including aviation, space flight, nuclear energy production, and long haul trucking.[32-36] Although there is no easy solution, until health care facilities recognize that there should be a combination of systems-based support and cultural change in medicine that embraces patient safety, they remain exposed to medical errors. The IOM has estimated that medical errors affect 1.5 million Americans annually, costing our health care system over 20.8 billion dollars.[37]

What has been called *normalization of deviance* is also known to occur in the health care setting. Normalization of deviance breaks the safety culture and provides a pattern of tolerating more and more errors and accepting more and more risks, always in the interest of efficiency and on-time schedules.[38] An example of normalization of deviance that could occur in the ambulatory sedation setting includes continually sedating high-acuity patients whose associated comorbidities (e.g., morbid obesity, history of sleep apnea) should clearly preclude them from moderate procedural sedation services in an outpatient setting. These cases eventually become classified as the norm in many outpatient facilities. The previous boundaries of only performing moderate procedural sedation and analgesia on medically well-managed patients are pushed to the extreme without understanding

---

⚡ PATIENT SAFETY SBAR FOCUS

The Competent Sedation Provider

Situation:
Our interventional platform is chronically short staffed.

Background:
The manager consistently reassigns staff from different areas of the facility to provide moderate procedural sedation and analgesia patient care. A significant patient complication recently occurred within the interventional platform. During the root cause analysis (RCA), it was recognized that many of the reallocated providers never received procedural sedation competency validation.

Assessment:
The validation of moderate procedural sedation competencies is a dynamic process. Mastery of baseline procedural sedation competencies should focus on evidence based clinical practice, patient centered care and effective inter-professional team dynamics. A variety of evaluation methods are available to document ongoing staff competencies. These methods include direct observation, structured interviews, simulation exercises,

case studies, role playing and development dialogue. Core sedation competencies should always be documented prior to providing direct sedation patient care.

Recommendation
It is incumbent upon all healthcare providers to demonstrate professional competence when providing patient care. It is the right of every patient to expect healthcare providers to demonstrate ongoing professional competence. Regardless of the employment setting, every healthcare provider is responsible and accountable for maintaining his/her own professional competence. In 2015, the *Scope of Nursing Practice Decision-Making Framework* was created to provide a standardized, decision-making framework for all licensed nurses in all settings with respect to their education, role, function and accountability within the scope of nursing practice. Prior to accepting patient care reassignment, nurses may use the decision-making algorithm (see below) to determine whether patient care activities are within the nurse's level of education, licensure, and competence.

Continued

⚡ **PATIENT SAFETY SBAR FOCUS—cont'd**

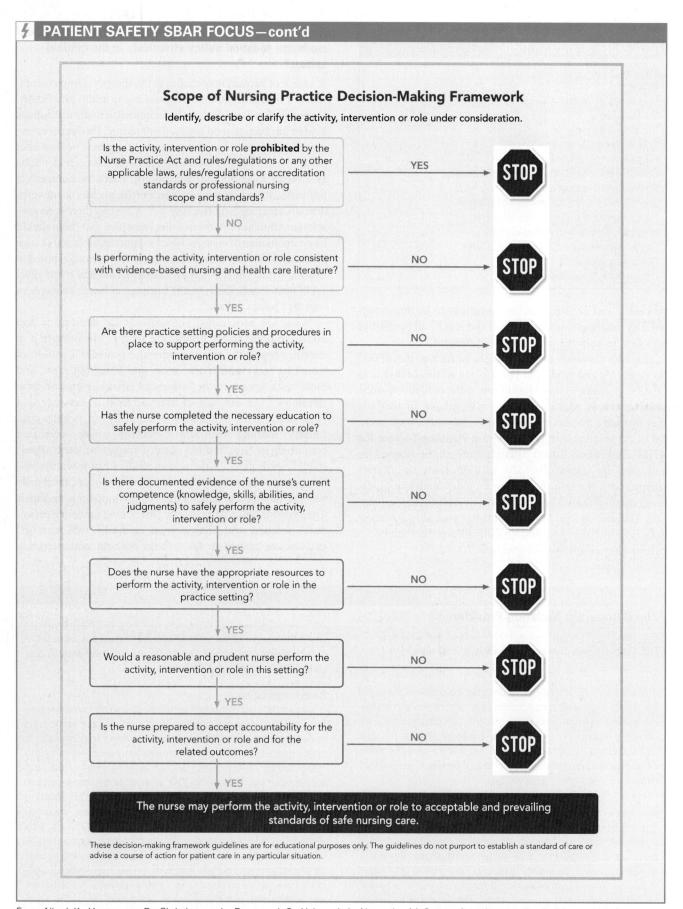

Scope of Nursing Practice Decision-Making Framework

Identify, describe or clarify the activity, intervention or role under consideration.

Is the activity, intervention or role **prohibited** by the Nurse Practice Act and rules/regulations or any other applicable laws, rules/regulations or accreditation standards or professional nursing scope and standards? — **YES** → STOP

↓ NO

Is performing the activity, intervention or role consistent with evidence-based nursing and health care literature? — **NO** → STOP

↓ YES

Are there practice setting policies and procedures in place to support performing the activity, intervention or role? — **NO** → STOP

↓ YES

Has the nurse completed the necessary education to safely perform the activity, intervention or role? — **NO** → STOP

↓ YES

Is there documented evidence of the nurse's current competence (knowledge, skills, abilities, and judgments) to safely perform the activity, intervention or role? — **NO** → STOP

↓ YES

Does the nurse have the appropriate resources to perform the activity, intervention or role in the practice setting? — **NO** → STOP

↓ YES

Would a reasonable and prudent nurse perform the activity, intervention or role in this setting? — **NO** → STOP

↓ YES

Is the nurse prepared to accept accountability for the activity, intervention or role and for the related outcomes? — **NO** → STOP

↓ YES

The nurse may perform the activity, intervention or role to acceptable and prevailing standards of safe nursing care.

These decision-making framework guidelines are for educational purposes only. The guidelines do not purport to establish a standard of care or advise a course of action for patient care in any particular situation.

From Allard, K., Haagenson, D., Christiansen, L., Damgaard, G., Halstead, J., Alexander, M. Scope of nursing practice decision-making framework. *Journal of Nursing Regulation* 2016; 7(3), 19–21.

exactly where and why the original limits were established—until an adverse event occurs.

Our GI physician attended a conference on propofol administration in the endoscopy setting recently. He is now requesting that we administer propofol to patients in our outpatient center. Our nurse manager approved the administration and enacted a new policy requiring all nurses in our center to comply. Is there any additional training required prior to administering propofol to our patients?

There have been many questions raised related to the administration of propofol by nonanesthesia-trained physicians and nurses. The administration of propofol by nonanesthesia providers in endoscopy, radiology, and emergency department settings has increased dramatically over the last decade, secondary to the rapid onset, short duration, and enhanced recovery profile associated with the sedative-hypnotics. However, prior to complying with your nurse manager's request to administer propofol, it is important to check with your state board of nursing to ensure that propofol administration by registered nurses for the purposes of procedural sedation is permitted in your state.

There have been multiple reports of adverse patient events related to the administration of propofol by nonanesthesia providers. Over a decade ago, the Pennsylvania Patient Safety Reporting System (PA-PSRS) received more than 100 reports in which propofol administration in untrained hands resulted in adverse patient events, and 16% of those reports were classified as serious events, including four patient deaths.[39] In 2009, Rex et al. reported that propofol is known to cause hypoventilation, hypotension, and bradycardia relatively frequently, but posited that severe adverse events are extremely rare.[40] Professional organizations that have endorsed nonanesthesiologist propofol administration or nurse-administered propofol sedation include the following:

- American College of Gastroenterology
- American Society for Gastrointestinal Endoscopy
- Society for Gastroenterology Nurses and Associates

Regardless of organizational position statements, the US Food and Drug Administration (FDA) has noted that Diprivan (propofol) injectable emulsion should be administered only by persons trained in the administration of general anesthesia and not involved in the conduct of the surgical or diagnostic procedure. In 2005, the American College of Gastroenterology petitioned the FDA to remove these warnings on propofol package labeling. In a letter dated August 11, 2010, the FDA denied the petition in its ruling stating that "For the reasons described, we conclude that you have not demonstrated that the warning is inappropriate or unwarranted. In fact, we conclude that both components of the warning are appropriate in light of the significant risks associated with propofol, and we further conclude that the warning should help ensure that propofol is used safely."[41] Nonanesthesia providers who administer or monitor patients receiving propofol in the endoscopy or emergency department setting must recognize that propofol is considered a high-risk medication by the Institute for Patient Safety.[42] Propofol is not a reversible medication and may produce rapid unpredictable effects, including respiratory arrest.

Is there anything specific I can do if I have questions regarding professional competence in my role as a sedation provider?

All health care providers must demonstrate professional competence when providing patient care. The American Nurses Association position statement on professional role competence has stated that "the public has a right to expect registered nurses to demonstrate professional competence throughout their careers. The registered nurse is individually responsible and accountable for maintaining professional competence."[43] Appendix C features an excellent competency verification resource from the Association of Operating Room Nurses.

SUMMARY

The administration of moderate procedural sedation and analgesia for diagnostic, therapeutic, or surgical procedures requires a highly specialized skill set. Clinicians engaged in the art and science of administering sedation and analgesia must be trained to recognize the fine line between a tranquil amnestic patient and an unconscious unresponsive patient. To achieve the objectives of moderate procedural sedation and analgesia satisfactorily and maximize patient safety, the following educational competencies must be clearly established:

- Knowledge of cardiovascular and pulmonary anatomy, physiology, cardiac dysrhythmia recognition, and complications related to the administration of sedation
- Knowledge of the pharmacokinetic and pharmacodynamic principles associated with sedation medications
- Demonstrated competence and training in presedation assessment, planning of sedation, and monitoring of physiologic parameters, including respiratory rate, oxygen saturation, blood pressure, cardiac rate and rhythm, and patient level of consciousness
- An understanding of the principles of oxygen delivery and the use of oxygen delivery devices
- The ability to assess, diagnose, and intervene rapidly in the event of an untoward reaction associated with the administration of sedative, hypnotic, and analgesic medications
- Proven skill in airway management
- Competence in the ability to rescue patients pharmacologically and physiologically from deep sedative states and general anesthesia
- Postsedation monitoring and discharge planning
- Ongoing competency validation for all aspects of sedation patient care

REFERENCES

1. Washington State Department of Health. Office of Nursing Care Quality Assurance Commission. In: *Administration of sedating, analgesic, and anesthetic agents* [Advisory opinion]: 2015

Retrieved from www.doh.wa.gov/Portals/1/Documents/6000/AdminOfSedating,AnalgesicAndAnestheticAgents.pdf.

2. Amornyotin S. Registered nurse-administered sedation for gastrointestinal endoscopic procedure. *World Journal of Gastrointestinal Endoscopy*. 2015; *7*:769–776.

3. Crego N. Procedural sedation practice: A review of current nursing standards. *Journal of Nursing Regulation*. 2015; *6*: 50–56.

4. Roback M, Carlson D, Babl F, Kennedy R. Update on pharmacological management of procedural sedation for children. *Current opinion in anaesthesiolog*. 2016; *29*:S21–S35. https://doi.org/10.1097/ACO.0000000000000316.

5. McQuaid K, Laine L. A systematic review for meta-analysis of randomized, controlled trials of moderate sedation for routine endoscopic procedures. *Gastrointestinal Endoscopy*. 2008; *67*:910–923.

6. Moon S. Sedation regimens for gastrointestinal endoscopy. *Clinical Endoscopy*. 2014; *47*:135–140. https://doi.org/10.5946/ce.2014.47.2.135.

7. Wilson TD, McNeil DW, Kyle BN, Weaver BD, Graves RW. Effects of conscious sedation on patient recall of anxiety and pain after oral surgery. *Oral Surgery Oral Medicine Oral Pathology Oral Radiology*. 2014; *117*:277–282. https://doi.org/10.1016/j.oooo.2013.11.489.

8. Atkinson P, French J, Nice A. Procedural sedation and analgesia for adults in the emergency department. *British Medical Journal*. 2014; *348*:35–37.

9. Becker D. Pharmacodynamic considerations for moderate and deep sedation. *Anesthesia Progress*. 2012; *59*:28–42.

10. Viana KA, Daher A, Maia LC, Costa PS, Martins CC, Paiva SM, Costa LR. What is the level of evidence for the amnestic effects of sedatives in pediatric patients? A systematic review and meta-analyses. *Public Library of Science ONE*. 2017; *12*. https://doi.org/10.1371/journal.pone.0180248.

11. Coble YD, Eisenbrey AB, Estes H. The use of pulse oximetry during conscious sedation. *Journal of the American Medical Association*. 1993; *270*:1463–1468. https://doi.org/10.1001/jama.1993.03510120085036.

12. Bennett C. *Conscious sedation in dental practice* (2nd ed.). St. Louis, MO. Mosby; 1978.

13. American Society of Anesthesiologists Task Force on Sedation and Analgesia by Non-Anesthesiologists. Practice guidelines for sedation and analgesia by non-anesthesiologists: An updated report. *Anesthesiology*. 2002; *96*:1004–1017.

14. Green SM, Krauss B. Procedural sedation terminology: Moving beyond "conscious sedation". *Annals of Emergency Medicine*. 2002; *39*:433.

15. American Society of Anesthesiologists. Practice Guidelines for Moderate Procedural Sedation and Analgesia 2018: A Report by the American Society of Anesthesiologists Task Force on Moderate Procedural Sedation and Analgesia, the American Association of Oral and Maxillofacial surgeons, American College of Radiology, American Dental Association, American Society of Dentist Anesthesiologists, and Society of Interventional Radiology. *Anesthesiology*. 2018; *128*(3): 437–479.

16. American Society of Anesthesiologists. *Continuum of depth sedation: Definition of general anesthesia and levels of sedation/analgesia*; 2014. Retrieved from http://www.asahq.org/~/media/sites/asahq/files/public/resources/standards-guidelines/continuum-of-depth-of-sedation-definition-of-general-anesthesia-and-levels-of-sedation-analgesia.pdf.

17. Cote CJ, Wilson S. Guidelines for monitoring and management of pediatric patients before, during, and after sedation for diagnostic and therapeutic procedures: Update 2016. *Pediatrics*. 2016; *138*. https://doi.org/10.1542/peds.2016-1212.

18. Bailey P, Pace N, Ashburn M. Frequent hypoxemia and apnea after sedation with midazolam and fentanyl. *Anesthesiology*. 1990; *73*:826.

19. Karamnov S, Sarkisian N, Grammer R, Gross W, Urman R. Analysis of adverse events associated with adult moderate procedural sedation outside the operating room. *Journal of Patient Safety*. 2017; *13*:111–121.

20. The Joint Commission. The joint commission standards and elements of performance standards for sedation and anesthesia care: Provision of care, treatment, and services PC.03.01.01. *2018 Comprehensive Accreditation Manual*. IL: Oakbrook Terrance; 2018.

21. Institute of Medicine. *Clinical practice guidelines we can trust*. Washington, DC: The. National Academies Press; 2011. https://doi.org/10.17226/13058.

22. American Academy of Pediatrics. Classifying recommendations for clinical practice guidelines. *Pediatrics*. 2004; *114*:874–877. https://doi: 10.1542/peds.2004-1260.

23. American Society for Gastrointestinal Endoscopy. Position statement: Nonanesthesiologist administration of propofol for GI surgery. *Gastrointestinal Endoscopy*. 2009; *70*:1053–1059. https://doi:10.1016/j.gie.2009.07.020.

24. Gunn I. The many issues regarding intravenous conscious sedation. *Specialty Nursing Forum*. 1990; *2*:3.

25. Sedation Certification. *Position statement by state*; 2017. Retrieved from https://sedationcertification.com/resources/position-statements/position-statements-by-state/.

26. Conscious Sedation Counseling. (2015). *Laws by state*. Retrieved from http://www.sedationconsulting.com/laws-by-state/.

27. The North Carolina Board of Nursing. (2018). Procedural Sedation and Analgesia, Position Statement for RN Practice. Retrieved from https://www.ncbon.com/vdownloads/position-statements-decision-trees/procedural-sedation.pdf.

28. O'Malley PA, Poling L. Finding a way through the sedation labyrinth: Is it conscious, moderate, deep, or procedural sedation? Emerging evidence for CNS practice. *Clinical Nurse Specialist: The Journal for Advanced Nursing Practice*. 2015; *29*(1):12–18.

29. Caparelli-White L, Urman R. Developing a moderate sedation policy: essential elements and evidence-based considerations. AORN Journal, 99(3), 416-430.

30. Helmreich RL, Merrit AC. *Culture at work in aviation and medicine: National, organizational, and professional influences*. Aldershot, UK: Ashgage Publishing Limited; 1998.

31. Agency for Healthcare Research and Quality. *Action planning tool for the AHRQ surveys on patient safety culture*. Rockville, MD: Agency for Healthcare Research and Quality; 2016. Retrieved from *https://www.ahrq.gov/sites/default/files/wysiwyg/professionals/quality-patient-safety/patientsafetyculture/planningtool.pdf*.

32. Hobbs A, Williamson A. Associations between errors and contributing factors in aircraft maintenance. *Human Factors*. 2003; *45*:186–201.

33. Perrow C. *Normal accidents*. New York, NY: Basic Books; 1984.

34. Lewis RS. *Challenger: The final voyage*. New York, NY: Columbia University Press; 1988.

35. Rasmussen J. Cognitive control and human error mechanisms. In: Rasmussen J, Duncan K, Leplat J, eds. *New Technology and Human Error.* Chichester: Wiley; 1987:53–61.
36. Reason J. The contribution of latent human failures to the breakdown of complex systems. *Philosophical Transactions of the Royal Society of London.* 1987; 327:475–484.
37. Perez K. The human and economic costs of medical errors. *HFM Blog*; 2016, (June 21). Retrieved from https://www.hfma.org/Content.aspx?id=48695.
38. Westgard JO, Westgard S. *It's not rocket science.* (2009). Retrieved from https://www.westgard.com/guest25.htm#refs.
39. Garment R. Data raises questions about who is administering sedation drug. *Health Care Business Daily News*: 2006, (April 6). Retrieved from https://www.dotmed.com/news/story/1574.
40. Rex DK, Deenadayalu VP, Eid E, Imperiale TF, Walker JA, Sandhu K, Meah N. Endoscopist-directed administration of propofol: A worldwide safety experience. *Gastroenterology.* 2009; 137:1229–1237. https://doi.org/10.1053/j.gastro.2009.06.042.
41. Department of Health and Human Services, Food and Drug Administration. Department of Drug Evaluation and Research. Re: Docket No. FDA-2005P-0059. August 11, 2010.
42. Institute for Safe Medication Practices. (2014). ISMP list of high-alert medications in acute care settings. Retrieved from https://www.ismp.org/Tools/highalertmedications.pdf.
43. American Nurses Association. *Professional role competence.* Silver Spring, MD: Nursebooks.org; 2014.
44. National Council State Boards of Nursing. Scope of nursing practice decision-making framework. *Journal of Nursing Regulation.* 2016; 19–21.

CHAPTER 1: REVIEW QUESTIONS

1. Which of the following is not an objective of moderate sedation?
   A. Guard the patient's safety and welfare
   B. Maintain adequate sedation with minimal risk
   C. Allay patient fear and anxiety
   D. Produce an unconscious patient

2. A drug-induced depression of consciousness during which patients respond purposefully to verbal commands, either alone or accompanied by light tactile stimulation, no interventions are required to maintain a patent airway, spontaneous ventilation is adequate, and cardiovascular function is usually maintained, is defined as which of the following states of sedation?
   A. Minimal sedation
   B. Moderate sedation
   C. Deep sedation
   D. General anesthesia

3. Which of the following states of sedation was formerly defined as conscious sedation?
   A. Minimal sedation
   B. Moderate procedural sedation
   C. Deep sedation
   D. General anesthesia

4. Which of the following characteristics best describes a patient in a state of deep sedation?
   A. Ventilation, adequate; cardiovascular function is usually maintained
   B. Ventilation, unaffected; cardiovascular function is unaffected
   C. Ventilation, may be inadequate; cardiovascular function is usually maintained
   D. Airway, unaffected; responsiveness is normal response to verbal stimulation

5. Which of the following states may predispose the patient to an increased incidence of respiratory depression, decreased response to the hypoxic drive, and cardiovascular depression?
   A. General anesthesia
   B. Deep sedation
   C. Moderate sedation
   D. Minimal sedation

6. Cardiovascular function may be impaired in which of the following states according to the term *continuum of sedation?*
   A. General anesthesia
   B. Deep sedation
   C. Moderate sedation
   D. Minimal sedation

7. Which of the following is the highest mandate for clinical behavior?
   A. Position statements
   B. Practice guidelines
   C. Practice standards
   D. Hospital policy

8. _____ generally represent emerging trends on a given topic and demonstrate less forceful criteria than practice standards.
   A. Position statements
   B. Practice guidelines
   C. Practice standards
   D. Hospital policy

9. Which of the following are potential barriers to the safe administration of moderate procedural sedation and analgesia? (Select two that apply.)
   A. The phenomenon known as *normalization of deviance*
   B. Professional organization practice standards or guidelines
   C. Production pressure
   D. Maintaining the patient in a state of moderate sedation
   E. Adhering to the goals and objectives of moderate sedation

10. The term *conscious sedation* was initially described in the _____ literature.
    A. Gastroenterology
    B. Pediatric
    C. Critical care
    D. Dental

11. _____ makes speed and output, not safety, the primary objective of personnel within a system.
    A. Maximal pressure
    B. Precision pressure
    C. Production pressure
    D. Primary pressure

12. _____ breaks the safety culture down and provides a pattern of tolerating more and more errors and accepting more and more risks, always in the interest of efficiency and on-time schedules.
    A. Impractical safety
    B. Normalization of deviance
    C. Variation of normalcy
    D. Patterned variation

Answers can be found in Appendix A.

Presedation Assessment and Patient Selection

At the completion of this chapter, the learner shall:
- Describe the goals of the presedation patient assessment.
- Identify two methods used to calculate ideal body weight.
- Differentiate the components of the patient's medical history and its impact on procedural care.
- Distinguish specific physiologic alterations in the cardiovascular, pulmonary, hepatic, renal, neurologic, and endocrine systems identified in the presedation patient assessment and their implications for procedural patient care.
- Propose the sedation plan of care based on the patient's past medical history.
- Discuss the treatment protocol for an allergic reaction.
- Describe the sedation patient population that requires presedation laboratory testing.
- State the sedation patient care considerations associated with positive findings on social history, including the following:
  - Tobacco use
  - Alcohol consumption
  - Substance abuse
  - Herbal product use
  - Pregnancy
- Identify the current recommended NPO guidelines for sedation patients.
- Implement the American Society of Anesthesiologists Physical Status Classification System of I, II, or III at the conclusion of the presedation patient interview.

COMPETENCY STATEMENT

The health care provider performs a comprehensive presedation assessment before administering moderate procedural sedation and analgesia based on evidence-based selection criteria established by professional organizations.

What are the goals of the preprocedure assessment for a patient presenting for moderate procedural sedation and analgesia?

There are a variety of goals and objectives for patients presenting for moderate procedural sedation and analgesia. These goals include the following:

1. Identify presedation risk factors.
2. Decrease the risk of adverse patient outcomes (e.g., apnea, airway obstruction, respiratory arrest, cardiac arrest, death).
3. Ensure that each patient's physiologic condition is optimized prior to the procedure.
4. Reduce patient anxiety through education and communication.
5. Ensure adequate presedation planning and patient education.
6. Obtain informed consent.
7. Optimize patient care, satisfaction, and comfort.
8. Evaluate the patient's health status.
9. Determine if any presedation specialty consultations are required.
10. Formulate a sedation plan of care.
11. Communicate patient management issues among providers.

Mechanisms whereby the presedation patient evaluation can influence and improve patient care are outlined in Fig. 2.1.

How do the goals of moderate procedural sedation and analgesia differ from those of a presedation patient assessment?

The goals of a presedation assessment focus on preparation of the patient to optimize safety during the moderate sedation and analgesia procedural phase of care. The goal of moderate procedural sedation and analgesia is to provide patient tolerance of unpleasant or prolonged procedures through the relief of anxiety, discomfort, and/or pain.[1]

What is the best process to prepare a patient optimally for a moderate sedation procedure?

Presedation patient assessment must be conducted in an unhurried and reassuring atmosphere. Adequate time must be allotted to alleviate the patient's anxiety while allowing sufficient time to gather data and answer the patient's questions. When feasible, presedation assessment should be conducted several days prior to the proposed procedure. Optimally,

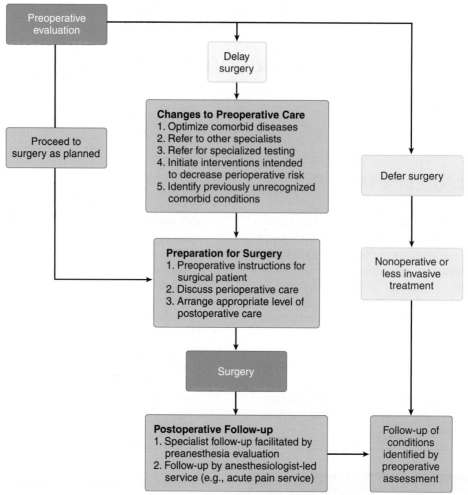

Fig. 2.1 Mechanisms whereby preoperative evaluation can help influence and improve perioperative care. (From Miller RD, ed. *Miller's Anesthesia*. 8th ed. Philadelphia: Saunders; 2015.)

the assessment is best conducted in conjunction with the health care provider who will administer the moderate procedural sedation and analgesia. Emergent cases may preclude the clinician's ability to obtain a presedation assessment in a relaxed atmosphere. Nonetheless, a complete assessment is still required prior to the administration of sedation. The assessment should be documented in the patient's record.

Presedation assessment allows the clinician time to gather additional data, order indicated laboratory and diagnostic tests, and implement a sedation plan of care. The presedation assessment period should attempt to identify patient risk factors that may lead to complications while affording the clinician the opportunity to ensure that the patient is in the best physical condition for the planned procedure. A comprehensive presedation assessment begins with a review of the medical record. Pertinent information recorded in the patient record offers insight into the patient's overall health status, as well as an opportunity to review the patient's past medical history. In some surgical centers, clinics, or physician offices, previous hospital records or access to the electronic medical record is not readily available. Therefore the patient, as the medical historian, is relied on to give an accurate past medical history.

In the presence of a well-documented past medical history recorded in the patient's record, the provider may use the presedation assessment period to confirm information with the patient. Patients with a significant medical history may require additional diagnostic testing and screening prior to the procedure. By performing a presedation assessment several days before the scheduled procedure, the provider may order the indicated tests, obtain specialty consultation, and request previous hospital records for review. To ensure that all presedation assessments are performed in a consistent manner and avoid the omission of key information, many clinicians follow a prescribed assessment format when interviewing patients. Components of this assessment format are outlined in Box 2.1.

Initial presedation assessment starts with a review of the planned procedure. By asking the patient to confirm the diagnostic or therapeutic procedure, the clinician verifies the scheduled procedure with the patient. A basic understanding of the procedure and anatomic area should be confirmed to ensure that the patient has been advised by the physician as to the nature of the planned intervention. Completion of the presedation assessment must be confirmed prior to the administration of any sedative agents. The Joint Commission

BOX 2.1   Components of Presedation Patient Assessment

Component
- Patient age, height, weight
- Proposed procedure
- Attending physician or service

Medical History

Cardiac
- Hypertension
- Coronary artery disease
- Angina
- Exercise tolerance
- Myocardial infarction
- Cardiac dysrhythmia
- Presence of pacemaker, AICD
- Valvular heart disease

Pulmonary
- Dyspnea
- Exercise tolerance
- Asthma
- Bronchitis
- Obstructive sleep apnea
- Tobacco use

Hepatic
- Enzyme induction
- Hepatitis
- Cirrhosis
- Ascites

Renal
- Renal insufficiency
- Renal failure
- Dialysis

Neurologic
- Cerebrovascular insufficiency
- Carotid artery and vertebral basilar disease
- Stroke
- Convulsive disorders
- Headaches
- Syncope
- Peripheral nervous system assessment

Endocrine
- Diabetes
- Hyper-, hypothyroidism
- Adrenal disease

Gastrointestinal
- Nausea
- Vomiting
- Recent weight loss
- Hiatal hernia

Hematology
- Anemia
- Aspirin, NSAID use
- Excessive bleeding

Musculoskeletal
- Arthritis
- Back pain
- Joint pain

Surgical History
- Anesthesia complications (e.g., nausea, vomiting, delayed emergence)
- Diagnostic procedures
- Family anesthesia history
- Operations

Medications
- Name
- Dosage
- Patient compliance

Allergies
- Anaphylactic
- Anaphylactoid
- Side effects

Laboratory Data
- Additional laboratory profiles
- Chest x-ray
- ECG
- Electrolytes

Dentition
- Capped teeth
- Loose or chipped teeth

Social History
- Tobacco use
- Alcohol use
- Illicit drug use
- Herbal use
- Possibility of pregnancy

NPO Status
- Instructions
- Liquids
- Solids

Informed Consent
- Patient questions answered
- Written consent obtained
- Patient instructions given

ASA Physical Status Classification
- ASA risk 1–3

AICD, Automatic implantable cardioverter-defibrillator; *ECG,* electrocardiogram; *NSAID,* nonsteroidal antiinflammatory drug.

⚡ PATIENT SAFETY SBAR FOCUS

Comprehensive Presedation Patient Assessment

Situation

We continue to see an increase in patients presenting to our ambulatory care unit for moderate procedural sedation and analgesia with complex medical histories and significant systemic disease states.

Background

Our ambulatory surgical facility is owned by a 'for profit' healthcare provider group. The providers refer their own patients to their facility for ambulatory procedures. During the last six months we have seen an increase in the patients presenting with significant hypertension, diabetes, obesity and cardiovascular disease. Last month's quality data also demonstrate prolonged discharge times and several unexpected hospital transfers.

Assessment

The continuing trend to 'push the outer edge of the envelope' has resulted in sicker patients presenting to ambulatory care facilities. Patient comorbidities offer a number of challenges to the sedation provider, including increased procedural risk. During the presedation patient assessment it is critically important to abide by clearly prescribed patient care criteria outlined in the ambulatory care policy and procedure manual. Patients that do not meet specific ambulatory care criteria should have their procedure completed at an inpatient facility.

Recommendation

The overarching goal of the presedation patient assessment is to minimize procedural risk, identify and optimize comorbidities, and decrease the risk for developing adverse outcomes secondary to moderate sedative agents administered. Completion of the presedation assessment is the first crucial step in identifying appropriate candidates for the outpatient setting. Use of the *A2, B2, C2, D2, E2, F2, G2* mnemonic allows the presedation provider the ability to exceed the goals of the presedation patient evaluation (thorough patient interview, physical examination, review of diagnostic data). This mnemonic is designed to follow the degree of significance of components of preanesthetic assessment:

A - Affirmative history: The history of present surgical condition with the details of progression to present state. Details of past illness and treatment should be elicited.

A - Airway: Perform detailed airway examination and have a plan for airway management. Always have plan B in case plan A fails.

B - Blood hemoglobin, blood loss estimation, and blood availability: Check for hemoglobin level and take measures to improve the same. Assess the requirement of blood based on expected blood loss and preoperative hemoglobin. Ensure availability of blood.

B - Breathing: Look for respiratory rate, pattern, and dyspnea.

C - Clinical examination: Assess pulse volume, rhythm, and blood pressure. Do detailed systemic examination. Assess effort tolerance.

C - Co-morbidities: Look for co-morbid diseases like diabetes, hypertension, asthma, and epilepsy and optimize the end organ problems.

D - Drugs being used by the patient: Elicit the details of current drug therapy and allergies to plan anesthesia.

D - Details of previous anesthesia and surgeries: Elicit the details of previous anesthesia and surgeries to anticipate anesthetic difficulty.

E - Evaluate investigations: Look for appropriate investigations that would guide anesthetic management.

E - End point to take up the case for surgery: End point to take up the case for surgery should be decided to avoid unnecessary postponement if further optimization is not possible.

F - Fluid status: Follow fasting guidelines appropriate to the age and surgery.

F - Fasting: Assess adequate duration of fasting for that particular age to prevent aspiration.

G - Give physical status: Assign a physical status classification.

G - Get consent: Discuss the surgical problems and the anesthetic risk with the patient and relatives to obtain appropriate consent.

Hemanth Kumar, V. R., Saraogi, A., Parthasarathy, S., & Ravishankar, M. (2013). A useful mnemonic for pre-anesthetic assessment. *Journal of Anaesthesiology, Clinical Pharmacology, 29*(4), 560–561. https://doi.org/10.4103/0970-9185.119127

Standards and Elements of Performance require that the patient be reevaluated immediately prior to the administration of sedation. The word *immediately* would mean when the patient is on the procedure table in the moments before the sedation is to be administered.[2]

How pertinent are age, height, and weight with regard to the presedation patient assessment?

The patient's age should be noted on the presedation assessment form. Although chronologic age does not necessarily correlate with physiologic age, it must be noted. Appreciation of patients' functional age (i.e., what are their physical capabilities?) is far more important than their chronologic age. It is equally important to ascertain the psychological state of the

patient at the time of the presedation assessment. Psychological characteristics and the anxiety level of the patient are assessed throughout the entire presedation process. During the initial phase of the presedation assessment, some patients may interject and ask, "What are you going to do to me?" or "What are you going to give me?" It is important to reiterate to the patient that once you conclude your assessment, you will answer questions related to the patient's upcoming plan of care. It is premature to comment or recommend a sedation plan before a complete and thorough presedation assessment has been conducted.

Body Mass Index. It is important to record an accurate height and weight prior to the planned procedure. Body mass index (BMI) measures the mass of the body in relation to height and weight. By making this calculation, one can make a relatively accurate assumption of body fat percentage. For example, if you calculate your own BMI, you will learn whether your current weight in relation to your height is considered underweight, normal, overweight, or obese. The formula for measuring BMI is as follows:

$$BMI = weight\,(lb)/[height\,(inches)]^2 \times 703$$

The BMI is calculated by dividing weight in pounds (lb) by height in inches (in) squared and then multiplying by a conversion factor of 703. For example, weight = 150 lb and height = 5'5" (65"):

$$\left[150 \div (65)^2\right] \times 703 = 24.96$$

So, the BMI in this case would be 24.96.

Body Mass Index Weight Status Categories. The following is how the BMI is categorized[3-5]:

- Below 18.5, underweight
- 18.5 to 24.9, normal or healthy weight
- 25.0 to 29.9, overweight
- 30.0 and above, obese

Another method used to calculate body weight is ideal body weight (IBW). Actual patient weight is compared to ideal body weight. Obesity = 20% excess of ideal body weight when using the IBW formula.

Ideal Body Weight.

- IBW (male): 105 lb + 6 lb for each inch > 5 feet
- IBW (female): 100 lb + 5 lb for each inch > 5 feet

What challenges does the obese patient present to the sedation provider?

Assessment of ideal body weight is important because obesity has a significant impact on the cardiovascular, pulmonary, gastrointestinal, endocrine, and hepatic systems. Obesity is defined as body weight greater than ideal weight. The multisystemic effects of obesity are listed in Table 2.1. To avoid the development of deep sedative states and respiratory depression, dosage requirements for sedative medications should be based on the ideal body weight and not the patient's actual weight.

TABLE 2.1 Multisystemic Effects of Obesity

Pulmonary	Cardiovascular	Gastrointestinal
Chest wall mass ↑	Cardiac output ↑	Intraabdominal pressure ↑
CO_2 production ↑	Hypertension	
Functional residual capacity ↓↓	Pulmonary hypertension	Intragastric pressure ↑
	Stroke volume ↑	Risk of aspiration ↑
Pulmonary compliance ↓		
Total oxygen consumption ↑		
Work of breathing ↑		

At times, management of the obese patient's airway during the administration of sedation may be challenging. Because of an increase in body mass and redundant oropharyngeal airway tissue, the patient should not be allowed to progress into a state of deep sedation. Heightened vigilance regarding titration of medications is required for the obese patient population. Obese patients are prone to pulmonary aspiration secondary to increased gastric volume. Treatment of gastric reflux symptoms may benefit from the presedation administration of H_2 blockers (e.g., ranitidine, famotidine), gastric stimulants (e.g., metoclopramide), and proton pump inhibitors (e.g., pantoprazole, lansoprazole) to decrease gastric volume and increase gastric acidity. Because of the significant challenges associated with the management of obese patients, presedation concerns may require consultation with a member of the anesthesia care team. Diagnostic tests indicated for the obese patient may include a complete blood count, radiograph of the chest, and baseline electrocardiogram (ECG) to rule out ventricular hypertrophy. Unless there is a specific contraindication, it is prudent to administer supplemental oxygen to all obese patients for sedation procedures. Postoperative administration of oxygen therapy should continue until the patient has fully recovered and there are no clinical signs of hypoxia. A plan of minimal sedation may be indicated when nonanesthesia clinicians are requested to administer sedation and analgesia to the obese patient population.

What is the purpose of the presedation cardiovascular assessment?

The purpose of the presedation cardiac assessment includes the following:

- Assessment for the presence of preexisting cardiovascular disease
- Assessment for disease severity, stability, and prior treatment
- Identification of comorbid states
  - Diabetes, chronic obstructive pulmonary disease (COPD)
- Identification of the type of procedure to be performed
  - Assessment of inherent procedural risks
- Identification of interventions that will decrease the incidence of complications

What considerations must be given to the patient presenting for moderate procedural sedation and analgesia with a history of hypertension?

Hypertension is defined as a systolic blood pressure greater than 130 mm Hg or a diastolic blood pressure greater than 80 mm Hg. People with readings of 130 as the top number, or 80 as the bottom number, are now considered to have high blood pressure, according to the latest 2017 guidelines from the American Heart Association (AHA) et al.[6]

High blood pressure used to be defined as 140 mm Hg/90 mm Hg. The new AHA guidelines are designed to help people take steps to control their blood pressure earlier in the disease process. High blood pressure is a major risk factor for heart disease and stroke, the two leading causes of death in the

TABLE 2.2   Classification of Systemic Blood Pressure (BP) in Adults

Category	Systolic (mm Hg)	Diastolic (mm Hg)	Recommendations
Normal	<120	<80	Healthy lifestyle choices and yearly checks
Elevated blood pressure	120–129 and	<80	Healthy lifestyle changes, reassessed in 3–6 mo
High blood pressure, stage 1	130–139 or	80–89	10-year heart disease and stroke risk assessment—if <10% risk, lifestyle changes, reassessed in 3–6 mo; if higher, lifestyle changes and medication with monthly follow-ups until BP controlled
High blood pressure, stage 2	≥140 or	≥90	Lifestyle changes and two different classes of medicine, with monthly follow-ups until BP is controlled

Adapted from https://www.heart.org/en/news/2018/05/01/nearly-half-of-us-adults-could-now-be-classified-with-high-blood-pressure-under-new-definitions

BOX 2.2   End-Organ Damage in Hypertension

Vasculopathy
Endothelial dysfunction
Remodeling
Generalized atherosclerosis
Arteriosclerotic stenosis
Aortic aneurysm

Cerebrovascular Damage
Acute hypertensive encephalopathy
Stroke
Intracerebral hemorrhage
Lacunar infarction
Vascular dementia
Retinopathy

Heart Disease
Left ventricular hypertrophy
Atrial fibrillation
Coronary microangiopathy
Coronary heart disease, myocardial infarction
Heart failure

Nephropathy
Albuminuria
Proteinuria
Chronic renal insufficiency
Renal failure

Data from Schmieder RE. End-organ damage in hypertension. Dtsch Arztebl Int. 2010;107:866–873.

world. The guideline change now recognizes that 46% of US adults are now identified as having high blood pressure, compared with 32% under the previous definition. Classification of systemic blood pressure for adults is presented in Table 2.2. Unfortunately, only about half (54%) of hypertensive patients have their condition under control.[7] End-organs affected by hypertension include the heart, brain, and kidneys. The heart is predisposed to hypertrophic changes secondary to increased vascular resistance associated with the hypertensive state. Hypertensive damage to the intracerebral vasculature may result in hemorrhage or stroke. End-organ renal damage secondary to hypertension reduces the glomerular filtration rate and renal blood flow.

Systemic hypertension is a significant risk factor for the development of vasculopathy, cerebrovascular damage, heart disease, and nephropathy. End-organ effects associated with chronic hypertension are identified in Box 2.2. Presedation concerns associated with the hypertensive patient presenting with a long-standing history of hypertension include the following:

- Duration of hypertension (when initially diagnosed)
- Effectiveness of prescribed treatment plan (e.g., diet, salt restriction, medication use)
- Identification of medication and dosage used to treat hypertension
- Identification of the patient's presedation anxiety level

How should the presedation patient assessment be conducted for the hypertensive patient?

Presedation assessment of the hypertensive patient should initially include documentation of the patient's baseline blood pressure. It is equally important to assess the patient's level of compliance with the prescribed treatment plan. During this portion of the cardiovascular assessment, dietary compliance (e.g., salt restriction, weight reduction) and antihypertensive medication efficacy should be ascertained. This assessment should identify all medications used to treat hypertension. Commonly used antihypertensive medications are shown in Table 2.3. Antihypertensive medications should be continued on the day of surgery. Angiotensin-converting enzyme inhibitors (e.g., lisinopril, captopril, enalapril) and angiotensin II receptor blockers (e.g., valsartan, eprosartan) are generally held for patients who have medical conditions in which hypotension is particularly dangerous or major fluid shifts are anticipated during the procedure. Hypertensive patients scheduled for moderate procedural sedation and analgesia should receive presedation medication instructions prior to the planned procedure from the physician's office or health care facility responsible for scheduling the procedure.

It is not uncommon for patients presenting for their procedure to be hypertensive on their initial presedation blood pressure screening. Presedation anxiety increases catecholamine release. At times, this patient population is

TABLE 2.3 Commonly Used Antihypertensive Medications

Class	Subclass	Generic Name	Trade Name
Diuretics	Thiazide	Chlorothiazide	Diuril
		Hydrochlorothiazide	HydroDIURIL, Microzide
		Indapamide	Lozol
		Metolazone	Zaroxolyn, Mykrox
	Loop	Bumetanide	Bumex
		Furosemide	Lasix
		Torsemide	Demadex
	Potassium-sparing	Amiloride	Midamor
		Spironolactone	Aldactone
		Triamterene	Dyrenium
Adrenergic antagonists	Beta blocker	Atenolol	Tenormin
		Bisoprolol	Zebeta
		Metoprolol	Lopressor
		Nadolol	Corgard
		Propranolol	Inderal
		Timolol	Blocadren
	Alpha-1 blocker	Doxazosin	Cardura
		Prazosin	Minipress
		Terazosin	Hytrin
	Combined alpha and beta blockers	Carvedilol	Coreg
		Labetalol	Normodyne, Trandate
	Centrally acting	Clonidine	Catapres
		Methyldopa	Aldomet
Vasodilators		Hydralazine	Apresoline
Angiotensin-converting enzyme inhibitors		Benazepril	Lotensin
		Captopril	Capoten
		Enalapril	Vasotec
		Fosinopril	Monopril
		Lisinopril	Prinivil, Zestril
		Moexipril	Univasc
		Quinapril	Accupril
		Ramipril	Altace
		Trandolapril	Mavik
Angiotensin receptor blockers		Candesartan	Atacand
		Eprosartan	Teveten
		Irbesartan	Avapro
		Losartan	Cozaar
		Olmesartan	Benicar
		Telmisartan	Micardis
		Valsartan	Diovan
Calcium channel blockers	Dihydropyridine	Amlodipine	Norvasc
		Felodipine	Plendil
		Isradipine	DynaCirc
		Nicardipine	Cardene
		Nifedipine	Adalat, Procardia
		Nisoldipine	Sular
		Clevidipine	Cleviprex
	Nondihydropyridine	Diltiazem	Cardizem, Dilacor, Tiazac
		Verapamil	Calan, Isoptin SR, Covera

From Hines RL, Marschall KE: *Stoelting's Anesthesia and Co-Existing Disease.* 7th ed. Philadelphia: Elsevier; 2018.

normotensive when presedation assessment is performed several days prior to the procedure and hypertensive on the day of the procedure. Management of patients in this group includes thorough patient preparation for the procedure, reassurance, and administration of the patient's morning antihypertensive medication. Once an IV line is established, the administration of small doses of a benzodiazepine may reduce the patient's anxiety level, with a resultant decrease in blood pressure. Elevated blood pressure does not necessarily require procedural cancellation. Procedural cancellation is generally reserved for marked hypertension when the systolic blood pressure exceeds 180 mm Hg and the diastolic readings exceed 110 mm Hg, or when there is evidence of end-organ damage. An altered baroreceptor reflex and intravascular volume depletion, which frequently accompany a chronic hypertensive state, may also manifest as labile blood pressure throughout the procedure.

What considerations must be given to the patient presenting for moderate procedural sedation and analgesia with a history of myocardial ischemia?

Atherosclerotic vascular disease increases directly with the aging process. Fig. 2.2 identifies the prevalence of coronary heart disease by age and gender in the United States.

Heart disease is the leading cause of death for both men and women.[8] Therefore it is vitally important to assess for the presence of myocardial ischemia in patients presenting for moderate procedural sedation and analgesia. Risk factors for the development of coronary artery disease and myocardial ischemia include the following:

- Male gender
- Increased age
- Hypercholesterolemia
- Systemic hypertension
- Cigarette smoking
- Diabetes mellitus
- Obesity
- Sedentary lifestyle
- Genetics, family history

Myocardial ischemia occurs when there is an imbalance between coronary blood flow and myocardial consumption. The imbalance in this supply and demand phenomenon results in the development of myocardial ischemia. The patient's cardiopulmonary status or fitness level must be assessed to ensure that there is no imbalance between supply and demand. The patient's actual exercise tolerance and work activity tolerance can be summarized by evaluating their metabolic equivalents of the task (METs). Table 2.4 provides a summary of METs of functional capacity related to the activities of daily living. Once metabolic equivalent assessment is completed, it is also important to ascertain a history of chest

TABLE 2.4	Metabolic Equivalents (METs)[a] of Functional Capacity
METs	**Equivalent Level of Exercise**
1	Eating, working at computer, or dressing
2	Walking down stairs, walking in your house, or cooking
3	Walking one or two blocks on level ground
4	Raking leaves or gardening
5	Climbing one flight of stairs, dancing, or bicycling
6	Playing golf or carrying clubs
7	Playing singles tennis
8	Rapidly climbing stairs or slowly jogging
9	Jumping rope slowly or cycling moderately
10	Swimming quickly, running, or jogging briskly
11	Skiing cross country or playing full court basketball
12	Running rapidly for moderate to long distances

[a]1 MET is equivalent to oxygen consumption of 3.5 mL/min per kg body weight.
Modified from Jette M, Sidney K, Blumchen G: Metabolic equivalents (METS) in exercise testing, exercise prescription, and evaluation of functional capacity, *Clin Cardiol.* 1990;13:555–565.

pain. Questions related to chest pain must attempt to identify the following parameters, including these:

- Character
- Frequency
- Location
- Duration
- Radiation
- Methods of relief

Physical assessment of the patient with coronary artery disease includes the assessment of skin color, presence of jugular venous distention, peripheral edema, assessment of baseline blood pressure, and auscultation of heart sounds. An electrocardiogram may reveal normal sinus rhythm, the presence of dysrhythmias, or signs of previous infarction. Previous ECGs should be available for comparison. Postoperative monitoring must also be continued until the patient is fully recovered and demonstrates no signs of cardiovascular instability. Patients with coronary artery disease should receive their prescribed nitrates, calcium channel blockers, beta blockers, and antihypertensive medications before the scheduled procedure.

What considerations must be given to the patient presenting for moderate procedural sedation and analgesia with a history of previous myocardial infarction?

Presedation assessment of patients with previous myocardial infarction must identify the length of time elapsed since the last myocardial infarction (MI). Questioning to elicit a history of angina, precipitating factors and cardiovascular instability, or shortness of breath is required. If the patient admits to a history of angina, mechanisms of relief must be ascertained. Identifying a history of MI is an important assessment factor when conducting the cardiac preprocedure patient assessment. Using a discharge database of more than 0.5 million

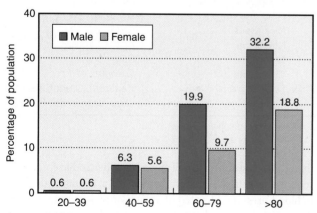

Fig. 2.2 Prevalence of coronary heart disease by age and gender. (From Hines RL, Marschall KE: *Stoelting's Anesthesia and Co-Existing Disease.* 7th ed. Philadelphia: Elsevier; 2018.)

patients, it was shown that the postoperative MI rate in patients with a recent MI decreased substantially as the length of time from the prior MI to the time of surgery increased:

- <1 month = 32%
- 1 to 2 months = 18.7%
- 2 to 3 months = 8.4%
- 3 to 6 months = 5.9%

The 30-day mortality rate also decreased as time since the recent MI increased.[9] Patients with a history of recent myocardial ischemia should be evaluated and managed by a member of the anesthesia care team. Anesthesia care team members can provide and more closely manage procedural events that influence the balance between myocardial oxygen delivery and myocardial oxygen requirements. Procedural events, including decreased oxygen delivery and increased oxygen requirements, are featured in Box 2.3.

What considerations must be given to the patient presenting for moderate procedural sedation and analgesia with a history of cardiac dysrhythmias?

Cardiac dysrhythmias may be caused by the following:

- Effects of medications administered
- Hypoxemia
- Hypercarbia
- Electrolyte abnormalities
- Alterations of the autonomic nervous system
- Procedural manipulations
- Presedation patient anxiety
- Hypovolemia
- Hypotension

In most patients with a normal cardiac reserve, dysrhythmias are generally well tolerated. Patients with limited cardiac

reserve, however, may not tolerate even the most benign dysrhythmias. Newly diagnosed dysrhythmias or those that impair myocardial performance require further evaluation and consultation. Cardiac dysrhythmias and treatment protocols are discussed in Chapter 8.

When are antibiotics indicated for the moderate procedural sedation patient with a history of cardiac valvular disease?

Patients at risk for infective endocarditis for scheduled moderate procedural sedation and analgesia procedures include the following:

- Valve replacements
- Complex congenital heart disease
- Previous endocarditis

Contemporary guidelines have dramatically scaled back conditions and procedures requiring antibiotic prophylaxis.[10] Procedures now requiring antibiotic prophylaxis are reserved for high-risk patients. Recommended antibiotic prophylaxis from the AHA is available at http://www.heart.org/en/health-topics/infective-endocarditis.

What are the components of the presedation cardiac evaluation?

Completion of the presedation cardiac evaluation should incorporate the findings of the patient's history, physical examination, and a review of recent laboratory data. Patients with a recent MI, unstable angina, poor exercise tolerance, cardiac dysrhythmias, dyspnea, fatigue, coronary artery disease, or hypertension may require further consultation and evaluation with a cardiologist. When indicated, additional cardiac testing (e.g., stress test, echocardiography, cardiac catheterization) may reveal valuable information that will alter presedation and procedural management of the sedation patient. The 2014 American College of Cardiology/AHA Task Force has a stepwise algorithm that can be adapted for clinical use in assessing the sedation patient with cardiovascular disease; it is shown in Fig. 2.3. Adequate time must be allotted for all nonemergent therapeutic and diagnostic procedures to ensure that the patient is thoroughly evaluated, as outlined by the American College of Cardiology and AHA guidelines, and is hemodynamically stable and in optimum cardiovascular condition prior to the planned procedure.

Which pulmonary parameters require assessment prior to administering moderate procedural sedation and analgesia?

Sedative and analgesic medications interfere with the regulation of spontaneous pulmonary ventilation. Patterns of respiration are identified in Fig. 2.4. Prevention of respiratory complications, including respiratory failure, atelectasis, and hypoxia, requires careful presedation assessment and planning. Presedation pulmonary assessment must address the type, severity, and reversibility of preexisting pulmonary disease. Symptoms of pulmonary disease must be ascertained

---

BOX 2.3 Procedural Events That Influence the Balance Between Myocardial Oxygen Delivery and Myocardial Oxygen Requirements

Decreased Oxygen Delivery
Decreased coronary blood flow
Tachycardia
Hypotension
Hypocapnia (coronary artery vasoconstriction)
Coronary artery spasm
Decreased oxygen content
Anemia
Arterial hypoxemia
Shift of the oxyhemoglobin dissociation curve to the left

Increased Oxygen Requirements
Sympathetic nervous system stimulation
Tachycardia
Hypertension
Increased myocardial contractility
Increased afterload
Increased preload

From Hines RL, Marschall KE: *Stoelting's Anesthesia and Co-Existing Disease.* 7th ed. Philadelphia: Elsevier; 2018.

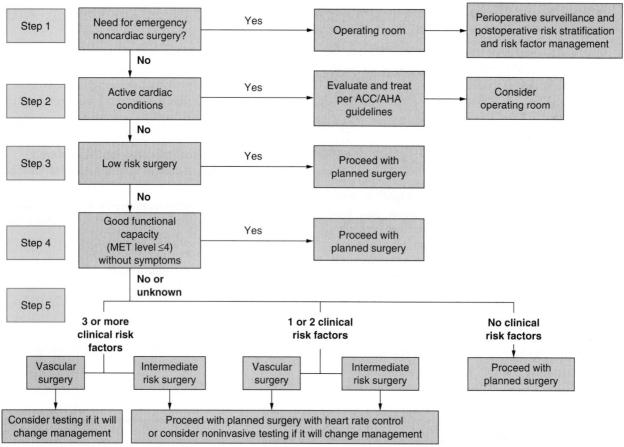

Fig. 2.3 2014 ACC/AHA guideline on perioperative cardiovascular evaluation. (Adapted from Fleisher LA, Fleischmann KE, Auerbach AD, et al; American College of Cardiology; American Heart Association. 2014 ACC/AHA guideline on perioperative cardiovascular evaluation and management of patients undergoing noncardiac surgery: a report of the American College of Cardiology/American Heart Association Task Force on practice guidelines. *Am Coll Cardiol.* 2014;64[22]:e77–e137.)

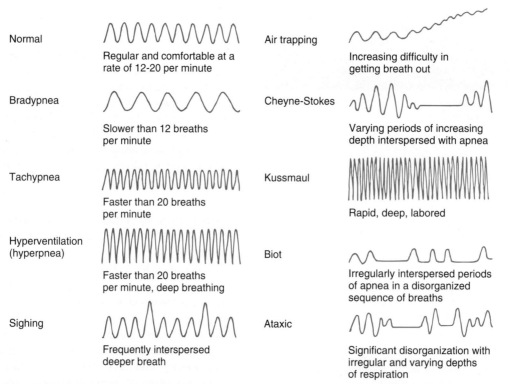

Fig. 2.4 Patterns of respiration. (From Ball JW, Dains JE, Flynn JA, et al, eds: *Seidel's Guide to Physical Examination.* 9th ed. St Louis: Elsevier; 2019.)

by the clinician before the anticipated procedure. Pulmonary symptoms that predispose the patient to increased risk include the following:

- Chronic cough
- Sputum production
- Rhinitis
- Sore throat
- Dyspnea
- Cigarette smoking
- Previous pulmonary complications
- Hemoptysis

What is the impact of preprocedure dyspnea on the moderate sedation patient?

Dyspnea is present when there is demonstrated difficult or labored breathing, with shortness of breath, and may be described by the patient as a subjective feeling of discomfort associated with breathing. Dyspnea may manifest as a symptom of obesity, deconditioning, and cardiac or pulmonary disorders. It generally increases with the severity of the underlying pathophysiologic condition. The presence of dyspnea on presedation evaluation may be an ominous sign. Dyspnea occurs when the requirement for oxygen is greater than the patient's ability to respond to the increased demand physiologically. Causes of dyspnea are listed in Box 2.4.[11-21] Patients with a history of dyspnea require further presedation pulmonary evaluation. Assessment of dyspnea at rest or at specific levels of exertion is an important indicator of the severity of preexisting pulmonary disease. It is important to assess the amount and type of effort that produces dyspnea. Identification of dyspnea at rest, walking (upstairs vs. level surface), and frequency of stopping for rest during the climb or walk, and determining with what other activities of daily life dyspnea occurs, are qualitative assessment tools used by the health care provider assessing the patient prior to moderate procedural sedation administration.

Regardless of the presence of preexisting pulmonary disease, the presedation pulmonary assessment should focus on the identification and treatment of acute infections with appropriate antibiotic therapy. Relief of bronchospastic disease using bronchodilators, implementation of mechanisms to improve sputum clearance (e.g., postural drainage, incentive spirometry), and cessation of cigarette smoking will help optimize the patient's presedation pulmonary condition. Patients presenting for moderate procedural sedation or analgesia must undergo a focused physical examination, including vital signs, auscultation of the heart and lungs, and evaluation of the airway.

Are there specific preprocedure assessment considerations for the sedation patient presenting with chronic obstructive pulmonary disease?

Patients with COPD frequently have a history of cigarette smoking. Dyspnea, cough, and wheezing may be present. As the disease progresses, a barrel chest may develop and use of accessory muscles for respiratory excursion and pursed

---

BOX 2.4   Causes of Dyspnea[11-21]

Acute Causes
- Asthma
- Carbon monoxide poisoning
- Cardiac tamponade
- Hiatal hernia
- Heart failure
- Hypotension
- Pulmonary embolism
- Pneumothorax
- Pneumonia
- Anemia
- Upper airway obstruction

Chronic Causes
- Asthma
- Chronic obstructive pulmonary disease
- Deconditioning
- Heart dysfunction
- Interstitial lung disease
- Obesity

Additional Causes
- Croup
- Lung cancer
- Pleurisy
- Pulmonary edema
- Pulmonary hypertension
- Sarcoidosis
- Tuberculosis
- Cardiomyopathy
- Dysrhythmias
- Heart failure
- Pericarditis
- Broken ribs
- Anxiety disorder
- Neuromuscular disease(s)

---

lip breathing may ensue. COPD encompasses asthma, chronic obstructive bronchitis (with obstruction of small airways), and emphysema—with enlargement of air spaces and destruction of lung parenchyma, loss of lung elasticity, and closure of small airways.[22]

Are there specific preprocedure assessment considerations for the sedation patient presenting with a history of asthma?

Asthma affects approximately 7.6% of the adult population, 8.4% of children in the United States, and 300 million people globally.[23] Asthma is a chronic condition characterized by airway inflammation and reversible expiratory airway obstruction owing to narrowing of the airway lumen and airway hyperreactivity. Asthma is accompanied by a combination of clinical features, which include the following:

- Wheezing
- Bronchial hyperreactivity with reversibility
- Increased airway responsiveness
- Decreased mucociliary clearance
- Increased mucus production

Stimuli that provoke symptoms and clinical features of asthma include the following:

- Pharmacologic agents, including aspirin, beta antagonists, some nonsteroidal antiinflammatory drugs, and sulfating agents in food preservatives
- Respiratory viral and bacterial infections
- Exercise in which attacks typically follow exertion, rather than occurring during exercise
- Emotional stress
- Vagal mediation

Prior to the administration of sedation, the asthmatic patient should exhibit no signs of respiratory infection (e.g., fever, productive cough). Eradication of acute and chronic infection with antibiotics is essential. The absence of wheezing, dyspnea, or recent attacks most likely indicates that the patient is in a stable phase of the disease. Presedation assessment must include pharmacologic evaluation of the asthmatic patient. Prior to the procedure, the asthmatic patient's response to short-acting bronchodilators—albuterol (Proventil), levalbuterol (Xopenex), metaproterenol, and pirbuterol (Maxair)—and asthmatic medications for long-term treatment of asthma, featured in Table 2.5, must be assessed prior to the administration of moderate procedural sedation and analgesia. Additional presedation assessment for asthma includes identifying the date of the last asthma attack, severity of the attack, and mechanisms used to relieve symptoms associated with the attack. The patient taking beta agonists should use his or her own metered-dose inhaler (MDI) before the planned procedure, as per physician orders.

TABLE 2.5   Drugs Used for Long-Term Treatment of Asthma

Class	Drug	Action	Adverse Effects
Inhaled corticosteroid	Beclomethasone Budesonide (Pulmicort) Ciclesonide Flunisolide Fluticasone (Flovent) Mometasone Triamcinolone	Decrease airway inflammation. Reduce airway hyperresponsiveness.	Dysphonia Myopathy of laryngeal muscles Oropharyngeal candidiasis
Long-acting bronchodilator	Arformoterol (Brovana) Formoterol Salmeterol	Beta-2 agonist stimulates beta-2 receptors in the tracheobronchial tree.	Therapy with just long-acting bronchodilators can cause airway inflammation and an increased incidence of asthma exacerbations; should not be used except with an inhaled corticosteroid
Combined inhaled corticosteroids + long-acting bronchodilators	Budesonide + formoterol (Symbicort) Fluticasone + salmeterol (Advair)	Combines long-acting bronchodilator and inhaled corticosteroid.	
Leukotriene modifier	Montelukast (Singulair) Zafirlukast (Accolate) Zileuton (Zyflo)	Reduce synthesis of leukotrienes by inhibiting 5-lipoxygenase enzyme.	Minimal
Anti-IgE monoclonal antibody	Omalizumab (Xolair)	Decreases IgE release by inhibiting binding of IgE to mast cells and basophils.	Injection site reaction Arthralgia Sinusitis Pharyngitis Headache
Methylxanthine	Theophylline Aminophylline	Increase cAMP by inhibiting phosphodiesterase, block adenosine receptors, and release endogenous catecholamines.	Disrupted sleep cycle Nervousness Nausea, vomiting, anorexia Headache Dysrhythmias
Mast cell stabilizer	Cromolyn	Inhibits mediator release from mast cells; membrane stabilization.	Cough Throat irritation

cAMP, Cyclic adenosine monophosphate; *IgE,* immunoglobulin E.
From Hines RL, Marschall KE: *Stoelting's Anesthesia and Co-Existing Disease.* 7th ed. Philadelphia: Elsevier; 2018

MDIs, oxygen, and breathing treatment equipment should also be available in the procedure room. Morphine sulfate is relatively contraindicated in the asthmatic patient population because of its histamine-releasing properties. An estimated 5% of patients with asthma are sensitive to bisulfite and metabisulfite, which are used for preservatives and antioxidants by the food processing industry. These substances are also present in a large number of medications used in health care today.[24] Fortunately, through identification of the last attack, assessing attack severity, determining the mechanism of relief, and continuation of the patient's prescribed pharmacologic protocol, many asthmatic patients tolerate the administration of moderate procedural sedation and analgesia without incident.

Are there specific preprocedure assessment considerations for the sedation patient presenting with a history of bronchitis?

Chronic bronchitis may occur secondary to prolonged exposure of the airways to nonspecific irritants. It is characterized by the hypersecretion of mucus and inflammatory changes in the bronchi. Bronchitis is a common cause of COPD and is manifested by permanent or minimally reversible obstruction to airflow during exhalation. Patients with cough, dyspnea, and sputum production may require supplemental oxygenation to avoid hypoxemia and allow the patient the ability to carry out the activities of daily living. Presedation assessment of the patient with bronchitis requires a determination of the severity of dyspnea, hypoxia, and infection. Supplemental oxygen is recommended during the procedure and should remain in place until all residual respiratory depressant effects have dissipated. Depending on the severity of the pathophysiologic disease process, pulmonary function tests, chest radiography, arterial blood gases, bronchodilators, and antibiotic therapy may be ordered by the physician prior to the planned sedation procedure.

What is the impact of a history of sleep apnea on a patient presenting for moderate procedural sedation?

A pulmonary disorder of significant concern for the sedation provider is sleep apnea. Sleep apnea affects up to 9% of middle-aged women and 24% of middle-aged men. However, less than 15% of these cases have been diagnosed. Sleep apnea occurs when there is cessation of airflow at the mouth for longer than 10 seconds. Central alveolar hypoventilation syndrome occurs when there is absence of the neural drive to ventilation when voluntary control of breathing is diminished by sleep. Central sleep apnea most likely reflects a defect in the function of the medullary ventilatory center. Obstructive sleep apnea is due to abnormal relaxation of the genioglossus muscle that normally holds the tongue forward and relaxation of the pharyngeal muscles. Obstructive sleep apnea may also occur secondary to decreased neural input to these muscles from the brain stem.

What is the cause of sleep apnea?

Regardless of the cause, sleep apnea is primarily a disorder of the upper airway at the level of the pharynx. Sleep apnea is characterized by episodes of apnea or hypopnea during sleep. Airway obstruction results in snoring and daytime somnolence. The upper airway obstruction leads to fragmented sleep, arterial hypoxemia, hypercarbia, polycythemia, systemic and pulmonary hypertension, and right ventricular failure.

The cause of obstructive sleep apnea (OSA) is associated with the dilator muscles responsible for maintaining increased airway tone to prevent collapse and obstruction. Relaxation of the dilator muscles during sleep results in decreased laminar flow, with resultant turbulent airflow and snoring. The decreased airflow and partial obstruction leads to sleep disturbances, arterial hypoxemia, and hypercarbia. This pattern ultimately results in arousal from the sleep state.

How is sleep apnea diagnosed?

Diagnosis of sleep apnea is confirmed by polysomnography in a designated sleep laboratory. Polysomnography sleep laboratory technicians monitor the patient for obstructive apneic episodes during sleep. An "episode" is defined as 10 seconds or longer of total cessation of airflow, despite continuous inspiratory effort against a partially or completely obstructed airway. Presedation patient assessment includes questioning for signs and symptoms associated with OSA. These signs and symptoms include the following:
- Morning headache
- Hypertension
- Stroke
- Ischemic heart disease
- Loss of initiative
- Lassitude
- Memory loss
- Cognitive dysfunction
- Overwhelming somnolence during normal waking hours

What is the optimal clinical management for a sleep apneic patient?

Patients presenting for sedation with OSA should be scheduled as early in the morning as possible. This patient population is sensitive to the respiratory depressant effects associated with the administration of central nervous (CNS) depressant medications. Clinical management includes careful assessment of the patient's airway prior to the commencement of the procedure. Titration to clinical effect is required to avoid the development of deep sedative states or general anesthesia. Institution of the patient's CPAP (continuous positive airway pressure), BIPAP (bilevel positive airway pressure), or ASV (adaptive servo-ventilation) immediately postprocedure should be ordered by the attending physician. Oxygen therapy is also beneficial during procedural and postprocedural patient care. It is imperative for the sedation provider to realize that patients with OSA are extremely sensitive to all CNS depressant medications. The administration of these medications increases the potential for increased airway obstruction or the development of apnea with minimal doses of these medications. For this reason, the prudent sedation practitioner should use minimal doses of sedation and analgesic medications to avoid unnecessary complications.

Should sedative dosages be reduced for the sleep apneic patient?

The dosage of sedative medications must be based on the patient's response to an initial low-dose sedative and analgesic medication test doses. Many prudent practitioners administer an initial test dose of sedative or analgesic agent to the sleep apneic patient that is reduced by as much as 50% to 70% to ascertain the ventilatory depressant effects associated with the medication(s), as well as the patient's response to this initial dose of sedation. The sleep apneic patient is also at high risk for developing arterial hypoxemia during the postprocedure period. For the reasons delineated, it is important to identify the sleep apneic patient prior to administering moderate procedural sedation. The STOP-Bang questionnaire, featured in Box 2.5, is a validated preanesthesia screening tool that provides the health care provider with an assessment score to identify the level of risk for the sleep apneic patient and the severity of sleep apnea.[25,26] The currently available data in the literature support the idea that a correlation exists between a higher STOP-Bang score and the severity of OSA. Accordingly, the STOP-Bang score can be used not only to identify cases with any degree of OSA but also prioritize those who are more likely to have moderate to severe disease. The STOP-Bang questionnaire should be considered the optimal screening tool at present; the score can be used for making more reasoned clinical decisions.[27] Regardless of clinical practice setting (e.g., hospital, surgery center, physician's office), a clearly written policy on managing the sleep apneic patient should be aligned with the guidelines from the American Society of Anesthesiologists Task Force on the Perioperative Management of Patients with Obstructive Sleep Apnea.[28] A summary of clinical considerations for the sleep apneic patient is presented in Table 2.6.

Are there specific preprocedure assessment considerations for the sedation patient presenting with a history of liver disease?

The liver is responsible for the synthesis of proteins and clotting factors and for the detoxification of pharmacologic agents and metabolic byproducts. The liver also excretes bodily waste products, stores iron and vitamins, and supplements the body's energy stores. It is the largest organ in the body and receives approximately 25% of the cardiac output, although it constitutes only 2.5% of the body weight.[29] Treatment of patients with impaired hepatic function should attempt to prevent further hepatic deterioration. Patients presenting for moderate procedural sedation and analgesia sedation services must be assessed for signs or symptoms associated with acute or chronic liver disease. These symptoms include the following:

- Ascites
- Portal hypertension
- Arteriolar vasodilation
- Arterial desaturation
- Decreased hematocrit
- Encephalopathy

BOX 2.5   STOP-Bang Questionnaire[a]

Height _____ cm/inches
Weight _____ lb/kg
Age _____
Male/Female
BMI _____
Collar size of shirt: S, M, L, XL or _____ cm/inches
Neck circumference_____ cm

1. Snoring
   Do you snore loudly (louder than talking or loud enough to be heard through closed doors)?
   Yes/No
2. Tired
   Do you often feel tired, fatigued, or sleepy during daytime?
   Yes/No
3. Observed
   Has anyone observed you stop breathing during your sleep?
   Yes/No
4. Blood Pressure
   Do you have or are you being treated for high blood pressure?
   Yes/No
5. BMI
   BMI more than 35 kg/m^2?
   Yes/No
6. Age
   Age over 50 years old?
   Yes/No
7. Neck circumference (measure with approved measuring tape)[b]
   Neck circumference greater than 40 cm?
   Yes/No
8. Gender
   Gender: male?
   Yes/No

BMI, Body mass index.
Modified from Chung F, Yang Y, Liao P. Predictive performance of the STOP-BANG score for identifying obstructive sleep apnea in obese patients. *Obes Surg,* 2013;23(12):2050–2057.
[a]Score of 4—high sensitivity of 88% for identifying severe obstructive sleep apnea (OSA); score of 5 or more—high risk of OSA; score of 6 is more specific.
[b]Neck circumference is measured by staff.

- Laboratory abnormalities
- Elevated ALT (alanine aminotransferase) level
- Elevated AST (aspartate aminotransferase) level

Are there pharmacologic considerations for the moderate sedation patient presenting with a history of hepatic disease?

An important pharmacologic function of the liver is the breakdown of lipid-soluble medications into water-soluble compounds via the hepatic cytochrome P-450 microsomal enzyme system. The degree of metabolism of pharmacologic compounds is dependent on hepatic blood flow and enzyme activity in the endoplasmic reticulum. In some cases, patients with significant liver impairment may exhibit resistance to

TABLE 2.6   Management of the Sedation Patient with Obstructive Sleep Apnea

Potential Sources of Perioperative Risk	Perioperative Risk Mitigation
Lack of institutional protocol for perioperative management of sleep apnea patients	Develop and implement institutional protocol for perioperative management of sleep apnea patients.
Patients with a known diagnosis of obstructive sleep apnea (OSA)	Know sleep study results. Know the therapy being used—oral appliance, positive airway pressure (PAP) with settings (mode, pressure level, supplemental oxygen, if any). Consult sleep medicine specialist as needed.
Patients without a diagnosis of OSA	Use a screening tool to determine the likelihood of OSA— AASM questionnaire, ASA checklist, Berlin questionnaire, or STOP-Bang questionnaire.
Inpatient versus outpatient surgery	Decisions based on institutional protocol containing factors related to (1) patient, (2) procedure, (3) facility, and (4) postdischarge setting.
Preoperative lack of optimization of therapy for OSA	Consult sleep medicine specialist to optimize therapy.
Preoperative sedative-induced airway compromise or respiratory depression	Use preoperative sedation only in a monitored setting.
Intraoperative sedative-, opioid-, anesthetic-induced upper airway compromise or respiratory depression during monitored anesthesia care (MAC)	Whenever possible, use topical, local, or regional anesthesia, with minimal to no sedation. Continuously monitor ventilation adequacy. Use the patient's OSA therapy device during MAC, with sedation. Consider general anesthesia with a secured airway versus deep sedation with an unsecured airway
At risk for oxygen desaturation	Elevate head of bed to facilitate spontaneous ventilation and oxygenation. Preoxygenate sufficiently. Maintain oxygen insufflation by nasal cannula during endotracheal intubation.
Possible difficult mask ventilation or endotracheal intubation	Apply ASA difficult airway algorithm, including the use of laryngeal mask airway, videolaryngoscope, fiberoptic bronchoscope, and transtracheal jet ventilation as indicated. Optimize head and neck position for mask ventilation and endotracheal intubation.
Potential difficulty with noninvasive blood pressure monitoring and/or increased risk for cardiovascular complications	Consider intraarterial catheter for blood pressure monitoring and blood sampling for arterial blood gases.
Postextubation airway obstruction in the operating room or postanesthesia care unit, with associated risk of negative pressure pulmonary edema	Elevate the head of the bed. Extubate only after patient clearly meets objective extubation criteria. Maintain readiness for re-intubation with the same device used during induction, and expect that the difficulty of intubation will be greater than previously.
At risk for postoperative oxygen desaturation	Use supplemental oxygen therapy. Consider nasal airway. Consider PAP therapy (this can be initiated de novo in the postoperative setting).
Communication failure during transfer of care	Identify the patient's diagnosis of sleep apnea and its therapy. Alert staff about expected problems and their management.
Perioperative opioid-related respiratory depression due to opioids administered by neuraxial route, intravenous route with bolus injection, or via IV patient-controlled analgesia (IV-PCA)	Give supplemental oxygen as needed. Continuous electronic monitoring of oxygenation and ventilation. Maintain patient's OSA therapy whenever possible; use home settings as a guide. Avoid background mode with IV-PCA. Consider opioid-sparing analgesic techniques (e.g., transcutaneous electrical nerve stimulation), and use nonopioid analgesics (e.g., NSAIDs, acetaminophen, tramadol, ketamine, gabapentin) whenever possible.
Postdischarge opioid-induced respiratory depression and/or exacerbation of OSA	Ensure companionship and a safe home environment for high-risk patients. Consult sleep medicine specialist to optimize sleep apnea therapy if needed.

AASM, American Academy of Sleep Medicine; *ASA,* American Society of Anesthesiologists; *NSAIDs,* nonsteroidal antiinflammatory drugs.
From Hines RL, Marschall KE: *Stoelting's Anesthesia and Co-Existing Disease.* 7th ed. Philadelphia: Elsevier; 2018.

sedative and analgesic medications because of the accentuated drug metabolism attributed to enzyme induction. Conversely, patients with liver disease may be extremely sensitive to pharmacologic medications because of a decrease in hepatic blood flow and destruction of hepatocytes, which contain the microsomal enzyme system. It is critically important for the sedation provider to recognize that patients with liver disease have diminished physiologic reserves. Therefore, with acute or chronic liver failure, careful titration and vigilance are required to assess a patient's response to the medications administered.

What are the presedation considerations associated with the patient presenting for moderate procedural sedation and analgesia with a history of hepatitis?

Hepatitis is characterized by inflammation of the hepatocytes. Characteristics of hepatitis are listed in Table 2.7 and Table 2.8. The diagnosis of hepatitis is often confirmed only after presentation with fatigue, anorexia, dark urine, fever, hepatomegaly, ascites, esophageal varices, and peripheral edema. A combination of these symptoms may signify severe hepatic disease. The treatment of hepatitis often focuses on the presenting symptoms. Attention to the nutritional support and hydration status of the patient is imperative. Presedation preparation of the patient with hepatitis should discourage the use of alcohol. Assessment of the

coagulation profile, nutritional status, and optimization of presenting symptoms is required before the planned procedure is performed.

What are the presedation considerations associated with the patient presenting for moderate procedural sedation and analgesia with a history of cirrhosis?

Cirrhosis is a liver disease that results in scarring and destruction of liver cells. Decreased hepatic blood flow occurs with increased resistance of flow through the portal system. Cirrhosis and portal hypertension also affect the cardiopulmonary system in the cirrhotic patient. The cardiovascular effects associated with cirrhosis include hyperdynamic circulation, cardiomyopathy, and portal vein hypertension. Pulmonary considerations associated with cirrhosis include decreased oxygen affinity for the hemoglobin molecule, accompanied by varying degrees of oxygen desaturation. This predisposition to desaturation and hypoxemia requires careful titration, with a dosage reduction of sedative and analgesic medications. In cases of advanced liver disease, ascites secondary to portal hypertension, hypoalbuminemia, and edema also predispose cirrhotic patients to hypoxemia. Patients presenting with hepatic disease require careful assessment to ascertain the magnitude of the disease. A predisposition to hypoxemia and decreased drug metabolism require attentive monitoring and careful titration and dosage reduction of all medications.

TABLE 2.7   The Hepatitis Viruses

Virus	Hepatitis A (HAV)	Hepatitis B (HBV)	Hepatitis C (HCV)	Hepatitis D (HDV)	Hepatitis E (HEV)
Viral genome	ssRNA	partially dsDNA	ssRNA	Circular defective ssRNA	ssRNA
Viral family	Hepatovirus; related to picornavirus	Hepadnavirus	*Flaviviridae*	Subviral particle in *Deltaviridae* family	Calicivirus
Route of transmission	Fecal-oral (contaminated food or water)	Parenteral, sexual contact, perinatal	Parenteral; intranasal cocaine use is a risk factor	Parenteral	Fecal-oral
Incubation period	2–6 weeks	2–26 weeks (mean 8 weeks)	4–26 weeks (mean 9 weeks)	Same as HBV	4–5 weeks
Frequency of chronic liver disease	Never	5%–10%	>80%	10% (coinfection); 90%–100% for superinfection	In immunocompromised hosts only
Diagnosis	Detection of serum IgM antibodies	Detection of HBsAg or antibody to HBcAg; PCR for HBV DNA	ELISA for antibody detection; PCR for HCV RNA	Detection of IgM and IgG antibodies, HDV RNA in serum, or HDAg in liver biopsy	Detection of serum IgM and IgG antibodies; PCR for HEV RNA

ssRNA, Single-stranded RNA; *dsDNA,* double-stranded DNA; *HBcAg,* hepatitis B core antigen; *HBsAg,* hepatitis B surface antigen; *HDAg,* hepatitis D antigen; *ELISA,* enzyme-linked immunosorbent assay.
From Washington K: Inflammatory and infectious diseases of the liver. In Iacobuzio-Donahue CA, Montgomery EA, editors: *Gastrointestinal and liver pathology,* Philadelphia, 2005, Churchill Livingstone.

TABLE 2.8   Characteristics of Hepatitis Viruses

Incubation Period and Mode of Transmission	Sources of Infection	Infectivity
Hepatitis A Virus (HAV) *Incubation:* 15-50 days (average 28) • Fecal-oral (primarily fecal contamination and oral ingestion)	• Crowded conditions (e.g., day care, nursing home) • Poor personal hygiene • Poor sanitation • Contaminated food, milk, water, shellfish • Persons with subclinical infections, infected food handlers, sexual contact, IV drug users	• Most infectious during 2 wk before onset of symptoms • Infectious until 1-2 wk after the start of symptoms
Hepatitis B Virus (HBV) *Incubation:* 45-180 days (average 56-96) • Percutaneous (parenteral) or permucosal exposure to blood or blood products • Sexual contact • Perinatal transmission	• Contaminated needles, syringes, and blood products • Sexual activity with infected partners. Asymptomatic carriers • Tattoos or body piercing with contaminated needles • HBV-infected mother (perinatal transmission)	• Before and after symptoms appear • Infectious for 4-6 mo • Carriers continue to be infectious for life
Hepatitis C Virus (HCV) *Incubation:* 14-180 days (average 56) • Percutaneous (parenteral) or mucosal exposure to blood or blood products • High-risk sexual contact • Perinatal contact	• Blood and blood products • Needles and syringes • Sexual activity with infected partners	• 1-2 wk before symptoms appear • Continues during clinical course • 75%-85% go on to develop chronic hepatitis C and remain infectious
Hepatitis D Virus (HDV) *Incubation:* 2-26 wk • HBV must precede HDV • Chronic carriers of HBV always at risk	• Same as HBV • Can cause infection only when HBV is present • Routes of transmission same as for HBV	• Blood infectious at all stages of HDV infection
Hepatitis E Virus (HEV) *Incubation:* 15-64 days (average 26-42 days) • Fecal-oral route • Outbreaks associated with contaminated water supply in developing countries	• Contaminated water, poor sanitation • Found in Asia, Africa, and Mexico • Not common in United States	• Not known • May be similar to HAV

From Lewis SL et al: *Medical-surgical nursing: Assessment and management of clinical problems,* ed 10, St Louis, 2017, Elsevier.

What are the presedation considerations associated with the patient presenting for moderate procedural sedation and analgesia with renal disease?

Presedation assessment of the renal system is required to assess for the presence of renal pathology prior to the scheduled sedation procedure. Functions of the kidney include the following:

• Regulation and maintenance of fluid status
• Acid-base maintenance system
• Excretion of waste products and electrolyte balance
• Detoxification of pharmacologic agents

The kidneys perform these tasks via filtration, reabsorption, and secretion. Presedation evaluation of renal function consists of assessment of the patient for a history of renal surgery or any degree of renal impairment. A history of minor urologic or renal impairment may include cystitis, incontinence, and benign prostatic disease. Hypertension is also commonly associated with renal disease. Hypertension secondary to renal disease is a result of hypervolemia or alterations in the renin-angiotensin mechanism. Hypertension associated with renal disease is often treated as essential hypertension until end-stage renal failure ensues. There are distinct groups of patients with renal impairment who require additional presedation evaluation.

What is optimal procedural management for the patient with renal disease?

For patients with renal insufficiency presenting for sedation services, optimization of hydration status is a priority. The goal of the provider is to preserve normal renal function throughout the procedure and in the immediate postprocedure period. Depending on the state of hypovolemia or hypervolemia, many authors advocate titration of chloride restrictive fluids.[30,31] Although it is not practical to measure urine output during short diagnostic procedures, urine output should be measured and documented before and after the procedure. Attention to volume status is ensured through adequate presedation assessment of skin turgor, weight, blood pressure, and heart rate. Patients who appear hypervolemic may also require diuretic therapy before the planned procedure.

For patients with little or no existing renal function, presedation assessment and planning should focus on preservation of the remaining organ systems in the body. The vascular cannulation site used for dialysis must be carefully guarded against insult. Blood pressure must not be measured on the side of the vascular access site. Infection is a leading cause of morbidity and death in patients with compromised renal function. Strict adherence to aseptic or sterile technique must be used for all invasive procedures and IV cannula insertion. Anephric patients may be anemic as a result of decreased erythropoietin secretion. Erythropoietin secreted by the kidney is required for the synthesis of hemoglobin molecules. This anemia predisposes the patient to the development of hypoxia. However, issues of anemia can be controlled by the injection of epoetin alfa (Epogen) to supplement lack of erythropoietin secretion, improving laboratory values in some renal patients. Presedation laboratory work may reveal hyperkalemia, increased blood urea nitrogen, calcium, and creatinine levels, and acidosis requiring dialysis. Dialysis before the procedure is beneficial for many patients. However, hypovolemia associated with dialysis performed within several hours of the planned procedure may predispose the patient to the development of procedural hypotension. Careful titration of sedative and analgesic medications is required to avoid hypotension and hypoxemia in this specific patient population.

Once presedation assessment is completed, treatment of renal disease must address presenting symptoms and focus on the following:
- Fluid volume
- Homeostasis
- Electrolyte balance
- Renal clearance
- Hormonal secretion
- Optimizing dialysis treatment (ideally within 24 hours of planned procedure) for the chronic renal patient

What are the pharmacologic considerations for the renal patient presenting for moderate procedural sedation and analgesia?

The presence of preexisting renal disease decreases protein binding, which results in accentuation of pharmacologic effects for highly protein-bound sedative and analgesic medications. Midazolam is 98% protein-bound. In the presence of renal failure and a decrease in protein binding, there is an increase in the active pharmacologic component of midazolam. Therefore, accentuation of benzodiazepine effects may

be greatly enhanced in patients with renal disease. Patients with renal impairment also have a greater risk of an adverse drug reaction.[32] As outlined earlier, pharmacologic effects are accentuated secondary to increased plasma levels of the drug, decreased protein binding, and drug accumulation. Titration and reduction of drug dose must be combined with careful assessment of the cardiopulmonary response to sedative medications in all settings, particularly in patients with preexisting renal dysfunction.

What are the presedation considerations associated with the patient presenting for moderate procedural sedation and analgesia with neurologic disease?

Presedation assessment of the patient with neurologic disease attempts to elicit a history of mental deficiency, cerebral vascular insufficiency, or intrinsic metabolic neurologic disease. The goal of a complete neurologic assessment is to ascertain and document presedation levels of consciousness while evaluating the patient for the presence of preexisting neurologic disease.

Transient ischemic attacks (TIAs) are temporary, reversible ischemic attacks with full recovery in periods ranging from minutes to 24 hours. Temporary interruption of cerebral blood flow may result from plaque or debris, with recovery occurring after dissolution of the debris. The finding of TIAs on presedation assessment may indicate impending severe neurologic dysfunction or stroke.

Cerebral ischemia may also result from insufficient blood flow to the circle of Willis. The circle of Willis receives blood flow for cerebral circulation from the internal carotid artery and the vertebral arteries, which converge to form the posterior basilar artery. Collection of arterial plaque in the carotid artery results in decreased cerebral circulation, with resultant neurologic symptoms, which include the following:
- Visual loss
- Paresis
- Numbness and tingling of the contralateral extremities

Documentation of the incidence, severity, and time to resolution of neurologic symptoms must be completed prior to administering moderate procedural sedation and analgesia. Specific documentation must address existing focal neurologic deficits and any functional neurologic limitations prior to the procedure. Complete documentation of neurologic limitations is important from a medicolegal perspective, particularly when a patient reports a new neurologic deficit postprocedure.

Patients with a history of convulsive disorder require a thorough assessment of their disease state to identify the type of seizure and specific symptoms. Epileptic seizures result from a discharge of abnormally excitable neurons. This excitation may be triggered by discontinuation of medications, infection, neoplasm, drug or alcohol use, electrolyte disturbance, and/or hypoxia. Presedation assessment must focus on the underlying cause of the seizure. Recommendations for anticonvulsant medications include maintenance of therapeutic plasma levels, with continued administration of the patient's medication regimen.

Evaluation of the peripheral nervous system includes assessment of extremity strength, color, temperature, capillary refill, and peripheral pulses. Sensory deficits and decreased reflexes may also signify peripheral sensory impairment. When the neurologic assessment reveals a peripheral neuropathy, the degree, any changes over time, and the exact nature of the specific neuropathy must be documented before the procedure or the administration of sedative or analgesic agents.

What are the presedation considerations associated with the patient presenting for moderate procedural sedation and analgesia with endocrine disease?

Presedation assessment of the endocrine system may reveal primary diseases associated with excess production or decreased production of hormones or by alterations in the stress response.

Diabetes is a chronic disease characterized by disruption of glucose metabolism. This altered glucose metabolism results in excessive plasma glucose levels. Hyperglycemia is a result of impaired synthesis, secretion, or use of endogenous insulin. The diagnosis of diabetes is indicated when a fasting blood glucose level $\geq$ 126 mg/dL after an 8-hour fast, a nonfasting glucose level $\geq$ 200 mg/dL along with symptoms of diabetes, a glucose level $\geq$ 200 mg/dL on a 2-hour glucose tolerance test, or a hemoglobin A1c $\geq$ 6.5%.[33] More than 30 million Americans have diabetes ($\approx$1 in 10), and 90% to 95% of them have type 2 diabetes. Type 2 diabetes usually develops in people older than 45 years, but more children, teenagers, and young adults are also developing it.[34] Type 2 diabetes is characterized by beta cell insufficiency and insulin resistance. Many type 2 diabetic patients do not require insulin and maintain adequate blood sugar levels through dietary restriction, exercise, and weight control. However, some patients may require oral medications to maintain glucose control. The oral and noninsulin injectable hypoglycemic therapies for diabetes are featured in Table 2.9. Glycemic goals and the algorithm for the treatment of the type 2 diabetic patient are featured in Fig. 2.5.

Type 1 diabetes is called insulin-dependent diabetes mellitus (IDDM) and occurs in the remaining 5% to 10% of diabetic patients. Type 1 patients tend to be younger and not predisposed to obesity. Type 1 diabetes occurs secondary to T cell–mediated destruction in the pancreas. Although the exact cause is unknown, possible causative factors include the following:

- Viruses
- Dietary proteins
- Autoimmune process initiation secondary to drugs or chemicals

Type 1 patients are predisposed to hyperglycemia, acidosis, and ketosis. Diabetes may result in end-organ impairment, including the following:

- Hypertension
- Coronary artery disease
- Nephropathy
- Retinopathy
- Neuropathy
- Peripheral vascular disease

TABLE 2.9 Oral and Noninsulin Injectable Hypoglycemic Therapy

Drug Class	Drug Name	Onset	Duration of Action
Oral Agents			
Second-generation sulfonylureas	Glyburide	30 min	24 h
	Glipizide	IR, 30 min ER, 2–4 h	IR, 24 h ER, 24 h
	Glimepiride	2–3 h	24 h
DPP-4 inhibitors	Sitagliptin	1 h	8 h
	Saxagliptin	1 h	8 h
	Linagliptin	1 h	8 h
GLP-1 analogues	Exenatide	1–2 h	24 h
	Liraglutide	1–2 h	24 h
Biguanides	Metformin	1–3 h	17 h
Thiazolidinediones	Rosiglitazone	1–3 h	4 h
	Pioglitazone	2 h	N/A
Nonsulfonylurea secretagogues (meglitinides [glinides])	Repaglinide	30–90 min	4 h
	Nateglinide	30–60 min	4 h
α-Glucosidase inhibitor	Acarbose	2 h	4 h
	Miglitol	1 h	4 h
Injectables			
Glucagon-like peptide 1 receptor agonists	Exenatide (Bydureon ER, once-weekly dosing)	2.1 h	Once weekly
	Byetta (shorter duration exenatide)	2.1 h	Every 12 h
	Liraglutide (Victoza)	8–12 h	Once daily
Amylin analogue	Pramlintide (Symlin)	Duration of action, 3 h	Prior to every major meal

DPP-4, Dipeptidyl peptidase-4; *ER*, extended release; *GLP-I*, glucagon-like peptide 1; *IR*, immediate release; *N/A*, not available.
Adapted from Drugs for type 2 diabetes. Treat Guide Med Lett. 2014;12(139):17–24; and Goldman L, Schafer AI, eds. Goldman's Cecil Medicine, 25th ed. Philadelphia: Elsevier; 2016,

Hypertension and coronary disease associated with diabetes mellitus may increase the incidence of cardiovascular complications (e.g., labile blood pressure, ischemic changes on the ECG, chest pain) during procedural sedation and analgesia. Autonomic neuropathy may present as silent myocardial ischemia and postural hypotension. Gastroparesis secondary to autonomic neuropathy increases the risk of aspiration and regurgitation.

What are the current medication management recommendations for the diabetic patient scheduled for moderate procedural sedation and analgesia?

The distinguishing features of diabetes are highlighted in Table 2.10. Oral and noninsulin injectable hypoglycemic

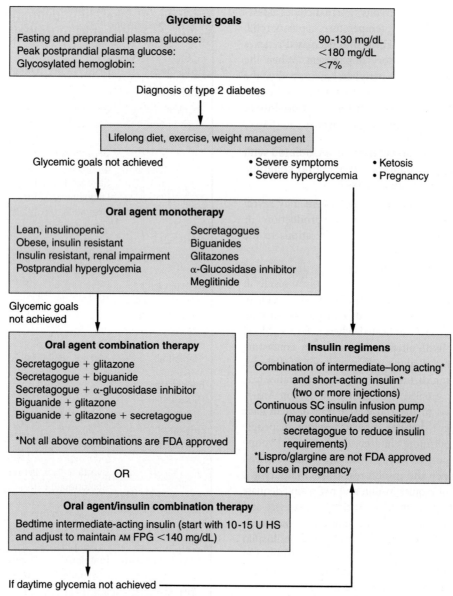

Glycemic goals

Fasting and preprandial plasma glucose:	90-130 mg/dL
Peak postprandial plasma glucose:	<180 mg/dL
Glycosylated hemoglobin:	<7%

Diagnosis of type 2 diabetes

Lifelong diet, exercise, weight management

Glycemic goals not achieved   • Severe symptoms   • Ketosis
• Severe hyperglycemia   • Pregnancy

Oral agent monotherapy

Lean, insulinopenic   Secretagogues
Obese, insulin resistant   Biguanides
Insulin resistant, renal impairment   Glitazones
Postprandial hyperglycemia   α-Glucosidase inhibitor
                              Meglitinide

Glycemic goals
not achieved

Oral agent combination therapy

Secretagogue + glitazone
Secretagogue + biguanide
Secretagogue + α-glucosidase inhibitor
Biguanide + glitazone
Biguanide + glitazone + secretagogue

*Not all above combinations are FDA approved

Insulin regimens

Combination of intermediate–long acting*
and short-acting insulin*
(two or more injections)
Continuous SC insulin infusion pump
(may continue/add sensitizer/
secretagogue to reduce insulin
requirements)
*Lispro/glargine are not FDA approved
for use in pregnancy

OR

Oral agent/insulin combination therapy

Bedtime intermediate-acting insulin (start with 10-15 U HS
and adjust to maintain AM FPG <140 mg/dL)

If daytime glycemia not achieved

Fig. 2.5 Algorithm for treatment of type 2 diabetes. *FDA,* US Food and Drug Administration; *FPG,* fasting plasma glucose. (From Hines RL, Marschall KE: *Stoelting's Anesthesia and Co-Existing Disease.* 7th ed. Philadelphia: Elsevier; 2018.)

agents are featured in Table 2.9. Common insulin preparations and guidelines for care are presented in Table 2.11. Procedural care should be coordinated with the physician managing the patient's diabetes to identify specific trends in blood glucose levels and compliance with prescribed diabetic treatment protocols. Procedures should be scheduled early in the day to prevent a prolonged overnight fast. Many physicians prefer the patient to be mildly hyperglycemic throughout the procedure, as opposed to hypoglycemic. Although there is no uniformly agreed-on procedural blood glucose level, many authors propose 180 mg/dL as a safe serum glucose level during the procedural period.[35] Procedural patient care for the diabetic patient treated with medication may be summarized as follows.[36]

Night Before the Procedure.

• Continue the usual dose of PM (afternoon, evening) glargine/NPH (neutral protamine Hagedorn) or mixture (can recommend two-thirds usual dose if tightly controlled), as long as the patient is allowed a usual diet.

Morning of the Procedure.

• Patients undergoing short simple procedures early in the morning, when preoperative fasting is required, can be managed by delaying the patient's normal diabetes treatments until the patient is ingesting food in the early postoperative period.

• Patients taking oral hypoglycemic agents should withhold the short half-life agents (e.g., repaglinide) on the day of surgery and withhold the longer lasting agents (e.g., chlor-propamide, glimepiride) for up to 48 hours.

- Fasting patients who are receiving insulin should have IV access established. A crystalloid solution containing 5% glucose should be available to infuse for the maintenance

of optimal blood glucose levels. The IV route still has the risk of making the patient hyperglycemic or hypoglycemic if the glucose or insulin infusions become unbalanced. The tighter the control of glucose levels, the more frequent the glucose monitoring. The subcutaneous route of insulin administration has been criticized as being too unpredictable in its absorption, especially perioperatively, with alterations in blood pressure and cutaneous blood flow.[37]

- Patients should not take short-acting insulin bolus the morning of the procedure, unless the blood glucose level is greater than 200 mg/dL, and more than 3 hours prior to the procedure.
- In the patient with type 1 diabetes, a common approach, especially for brief procedures, is to administer a fraction (50% of the usual dose) of the patient's usual morning dose of intermediate or long-acting insulin subcutaneously and institute continuous 5% glucose infusion.

Perioperative management of patients with an insulin pump is presented in Table 2.12.[38] Additional key points for the procedural management of the diabetic patient are identified in Box 2.6.

TABLE 2.10 Distinguishing Features of Diabetes Mellitus

Parameter	Type 1	Type 2
Previous name	Insulin-dependent diabetes	Noninsulin-dependent diabetes
Age of onset	Childhood	Middle age or elderly
Timing of onset	Abrupt	Gradual
Predisposing factors	Genetic	Obesity, pregnancy, drugs
Prevalence	0.2%–0.3%	2%–4%
Insulin requirement	Always	Infrequent
Ketoacidosis	Common	Rare
Systemic complications	Frequent	Frequent

Modified from Goldman L, Schafer AI, eds. *Goldman's Cecil Medicine.* 25th ed. Philadelphia: Elsevier; 2016,

TABLE 2.11 Insulin Preparations and Guidelines

Insulin Type	Onset	Peak (h)	Duration (h)	Comments
Very Rapid				
Lispro; Aspart	IV, immediate; SC, 5–15 min	SC, 0.5–1.5	SC, 3–4	Usually administered immediately prior to a meal; use SC, or via an insulin pump, but not recommended for continuous infusion
Short-Acting				
Regular	IV, immediate; SC, 30–60 min	SC, 2–3	SC, 3–6	Usually administered 30–60 min before meals; most common in continuous IV infusions
Intermediate-Acting				
NPH	SC, 2–4 h	SC, 6–10	SC, 10–16	Often combined with regular insulin
Lente	SC, 3–4 h	SC, 6–12	SC, 12–18	
Long-Acting				
Ultralente	SC, 6–10 h	SC, 10–16	SC, 18–20	Perioperative use uncommon
Glargine	SC, 4 h	Minimal peak activity	SC, 24	May be administered as usual to provide basal insulin levels during surgery
Combinations				
75/25 (75% protamine lispro, 25% insulin lispro)	SC, 30–60 min	Dual	10–14	
70/30 (70% NPH, 30% regular)	SC, 30–60 min	Dual	10–16	Usually given before breakfast
50/50 (50% NPH, 50% regular)	SC, 30–60 min	Dual	10–16	Usually given before dinner

IV, Intravenous; *NPH,* neutral protamine Hagedorn; *SC,* subcutaneous.
From Nagelhout JJ, Elisha S. *Nurse Anesthesia.* 6th ed. St Louis: Elsevier; 2018.

TABLE 2.12 Perioperative Management of the Patient with an Insulin Pump

Key Points	Comments
Preoperative preparation—topics to discuss with patient	Choice to continue pump during surgery
	Ensure adequate supply of pump consumables for entire surgical stay
	Re-site infusion set day before surgery; monitor blood glucose level
	Position infusion site away from operative field and cautery, accessible to anesthetist
	Overnight basal assessment prior to surgery
	Consultation with management team and patient to confirm self-management competency
Perioperative management	Assessment of glucose level hourly
	If glucose level not controlled, switch to IV infusion
	Disconnect pump in emergency surgery, switch to IV insulin
	Not to be used in radiology procedures
Postoperative management	Check capillary glucose hourly until the patient can self-manage
	Increase frequency of testing for 48 h postoperatively

Adapted from Partridge H, Perkins B, Mathieu S, et al. Clinical recommendations in the management of the patient with type 1 diabetes on insulin pump therapy in the perioperative period: a primer for the anaesthetist. *Br. J Anaesth.* 2016;116(1):18–26.

What are the presedation considerations associated with the patient presenting for moderate procedural sedation and analgesia with a history of hyperthyroidism?

The thyroid gland is responsible for regulation of the thyroid hormone. It responds to the pituitary gland's production of thyroid-stimulating hormone (TSH). Increased TSH results in an increase in thyroxine (T_4), which operates through a negative feedback loop. This negative feedback process decreases the release of TSH from the anterior pituitary gland. It is important to ascertain the status of thyroid function secondary to the thyroid hormone's function of regulating metabolic activity.

Hyperthyroidism produces an increased basal metabolic rate (BMR) secondary to increased secretion of the thyroid hormone. Symptoms of hyperthyroidism include weight loss, heat intolerance, tachycardia, nervousness, tremors,

BOX 2.6 Perioperative Diabetic Management Goals

These include broad management goals across the perioperative timeline. Overall goals include the following:
1. Reduce patient morbidity and mortality.
2. Avoid clinically significant hyper- or hypoglycemia.
3. Maintain acid-base, electrolyte, and fluid balance.
4. Prevent ketoacidosis.
5. Establish blood glucose measurements: <180 mg/dL in critical patients and <140 mg/dL in stable patients.

Preoperative Management Key Points	Intraoperative Management Key Points	Postoperative Management Key Points
1. Verify target blood glucose concentration with frequent glucose monitoring	1. Aim to maintain intraoperative glucose levels between 140 and 170 mg/dL	1. Target postoperative glycemic range between 140 and 180 mg/dL
2. Use insulin therapy to maintain glycemic goals	2. Physicians must take length of surgery into account when determining an intraoperative glucose management strategy	2. In the event a patient is hypoglycemic after surgery, begin a dextrose infusion at approximately 5–10 g/hour
3. Discontinue biguanides, alpha glucosidase inhibitors, thiazolidinediones, sulfonylureas, and GLP-1 agonists	3. For minor surgery, preoperative glucose protocols may be continued	3. Ensure basal insulin levels are met, especially in type 1 diabetic patients
4. Consider cancelling nonemergency procedures if patient presents with metabolic abnormalities (DKA, HHS, etc.) or glucose reading above 400–500 mg/dL	4. IV insulin infusion is being promoted as a more efficient method of glycemic control for longer or more complex surgeries	4. Postprandial insulin requirements should be tailored according to the mode in which the patient is receiving nutrition
		5. Supplemental insulin can be used to combat hyperglycemia and restore blood glucose values back to target range

From Salim S, Surani SR. Guidelines for perioperative management of the diabetic patient. *Surg Res Pract.* 2015; 2015;2015:284063.

and warm moist skin. This increase in thyroid hormone production may result from thyroiditis, adenoma, or dysfunction of the pituitary gland. Presedation management must focus on return of the patient to a euthyroid state. Procedures on a hyperthyroid patient should be postponed until the patient becomes euthyroid. It may take 6 to 8 weeks of methimazole or propylthiouracil therapy to decrease the overall synthesis of thyroxine, followed by 7 to 14 days of iodine.[39]

The presedation examination must assess the prescribed hyperthyroid treatment protocol, cardiovascular status, and state of patient anxiety. Beta-adrenergic antagonists such as propranolol and atenolol may be continued up to and including the day of surgery to control signs and symptoms (e.g., tachycardia, diaphoresis, tremors) associated with overstimulation of the sympathetic nervous system. During presedation assessment, it is important to assess the size of the thyroid gland. Visual assessment of gland size is recommended because frequent manual palpation of the gland releases thyroxine into the bloodstream. The T_4 produces an increase in the basal metabolic rate, heart rate, and blood pressure. Additional considerations related to the enlarged thyroid gland include difficult airway management because of increased tissue mass. Because of the increased basal metabolic rate, the pharmacologic effects of IV sedatives and analgesics may be reduced in the presence of hyperthyroidism, which leads to a hypermetabolic state in the patient.

What are the presedation considerations associated with the patient presenting for moderate procedural sedation and analgesia with a history of hypothyroidism?

Hypothyroidism results from insufficient circulating thyroid hormone. Symptoms of hypothyroidism include intolerance to cold, bradycardia, cardiomegaly, dry skin, hair loss, fatigue, congestive heart failure, decreased mentation, and periorbital edema. Causes of hypothyroidism include surgical ablation, pituitary or hyperthermic dysfunction, and decreased hormonal biosynthesis. Diagnosis of hypothyroidism includes decreased T_4 and increased TSH levels on a presedation thyroid serum panel. Treatment of hypothyroidism consists of supplemental thyroid medication. Levothyroxine is often used as an exogenous replacement because of its long half-life and its ability to produce consistent plasma T_4 levels.

Hypothyroid patients generally have a marked sensitivity to IV sedatives, analgesics, and hypnotics. Hypothyroidism also reduces the ventilatory response to $Paco_2$ and Pao_2. This marked sensitivity requires a reduction in the dose of sedative and analgesic medications administered to the patient. Careful titration of sedatives, analgesics, and hypnotics is required, because even markedly reduced doses have resulted in profound CNS and respiratory depression. Patients with hypothyroidism may also have macroglossia (large tongue) secondary to the increased accumulation of subcutaneous mucopolysaccharides.[40] This increase in tissue mass, coupled with the marked sensitivity to pharmacologic medications, requires careful attention to airway management. Airway obstruction is not well tolerated in the hypothyroid patient population.

What are the presedation considerations associated with the patient presenting for moderate procedural sedation and analgesia with Cushing disease (glucocorticoid overproduction)?

The adrenal cortex produces glucocorticosteroids, mineralocorticoids, and androgens. These hormones are under the control of the anterior pituitary gland through the secretion of adrenocorticotropic hormone (ACTH). Adrenocortical disease may occur from decreased or increased production of these hormones. The following conditions may be encountered on presedation assessment of the patient presenting for sedation services.

Glucocorticoid steroids regulate protein, carbohydrate, and nucleic acid metabolism. Under normal conditions, approximately 20 to 30 mg of cortisol is produced each day. Cortisol production is significantly increased in the presence of stress, infection, and anxiety. During periods of extreme stress, the adrenal gland secretes 200 to 500 mg/dL. Cushing disease may be caused by the increased production of ACTH, malignant tumors, or exogenous steroid administration. Glucocorticoid steroids also antagonize the effects of antidiuretic hormone (ADH). As a result of excess cortisol production, the symptoms of Cushing disease include the following:

- Hypertension
- Hyperglycemia
- Polyuria
- Osteoporosis
- Hypokalemia
- Truncal obesity
- Moon face
- Skin striations
- Hypovolemia
- Plethora

Presedation preparation of the patient with Cushing disease must focus on the correction of fluid and electrolyte abnormalities, treatment of hypertension, and regulation of blood sugar levels prior to the anticipated procedure.

What are the presedation considerations associated with the patient presenting for moderate procedural sedation and analgesia with Addison disease (decreased cortisol production)?

Decreased cortisol production may result from hemorrhagic destruction of the adrenocortical cells, carcinoma, or adrenocortical suppression secondary to the use of exogenous steroids. Exogenous steroid use to treat asthma, allergy, or associated inflammatory conditions leads to adrenal cortisol suppression. The administration of an exogenous steroid on a short-term basis (7–10 days) decreases cortisol-releasing hormone and ACTH release. This decreased hormone release generally returns to normal within several days after cessation of exogenous steroid therapy. However, long-term exogenous steroid supplementation in the presence of inflammatory bowel disease, asthma, and associated inflammatory conditions of more than 10 days' duration may result in adrenocortical insufficiency. The presenting symptoms of adrenal insufficiency mimic those of hypovolemic shock. Additional symptoms include hypovolemia, hypoglycemia, nausea, vomiting, hypotension, and hemoconcentration. The use of supplemental exogenous steroids has been advocated to prevent an intraoperative adrenal crisis. There are few documented cases in the anesthesia literature of acute adrenal crisis in the perioperative setting. However, because of the significant morbidity and mortality associated with adrenal crisis and the minimal side effects associated with exogenous steroid supplementation, many practitioners advocate the use of exogenous steroid supplementation to prevent the development of adrenal insufficiency. The decision to provide presedation steroid replacement should be based on the degree of stress and the magnitude of the procedure. An example of perioperative steroid supplementation recommendations is highlighted in Table 2.13.

What are the presedation considerations associated with the patient presenting for moderate procedural sedation and analgesia with Conn syndrome?

Conn syndrome results from the excess production of mineralocorticosteroids. Mineralocorticosteroids regulate extracellular fluid volume and potassium balance. Increased mineralocorticosteroid production may result from an adenoma or adrenal hyperplasia. Symptoms associated with hyperaldosteronism (Conn syndrome) include hypokalemia, hyponatremia, muscle weakness, hypertension, tetany, and polyuria. Hypokalemia is responsible for the kidney's inability to concentrate urine, polyuria, and muscle weakness associated with Conn syndrome. Presedation preparation of the patient with Conn disease includes replacement of potassium, administration of antihypertensive agents, and correction of fluid volume status. Determination of presedation serum electrolyte levels is also warranted.

TABLE 2.13 Perioperative Steroid Supplementation

Recommendation	Dosage
Superficial surgery (e.g., dental surgery, biopsy)	None
Minor surgery (e.g., inguinal hernia repair)	25 mg IV
Moderate surgery (e.g., cholecystectomy, colon resection)	50–75 mg IV, taper 1–2 days
Major surgery (e.g., cardiovascular surgery, Whipple procedure)	100–150 mg IV, taper 1–2 days
Intensive care unit (e.g., sepsis, shock)	50–100 mg q6–8h for 2 days–1 wk, followed by slow taper

From Hines RL, Marschall KE: *Stoelting's Anesthesia and Co-Existing Disease.* 7th ed. Philadelphia: Elsevier; 2018.

What are the presedation considerations associated with the patient presenting for moderate procedural sedation and analgesia with hypoaldosteronism?

Hypoaldosteronism results in hyperkalemia, with resultant heart block, cardiac conduction defects, hyponatremia, and hypotension. Causes of decreased aldosterone secretion include diabetes, renal failure, and adrenalectomy. Presedation treatment of decreased aldosterone secretion includes return of the patient to a eukalemic state, liberal fluid and sodium intake, and administration of exogenous mineralocorticosteroids (e.g., fludrocortisone).

What are the presedation considerations associated with the patient presenting for moderate procedural sedation and analgesia with a pheochromocytoma?

Catecholamine-secreting tumors located in the adrenal medulla or chromaffin tissue are termed *pheochromocytomas*. Additional sites of these catecholamine-secreting tumors include the spleen, ovary, bladder, and right atrium. Symptoms associated with pheochromocytoma are related to an increase in catecholamine release and include palpitations, headache, weight loss, diaphoresis, hypertension, flushing, and hyperglycemia. The main catecholamine released by pheochromocytoma is norepinephrine (80%). Diagnosis of pheochromocytoma is made after a 24-hour urine collection reveals excess catecholamines and metanephrines. Measurement of the plasma free metanephrine level, however, is a more sensitive test for patients at high risk of pheochromocytoma.

The combination of diaphoresis, tachycardia, and headache, particularly in young to middle-aged patients, is highly suggestive of the presence of pheochromocytoma. Its presence requires further consultation concerning surgical excision of the catecholamine-producing tumor prior to performing diagnostic, therapeutic, or minor surgical procedures. Before tumor resection, antihypertensive treatment with alpha blockers is required to lower blood pressure, promote vasodilation, increase intravascular volume, allow resensitization of adrenergic receptors, and decrease myocardial dysfunction. Phenoxybenzamine (Dibenzyline) is the most commonly prescribed alpha blocker for preoperative preparation of the patient. Cardiac dysrhythmias may be controlled with beta blockers. Correction of hypertension with a return of controlled heart rate facilitates a return of volume status. Patients presenting for sedation should be hemodynamically stable prior to the start of the diagnostic or therapeutic procedure.

What are the presedation considerations associated with the patient presenting for moderate procedural sedation and analgesia with a history of gastrointestinal issues?

Gastrointestinal assessment includes evaluation for the following conditions:

- Obesity
- Nausea
- Vomiting
- Diarrhea

- Gastrointestinal (GI) bleeding
- Gastric reflux

The presence of persistent nausea, vomiting, or diarrhea predisposes the patient to electrolyte abnormalities. Correction of electrolyte status and fluid volume is required before the initiation of sedation. Dryness of mucous membranes, decreased skin turgor, and a large swollen tongue may indicate significant hypovolemia. The hematocrit, serum osmolality, blood urea nitrogen level, electrolyte profile, and urine output are indicators to quantify volume deficit. Anemia secondary to diarrhea, nausea, vomiting, or GI bleeding requires careful assessment of hemoglobin and hematocrit levels. Risks and benefits of transfusion must be examined before the procedure. Severe diarrhea results in the excretion of large amounts of water, sodium, and potassium through the colon. In severe cases, shock and cardiovascular compromise may occur. Emergent colonoscopy or endoscopic examination raises several concerns. Bleeding into the stomach or upper GI tract increases gastric volume and the incidence of regurgitation. Anemia and a decreased oxygen-carrying capacity of the hemoglobin molecule also increase the risk of hypoxemia. Presedation assessment of GI bleeding must focus on restoration of blood volume, supplemental oxygenation, and a potential plan to use minimal sedation.

Why are anesthesia and the surgical history important aspects of the presedation patient assessment?

Presedation assessment of the patient's anesthesia and surgical history should be conducted to ascertain patient recollection of past anesthesia, surgical procedures, and complications related to these procedures. Because medical records and charts may not be readily available from other institutions or physician offices, it is important to obtain an accurate surgical and anesthesia history. Questions related to anesthetic and surgical history may be asked: "What operations have you had in the past?" and "Do you recall what type of anesthesia you had?" This question is generally answered with "I went to sleep." It is important to consider the amnestic effects of the benzodiazepines and sedatives used in the operating room. Many patients are under the impression that they received a general anesthetic when they actually received a local anesthetic with sedation or a regional anesthetic with sedation and monitoring. Adequate time should be allotted to allow the patient to answer questions related to his or her recollection of any complications associated with prior surgical procedures and anesthesia. Additional questioning related to past surgery and anesthesia include the following: "Has anyone in your family ever had any anesthesia complications?" An initial response to this question may be an immediate, "No." However, with some prompting, patients may recall a negative past anesthetic experience. This prompting includes "Have you ever had nausea or vomiting after any past surgical or diagnostic procedures or been admitted to the intensive care unit unexpectedly?" Affirmative responses may

require an additional medical record review to assess the following parameters:

- Response to preoperative sedative medications
- Presence of difficult airway management issues
- Vascular access
- Intraoperative complications
- Drug reactions
- Hemodynamic parameters
- Documented postoperative complications

Which patient medications are important to identify during the presedation assessment?

The purpose of the presedation evaluation is to decrease morbidity and optimize the patient's condition before the proposed procedure. During the presedation assessment, it is important for the health care provider to identify prescribed medication protocol, treatment efficacy, and patient compliance. A medication review during presedation assessment includes asking the patient, "What medications are you currently taking?" This question allows the patient to answer with prescription drugs, over-the-counter medications, or herbal preparations that they may be taking. It is also important to evaluate and ascertain drug dosage and last dose of medication administered. Once the medication history is complete, it is important to give the patient accurate presedation instructions related to their current medication regimen. Rarely, a patient may not be sure which medication he or she is taking. It is important to identify the name, dosage, and last ingestion of these medications. Fortunately, many patient medications are now listed in the electronic medical record of the facility. The preoperative management for a wide variety of medications and their dosing on the day of the procedure is featured in Box 2.7.

What is the best way to elicit information about patient allergies during the presedation assessment?

To avoid administering a medication that elicits an allergic response, the presedation medication assessment proceeds with an inquiry into the patient's allergy history. Questions related to an allergy history include "Are you allergic to any medication?" Allergies reported may include nausea associated with the use of analgesics or GI upset with the use of antibiotics. The side effects associated with the use of pharmacologic agents are separate and distinct from an allergic reaction. Side effects may be classified as unpleasant reactions or adverse reactions to prescribed drugs. True allergies to pharmacologic agents occur with less frequency and are manifested by the following conditions:

- Bronchospasm
- Circulatory collapse
- Edema
- Hives
- Hypotension
- Pruritus
- Skin wheals
- Wheezing

BOX 2.7   Preoperative Management of Medications

Instruct patients to take these medications with a small sip of water, even if fasting.

1. Antihypertensive medications: Continue on the day of surgery.
   a. Possible exception—for patients undergoing procedures with major fluid shifts, or for patients who have medical conditions in which hypotension is particularly dangerous, it may be prudent to discontinue ACEIs or ARBs before surgery.
2. Cardiac medications (e.g., beta blockers, digoxin): Continue on the day of surgery.
3. Antidepressants, anxiolytics, and other psychiatric medications: Continue on the day of surgery.
4. Thyroid medications: Continue on the day of surgery.
5. Birth control pills: Continue on the day of surgery.
6. Eye drops: Continue on the day of surgery.
7. Heartburn or reflux medications: Continue on the day of surgery.
8. Narcotic medications: Continue on the day of surgery.
9. Anticonvulsant medications: Continue on the day of surgery.
10. Asthma medications: Continue on the day of surgery.
11. Steroids (oral and inhaled): Continue on the day of surgery.
12. Statins: Continue on the day of surgery.
13. Aspirin: Consider selectively continuing aspirin in patients for whom the risks of cardiac events are thought to exceed the risk of major bleeding. Examples would be patients with high-grade CAD or CVD. If reversal of platelet inhibition is necessary, aspirin must be stopped at least 3 days before surgery. Do not discontinue aspirin in patients who have drug-eluting coronary stents until they have completed 12 months of dual-antiplatelet therapy, unless patients, surgeons, and cardiologists have discussed the risks of discontinuation. The same applies to patients with bare metal stents until they have completed 1 month of dual-antiplatelet therapy. In general, aspirin should be continued in any patient with a coronary stent, regardless of the time since stent implantation.
14. Thienopyridines (e.g., clopidogrel, ticlopidine): Patients having cataract surgery with topical or general anesthesia do not need to stop taking a thienopyridine. If reversal of platelet inhibition is necessary, then clopidogrel must be stopped 7 days before surgery (14 days for ticlopidine). Do not discontinue thienopyridines in patients who have drug-eluting stents until they have completed 12 months of dual-antiplatelet therapy, unless patients, surgeons, and cardiologists have discussed the risks of discontinuation. The same applies to patients with bare metal stents until they have completed 1 month of dual-antiplatelet therapy.
15. Insulin: For all patients, discontinue all short-acting (e.g., regular) insulin on the day of surgery (unless insulin is administered by continuous pump). Patients with type 2 diabetes should take none or up to half of their dose of long-acting or combination (e.g., 70/30 preparations) insulin on the day of surgery. Patients with type 1 diabetes should take a small amount (usually one-third) of their usual morning long-acting insulin dose on the day of surgery. Patients with an insulin pump should continue their basal rate only.
16. Topical medications (e.g., creams and ointments): Discontinue on the day of surgery.
17. Oral hypoglycemic agents: Discontinue on the day of surgery.
18. Diuretics: Discontinue on the day of surgery (exception: thiazide diuretics taken for hypertension, which should be continued on the day of surgery).
19. Sildenafil (Viagra) or similar drugs: Discontinue 24 hours before surgery.
20. COX-2 inhibitors: Continue on the day of surgery unless the surgeon is concerned about bone healing.
21. Nonsteroidal antiinflammatory drugs: Discontinue 48 hours before the day of surgery.
22. Warfarin (Coumadin): Discontinue 4 days before surgery, except for patients having cataract surgery without a bulbar block.
23. Monoamine oxidase inhibitors: Continue these medications and adjust the anesthesia plan accordingly.

ACEI, Angiotensin-converting enzyme inhibitor; *ARB,* angiotensin receptor blocker; *CAD,* coronary artery disease; *COX-2,* cyclooxygenase-2; *CVD,* cerebrovascular disease.
Source: Miller's Anesthesia, 8th Edition, Chapter 38, Box 38-3, page 1098, Preoperative Management of Medications.

What is the difference between an anaphylactic versus an anaphylactoid reaction?

Anaphylaxis refers to a life-threatening drug reaction of severe magnitude. Anaphylactic drug reactions are mediated via the immunoglobulin E (IgE) in the immune system. Therefore, anaphylactic reactions are life-threatening drug reactions mediated by antibodies. The term *anaphylactoid* applies when there is no antibody involvement in the reaction. Differentiation of an anaphylactic from an anaphylactoid reaction during the procedure is not important. What is important is the identification of an allergic response.

Presenting symptoms of an allergic reaction include urticaria, hypotension, oropharyngeal edema, hives, wheezing, bronchoconstriction, and cardiovascular compromise requiring immediate diagnosis and treatment. The treatment protocol for an allergic reaction includes the following:

- Discontinue the suspected allergen
- Secure the airway
- IV volume (several liters, 20 mL/kg, may be required if there is massive vasodilation)
- Epinephrine (in the presence of cardiovascular collapse)
- Diphenhydramine
- Terbutaline
- Aminophylline
- Corticosteroids

Presedation assessment of the patient with multiple allergies or documentation of a true anaphylactic or anaphylactoid reaction requires careful preparation prior to the planned procedure. The initial step in the prevention of an allergic reaction includes identification of the allergen. It may be difficult to identify an allergen in the patient's history or previous anesthesia and sedation records. When antibiotics, local anesthetics, sedatives, hypnotics, and analgesics are combined and administered throughout the procedure, it may be extremely difficult to specify which medication precipitated the allergic response. The patient's presedation record must include careful documentation of any allergies or adverse reactions.

Although the incidence of latex allergy sensitization has continued to increase, the development of better ways to identify at-risk patients has led to a decreased incidence of latex-induced anaphylaxis.[41] Those at risk for developing latex allergy include patients who have had multiple surgical procedures, those with atopic histories, and health care workers. When latex allergy is identified during the presedation patient assessment, the procedural team must be notified and instructed to follow the facility's latex allergy protocol. The American Association of Nurse Anesthetists Latex Allergy Management Guidelines identified in Appendix D can serve as a model template for facility policy and procedure creation for a latex allergy protocol.

What laboratory test(s) should be ordered for patients prior to the administration of moderate sedation and procedural analgesia?

The current state of health care reimbursement dictates conscientious, efficient presedation laboratory testing and screening. In the past, laboratory or diagnostic testing was reimbursed on a fee for service basis. As reimbursement continues to evolve into a capitated system, the clinician must focus on specific laboratory or diagnostic tests that yield beneficial information about the patient. Medicare and most private insurance companies no longer reimburse routine preoperative screening tests without documentation of pre-existing disease that warrants diagnostic testing. In addition, random laboratory testing in the absence of suspicious clinical features or symptoms is not only expensive, but it is time-consuming and inconvenient for the patient and could result in patient harm. It has been clearly established that routine preoperative testing in asymptomatic healthy patients has a very poor diagnostic yield, provides little to no additional prognostic information, and has not shown any beneficial effect on outcomes.[42-45] Therefore, presedation diagnostic testing criteria for moderate procedural sedation are based on the patient's past medical history, presence of comorbidities, and proposed diagnostic or therapeutic procedure. A framework that can serve as a guideline for ordering preoperative diagnostic testing based on the patient's medical history is featured in Table 2.14. These recommendations may prove beneficial for the attending physician who is ordering presedation laboratory and diagnostic testing.

What dental parameters should be documented prior to the procedure?

Dental damage is the most common of all claims associated with the administration of anesthesia. Laryngoscopy is the major causative factor that causes dental damage. Although moderate procedural sedation and analgesia patients are not subjected to direct vision laryngoscopy, it is important to assess their dentition and oropharynx during the preprocedure patient assessment. The initial assessment includes examination of the patient's oral cavity and documentation of any missing, loose, or damaged teeth. Fig. 2.6 identifies tooth numbering for documentation purposes in the patient's medical record prior to the procedure.

Does the patient's social history affect the moderate procedural sedation plan of care?

During presedation assessment, it is important to obtain a social history from the patient. Components of the social history include inquiry and assessment for tobacco use, alcohol ingestion, illicit substance use, and the possibility of pregnancy. Additionally, patients should be assessed for over-the-counter medication use and/or use of herbal preparations. When soliciting a patient's social history, it is important to use a nonjudgmental approach when posing all questions related to illicit substance use. Any attempts to belittle or pressure the patient will result in patient withdrawal and, most likely, an inaccurate history. A variety of mechanisms may be used to elicit this information in a diplomatic and tactful manner. Patients with a history of addiction are at risk for a myriad of perioperative complications, including withdrawal, acute intoxication, infections, end-organ damage, and altered tolerance of anesthetic or opioid medications.

What is the impact of smoking on the patient presenting for sedation services?

A tobacco use history is best quantified in pack-years and documented on the presedation assessment form, as follows:

$$\text{Pack years} = (\text{number of packs smoked/day}) \times (\text{number of years smoked})$$

The inhaled components of smoke are associated with the development of coronary artery disease, peripheral vascular disease, cerebrovascular disease, stroke, COPD, peptic ulcer disease, esophageal reflux, and lung cancer.[46] Nicotine produces an increase in heart rate, blood pressure, myocardial contraction, myocardial oxygen consumption, and myocardial excitement. These sympathetic nervous system changes are undesirable in a patient presenting for moderate procedural sedation who may already be apprehensive and anxious. Therefore, patients should be counseled to consider cessation of smoking 12 to 48 hours prior to the procedure. Even short-term smoking cessation (12 hours) prior to the planned procedure has been shown to reduce the deleterious effects of nicotine and carbon monoxide on

TABLE 2.14   Framework for Diagnostic Testing Based on Patients' Medical History

Preoperative Diagnosis	ECG	Chest Radiograph	Hct/Hb	CBC	Electrolytes	Creatinine	Glucose	Coagulation	LFTs	Drug Levels	Calcium
Cardiac disease											
History of MI	X			X	±						
Chronic stable angina	X			X	±						
CHF	X	±									
HTN	X	±			X[a]	X					
Chronic atrial fibrillation	X									X[b]	
PAD	X										
Valvular heart disease	X	±									
Pulmonary disease											
COPD	X	±		X						X[c]	
Asthma	(PFTs only if symptomatic; otherwise, no tests required)										
Diabetes	X				±	X	X				
Liver disease											
Infectious hepatitis								X	X		
Alcohol or drug-induced hepatitis								X	X		
Tumor infiltration								X	X		
Renal disease			X		X	X					
Hematologic disorders				X							
Coagulopathies				X				X			
CNS disorders											
Stroke	X			X	X		X				
Seizures	X			X	X		X			X	
Tumor	X			X						X	

Vascular disorders or aneurysms	X		X								
Malignant disease				X							
Hyperthyroidism	X		X		X						X
Hypothyroidism	X		X		X						
Cushing disease				X	X		X				
Addison disease				X	X		X				
Hyperparathyroidism	X		X		X						X
Hypoparathyroidism	X				X						X
Morbid obesity	X	±					X				
Malabsorption or poor nutrition	X			X	X	X	X				
Select drug therapies											
Digoxin (digitalis)	X				±					X	
Anticoagulants			X					X			
Phenytoin (Dilantin)										X	
Phenobarbital										X	
Diuretics					X	X					
Corticosteroids				X			X				
Chemotherapy				X		±					
Aspirin or NSAID											
Theophylline										X	

±, ; *CBC,* complete blood count; *CHF,* congestive heart failure; *CNS,* central nervous system; *COPD,* chronic obstructive pulmonary disease; *ECG,* electrocardiogram; *Hb,* hemoglobin; *Hct,* hematocrit; *HTN,* hypertension; *LFTs,* liver function tests; *MI,* myocardial infarction; *NSAID,* nonsteroidal antiinflammatory drug; *PAD,* peripheral arterial disease; *PFT,* pulmonary function test; *X,* obtain.

[a]If the patient is taking diuretics.

[b]If the patient is taking digoxin.

[c]If the patient is taking theophylline.

Adapted from Miller RD, ed: *Miller's Anesthesia.* 8th ed. Philadelphia: Saunders; 2015.

Maxillary

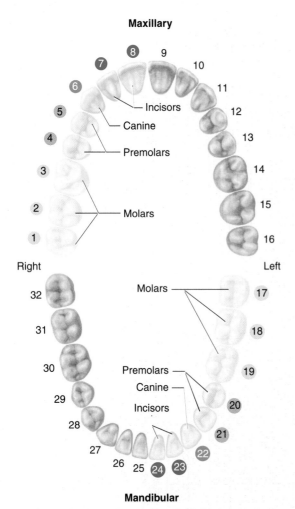

Mandibular

Fig. 2.6 Oral cavity inspection. (© Elsevier Collections.)

cardiopulmonary function resulting in a reduced heart rate, blood pressure, and circulating catecholamine levels.[47,48] The moderate procedural sedation practitioner caring for the pediatric patient subjected to second-hand smoke must be prepared to handle complications associated with children who are exposed to passive smoke.[49,50] These complications include the following:

- Increased reactive airway disease
- Abnormal pulmonary function tests
- Increased respiratory tract infection
- Laryngospasm
- Postsedation oxyhemoglobin desaturation
- Hypersecretion

What is the impact of chewing tobacco on the patient presenting for sedation services?

The chronic use of chewing tobacco or snuff can lead to significant pathologic changes that affect the oral cavity. Submucosal fibrosis associated with long-term use limits the patient's ability to open the mouth and can lead to dysphagia. Therefore, it is important to complete and document a thorough oral cavity inspection during the presedation assessment to identify any potential limitations accurately that would impede airway maneuvering should an emergency situation arise in the sedation setting.

What is the impact of vaping on the patient presenting for sedation services?

Despite being perceived as a "healthier" alternative to the use of tobacco cigarettes, vaping liquid contains nicotine, which may significantly increase the risk for complications related to surgery and anesthesia. In a report from the US Surgeon General, e-cigarette use has risen to the level of a public health concern. The report uses the term *e-cigarette* to refer to the many different products that deliver nicotine electronically. Consumers and marketers call them by many names, including *e-cigarettes, e-cigs, cigalikes, e-hookahs, mods, vape pens, vapes,* and *tank systems.* Most e-cigarettes contain nicotine, which can cause addiction.

The nicotine found in vapes and tobacco results in poor wound healing, increases anesthesia risk, and may lead to a host of other potential complications. Despite being perceived as a better alternative to tobacco cigarettes, vaping liquid contains nicotine, which significantly increases the risk for complications during and after surgery. The liquids used for vaping also contain a high concentration of diacetyl and 2,3-pentanedione. These compounds destroy the lungs' tiniest airways, leading to scar tissue buildup that blocks airflow. Inhaling the chemicals found in vaping liquids can lead to a permanent and sometimes fatal lung condition known as *bronchiolitis obliterans.* It is common knowledge that patients should quit smoking cigarettes at least a few weeks before and after surgery. For those who refuse to quit vaping, they should also discontinue using their devices for several weeks prior to the procedure.

Nicotine can lower the effectiveness of certain medications or interfere with how drugs work; it can also affect healing and lead to infection and greater discomfort after surgery. Although a longer period of cessation around anesthesia and surgery is most beneficial, even 12 to 24 hours can significantly increase the body's ability to deliver oxygen to vital organs and tissues. Quitting vaping and smoking has immediate and long-term benefits at any age. Studies have shown that the more times vapers or smokers stop using nicotine, the better chance they have of stopping their addiction.[51]

What is the best method of inquiry during the presedation assessment to identify patient alcohol consumption?

Traditional questions to elicit the type and amount of alcohol ingestion may be as direct as asking the patient "Have you ever had a drinking problem?" or "Have you had any alcohol in the last 24 hours?" Aside from their abrupt nature, these questions are also closed-ended. An alternative approach during the presedation assessment is to incorporate broader, more open-ended question. An example is, "How much alcohol do you generally consume in 1 week?" The patient can respond in a variety of ways, such as "I have wine with dinner every night," "None," "A couple of beers on the weekend," or "Two or three scotches every evening." These comments generally lead to further discussion of alcohol history and intake. The CAGE approach in evaluating a patient's alcohol consumption has been reported in the literature.[52] The CAGE approach uses the following four questions to solicit information related to alcohol use:

- Do you feel you should cut down on your alcohol consumption?
- Have people ᴀnnoyed you by criticizing your drinking?
- Have you ever felt ɢuilty about your drinking?
- Have you ever had a drink first thing in the morning to steady your nerves or get rid of a hangover (ᴇye opener)?

Two or more affirmative responses from the patient signify a high risk for alcoholism and an increased likelihood for experiencing withdrawal symptoms.[53]

What are the systemic effects associated with excess alcohol use?

Patients with rare social alcohol use afford minimal concern for multisystemic disease states. However, patients that admit to significant alcohol ingestion may demonstrate tolerance to sedative medications requiring additional sedative and opioid medication administration. This tolerance occurs secondary to stimulation of the cytochrome P-450 system located in the smooth endoplasmic reticulum in the liver. Additionally, alcoholism is associated with multisystem symptoms. Box 2.8 identifies the multitude of medical problems related to alcoholism. Patients with a history of chronic alcohol use require presedation preparation that addresses any presenting symptoms. Chronic alcoholism may lead to cirrhosis, elevated liver enzyme levels, esophageal varices, nutritional disorders, gastritis, psychiatric disorders, cardiac myopathy, electrolyte disturbances, and cerebral atrophy. These symptoms predispose patients to an increased risk during the administration of sedation. As opposed to chronic alcohol ingestion, a general rule of thumb when dealing with acute alcoholism is to anticipate a decrease in anesthetic requirements.

A full stomach and a lack of patient cooperation are also additional risk factors associated with acute alcohol intoxication. If morning presedation assessment reveals the odor of alcohol on the patient's breath, serum alcohol levels should be drawn immediately after patient consent is obtained. If the patient refuses consent or the blood level returned is indicative of recent alcohol ingestion, many practitioners will cancel the procedure to diminish risks associated with NPO noncompliance issues and the potential increase in gastric volume.

What is the impact of stimulant medications on the patient presenting for sedation services?

Stimulants, weight reduction medications, and designer drugs can be ingested orally, inhaled, or used intravenously. Amphetamines cause CNS stimulation and may predispose the patient to dilated pupils, dizziness, weight loss, anxiety, headaches, irritability, and cardiac dysrhythmias, including palpitations and tachycardia. Amphetamine abuse increases the release of catecholamines. Amphetamines are often used in patients with weight disorders, narcolepsy, or attention-deficit hyperactivity disorder (ADHD) and as recreational

---

BOX 2.8 Medical Problems Related to Alcoholism

Central Nervous System Effects
Psychiatric disorders (depression, antisocial behavior)
Nutritional disorders (Wernicke-Korsakoff syndrome)
Withdrawal syndrome
Cerebellar degeneration
Cerebral atrophy

Cardiovascular Effects
Cardiomyopathy
Cardiac dysrhythmias
Hypertension

Gastrointestinal and Hepatobiliary Effects
Esophagitis
Gastritis
Pancreatitis
Hepatic cirrhosis
Portal hypertension

Skin and Musculoskeletal Effects
Spider angiomata
Myopathy
Osteoporosis

Endocrine and Metabolic Effects
Decreased serum testosterone concentrations (impotence)
Decreased gluconeogenesis (hypoglycemia)
Ketoacidosis
Hypoalbuminemia
Hypomagnesemia

Hematologic Effects
Thrombocytopenia
Leukopenia
Anemia

From Hines RL, Marschall KE: Stoelting's Anesthesia and Co-Existing Disease. 7th ed. Philadelphia: Elsevier; 2018.

---

substances. Chronic abuse of amphetamines can lead to decreased anesthetic requirements secondary to depleted body catecholamine stores in the CNS. Patients prescribed amphetamines for narcolepsy or ADHD can be instructed to continue their medication regimen up to and including the day of the procedure. However, patients ingesting amphetamines for rapid weight reduction over short periods of time may require additional laboratory data review. A 12-lead ECG, comprehensive metabolic profile, and complete blood cell count should be considered to assess electrolyte and hematologic abnormalities and to rule out the presence of cardiac conduction abnormalities before the administration of sedation.

Addiction, life-threatening events, and multiple deaths have been reported as a result of designer drug use. The best known and most widely used designer drug is 3,4-methylenedioxymethamphetamine (MDMA [Ecstasy]). The drug chemically resembles a combination of amphetamine and mescaline and can be taken orally, injected, smoked, or snorted. Onset is generally within 20 to 45 minutes and effects may last up to 6 hours.[54] The recreational use of Ecstasy began to emerge in the mid-1980s and was commonly used during raves (large dance parties numbering in the thousands, often in abandoned warehouses).[55] The most common complications associated with its use include hyperthermia and idiosyncratic reactions. Physiologic symptoms associated with the use of Ecstasy include altered mental status, tachycardia, tachypnea, profuse sweating, and hyperthermia.[56] Clinical management is directed at controlling presenting symptomatology. Treatment includes fluids for hypotension, benzodiazepines for agitation and seizures, dopamine or norepinephrine for hypotension unresponsive to fluid challenges, phentolamine or nitroprusside for hypertension, and nitroglycerin for myocardial ischemic pain.

What is the impact of cocaine on the patient presenting for sedation services?

In 2018, there were an estimated 2 million current (past-month) cocaine users aged 12 years or older (0.8% of the population). Adults aged 18 to 25 have a higher rate of current cocaine use than any other age group, with 1.9% of young adults reporting past-month cocaine use.[57] Cocaine is an ester-based local anesthetic with vasoconstrictive properties. Its alkaloid derivative from the leaves of the *Erythroxylon coca* plant is prepared by dissolving the alkaloid base to form a water-soluble salt (cocaine hydrochloride). It can be sold as crystals, granules, or white powder. Cocaine can be ingested orally (chewing coca leaves), intravenously, intranasally (snorting), or smoked as free base cocaine (crack cocaine). Cocaine can produce negative inotropic and chronotropic effects on the heart muscle. In addition, cocaine impairs neural reuptake of dopamine, serotonin, and tryptophan. Illicit use results in a euphoric sensation. Through its vasoconstricting properties, it leads to hypertension, myocardial ischemia, myocardial infarction, dysrhythmias, cerebral hemorrhage, and seizures. Electrocardiographic evidence of silent ischemia persists for up to 6 weeks in humans after discontinuing cocaine use. In addition, the chronic alteration in cerebral blood flow that cocaine produces in people does not return to normal, even after 30 days of cocaine abstinence. Pulmonary effects include cocaine-induced asthma, hypersensitivity pneumonitis, chronic cough, pulmonary edema, pneumopericardium, and pulmonary hemorrhage. Patients suspected of cocaine abuse should also be carefully assessed in the following areas prior to the procedure:

- Deterioration of nasal mucosa
- Assessment of all extremities for the presence of needle marks
- Auscultation of the lungs to exclude asthma or barotraumas
- Careful cardiovascular and neurologic examination
- Chest radiograph to rule out pulmonary involvement
- Electrocardiography to identify signs of rhythm disturbance and presence of ischemia, injury, or previous MI

As noted, complications associated with the procedure secondary to cocaine abuse include cardiac dysrhythmias, tachycardia, and increased myocardial oxygen consumption.

Therefore, ketamine should be avoided or used with extreme caution in this patient population because it can markedly potentiate the cardiovascular toxicity of cocaine. Additional pharmacologic concerns include using ester-type local anesthetic solutions with caution secondary to their metabolism by plasma cholinesterase. These drugs may compete with cocaine for this metabolic pathway and result in decreased metabolism of both the cocaine and local anesthetic. Naloxone may intensify the actions of cocaine and thus should be used carefully in this patient population.

What is the impact of opioid abuse on the patient presenting for sedation services?

Opioids are abused via the oral, subcutaneous, or IV routes of administration. Opioid ingestion produces a euphoric state, with resultant analgesia. Tolerance of the effects of opioids occurs with chronic ingestion. Patients with a history of chronic opioid abuse generally require increased doses of sedative medications during the administration of sedation.[58] It is important to remember that the procedural period is not the time to withdraw an addict from opioid abuse.

Heroin was first introduced in the late 1800s and described as a "less addicting morphine substitute." Chemical alteration of the morphine molecule yields heroin, which is three to four times more potent than morphine. An intense rush is achieved with smoking or injection. Withdrawal symptoms begin approximately 8 to 24 hours after the last use of heroin. Characteristic withdrawal symptoms include the following[59]:

- Influenza-like syndrome
- Drug craving
- Anxiety
- Sweating
- Tremors
- Rhinorrhea
- Muscle aches
- Sympathetic nervous system discharge

Presenting symptoms should be controlled through the use of benzodiazepines to control anxiety and agitation and beta blockers for tachycardia and hypertension. Medical problems associated with heroin abuse include malnutrition, chronic anemia, cellulitis, bacterial endocarditis (tricuspid valve), pulmonary and systemic septic emboli and infarctions, aspiration pneumonitis, atelectasis, hepatitis, hepatomegaly, and sclerosing glomerulonephritis.[60] Presedation patient optimization is directed to the organ system affected. Laboratory testing (e.g., blood count, liver function tests) is indicated based on the presenting pathophysiology associated with opioid abuse. A baseline ECG is advised secondary to the enhanced automaticity of the heart associated with the heroin-addicted patient. The widespread effects of the current opioid epidemic are featured in Chapter 4.

What is the impact of marijuana abuse on the patient presenting for sedation services?

The most common means of ingestion of marijuana is smoking. Smoking marijuana increases the level of tetrahydrocannabinol

(THC), producing a postinhalation euphoric state from its primary psychoactive component, THC. Increased sympathetic stimulation increases the heart rate and myocardial oxygen consumption and produces orthostatic hypotension in some persons. Patients with a history of chronic marijuana use characteristically present with the following symptoms:

- Chronic sinusitis
- Tar deposit in the lung
- Pulmonary impairment
- Conjunctival irritation

The effects of inhaled marijuana last for only several hours. Therefore, it is rare to encounter patients who are acutely intoxicated secondary to marijuana ingestion. Patients who admit to marijuana ingestion should have resting heart rate and blood pressure documented before initiation of the procedure. Severe tachycardia should be controlled with beta blockers. To decrease the incidence of pulmonary complications, symptoms of pulmonary impairment should be resolved before the administration of sedation.

What is the best method to approach a patient with a history of suspected substance abuse?

It is important to approach patients with a history of substance abuse diplomatically on the basis of the drug abused, time of last ingestion, and presenting symptoms. Symptoms associated with drug abuse may be life-threatening and include the following:

- Cellulitis
- Abscess of the skin
- Cardiomyopathy
- Psychotic behavior
- Aspiration with overdose
- Hepatitis
- Acquired immunodeficiency disease
- Sepsis
- Endocarditis

Counseling and social service support are important for this patient population. It is important to approach these patients individually and to realize that they have a disease of addiction, which requires specific treatment and therapy.

What is the impact of herbal use for a patient presenting for sedation services?

During the social and medication history assessment, it is important for the clinician to identify the patient's use of herbal preparations. The use of herbal preparations has grown in popularity over the last decade. A 2012 report by the American Botanical Council has disclosed that herbal products sales exceeded 5.3 billion dollars in the United States in 2011, a 4% growth compared to 2010. In 2013, sales increased by 8%, reaching approximately 6 billion dollars.[61] Sedation patients may use herbal preparations for chronic conditions (e.g., arthritis, depression, diabetes) or dissatisfaction with traditional medical treatment. Although many of these products are recommended or prescribed by conventional medical practitioners, these drugs carry a potential to increase bleeding and can alter the patient's response to sedative, analgesic, and anesthetic agents. Health care providers need to focus on patient use of herbal preparations and document their use during the presedation patient assessment. Table 2.15 identifies the clinically important effects and concerns of selected herbal medicines and recommendations for discontinuation of use before surgery.

Is pregnancy testing required for patients of childbearing age presenting for moderate procedural sedation and analgesia?

Routine preoperative pregnancy testing remains a controversial topic. Indications for pregnancy testing that may become evident during the preprocedure interview and patient assessment include the following:

- Sexually active status
- Date of the last menstrual period
- Presence or absence of birth control methods

In case a pregnancy test is ordered based on the patient's history, it should be completed immediately prior to the diagnostic or therapeutic procedure after obtaining patient consent.[62] A serum level hCG (human chorionic gonadotropin) determination should be considered for patients who may be less than 4 weeks pregnant secondary to the potential for false-negative or false-positive results until week 5 of the pregnancy.[63] Additional issues that must be addressed when deciding whether to order a pregnancy test include the following:

- Policies of the hospital or health care facility based on medical staff bylaws. The medical facility should have established guidelines that indicate when testing for pregnancy is appropriate.
- The patient should be advised of the fetal risk (e.g., spontaneous abortion) if anesthesia is administered during pregnancy. The incidence of congenital abnormalities is no greater for the pregnant woman undergoing surgery than for the woman with a surgery-free pregnancy.[64,65] Despite these data, many patients are advised to postpone elective surgery until well after the first trimester, when fetal organogenesis is complete.
- The patient should be privately questioned about the possibility of being pregnant. Female staff should interview the adolescent patient in the absence of family members.

How long should the patient be NPO prior to the procedure?

Nil per os (NPO) is the Latin term for nothing by mouth. The NPO principle has been used by anesthesia clinicians and surgeons for years to decrease the risk of gastric acid aspiration.

Patients at risk for the development of pulmonary aspiration are identified in Box 2.9. The American Society of Anesthesiologists has recently updated its practice guidelines for

TABLE 2.15   Clinically Important Effects and Perioperative Concerns of Selected Herbal Medicines

Herb: Common or Latin Name(s)	Relevant Pharmacologic Effects	Perioperative Concerns	Preoperative Discontinuation
Echinacea: purple coneflower root	Activation of cell-mediated immunity	Allergic reactions; decreased effectiveness of immunosuppressive actions of corticosteroids and cyclosporine; potential for immunosuppression with long-term use; inhibition of hepatic microsomal enzymes may precipitate toxicity of drugs metabolized by the liver (e.g., phenytoin, rifampin, phenobarbital)	No data
Ephedra: ma huang	Increased heart rate and blood pressure through direct and indirect sympathomimetic effects	Risk of myocardial ischemia and stroke from tachycardia and hypertension; ventricular arrhythmias with halothane; long-term use depletes endogenous catecholamines and may cause intraoperative hemodynamic instability (control hypotension with direct vasoconstrictor, e.g., phenylephrine); life-threatening interaction with monoamine oxidase inhibitors	At least 24 hours before surgery
Garlic: *Allium sativum*	Inhibition of platelet aggregation (may be irreversible); increased fibrinolysis; equivocal antihypertensive activity	Potential to increase risk of bleeding, especially when combined with other medications that inhibit platelet aggregation	At least 7 days before surgery
Ginkgo: duck foot tree, maidenhair tree, silver apricot	Inhibition of platelet-activating factor	Potential to increase risk of bleeding, especially when combined with other medications that inhibit platelet aggregation	At least 36 hours before surgery
Ginseng: American ginseng, Asian ginseng, Chinese ginseng, Korean ginseng	Lowers blood glucose; inhibition of platelet aggregation (may be irreversible); increased PT-PTT in animals; many other diverse effects	Hypoglycemia; potential to increase risk of bleeding; potential to decrease anticoagulation effect of warfarin	At least 7 days before surgery
Kava: awa, intoxicating pepper, kawa	Sedation, anxiolysis	Potential to increase sedative effect of anesthetics; potential for addiction, tolerance, and withdrawal after abstinence unstudied	At least 24 hours before surgery
St. John's wort: amber, goat weed, hardhay, *Hypericum*, klamath weed	Inhibition of neurotransmitter reuptake, monoamine oxidase inhibition is unlikely	Induction of cytochrome P-450 enzymes, affecting cyclosporine, warfarin, steroids, protease inhibitors, and possibly benzodiazepines, calcium channel blockers, and many other drugs; decreased serum digoxin levels	At least 5 days before surgery
Valerian: all-heal, garden heliotrope, vandal root	Sedation	Potential to increase sedative effect of anesthetics; benzodiazepine-like acute withdrawal; potential to increase anesthetic requirements with long-term use	No data

PT-PTT, Prothrombin time–partial thromboplastin time.
Modified from Ang-Lee MK, Moss J, Yuan CS. Herbal medicines and perioperative care. JAMA. 2001;286:208–216; Kaye AD, Kucera I, Sabar R. Perioperative anesthesia clinical considerations of alternative medicines. *Anesthesiol Clin North America.* 2004;22:125–139; Hogg LA, Foo L. Management of patients taking herbal medicines in the perioperative period: a survey of practice and policies within anaesthetic departments in the United Kingdom. *Eur J Anaesthesiol.* 2010;27(1):11–15.

preoperative fasting and the use of pharmacologic agents. The ASA NPO guidelines for healthy patients are featured in Table 2.16.[66] Historically, patients have been instructed to have nothing to eat or drink after midnight. These NPO practice recommendations have become more liberal over the last several years. Studies that have been conducted challenging traditional fasting times ($\geq$7 hours) for clear liquids appeared to show that a reduced fasting interval did not

BOX 2.9 Conditions That Increase the Risk of Regurgitation and Pulmonary Aspiration During Anesthesia

- Age extremes (<1 yr or >70 yr)
- Anxiety
- Ascites
- Collagen vascular disease (e.g., scleroderma)
- Depression
- Esophageal surgery
- Exogenous medications (e.g., opioids, premedication)
- Failed intubation or difficult airway history
- Gastroesophageal junction dysfunction (e.g., hiatal hernia)
- Mechanical obstruction (e.g., pyloric stenosis, duodenal ulcer)
- Metabolic disorders (e.g., hypothyroidism, chronic diabetes, hepatic failure, hyperglycemia, obesity, renal failure, uremia)
- Neurologic sequelae (e.g., those of developmental delays, head injury, hypotonia, seizures)
- Pain
- Pregnancy
- Prematurity with respiratory problems
- Smoking
- Type and composition of gastric contents (e.g., solid foods and milk products)

From Nagelhout JJ, Elisa S: Nurse Anesthesia. 6th ed. St. Louis: Elsevier; 2018.

TABLE 2.16 ASA Fasting Guidelines[a]

Ingested Material	Minimum Fasting Period[b]
Clear liquid[c]	2 h
Breast milk	4 h
Infant formula	6 h
Nonhuman milk[d]	6 h
Light meal[e]	6 h
Fried foods, fatty foods, or meat	Additional fasting time (e.g., ≥8 h) may be needed.

[a]These recommendations apply to healthy patients who are undergoing elective procedures. They are not intended for women in labor. Following the guidelines does not guarantee complete gastric emptying.

[b]The fasting periods noted above apply to all ages.

[c]Examples of a clear liquid include water, fruit juices without pulp, carbonated beverages, clear tea, and black coffee.

[d]Because nonhuman milk is similar to solids in gastric emptying time, the amount ingested must be considered when determining an appropriate fasting period.

[e]A light meal typically consists of toast and clear liquids. Meals that included fried or fatty foods or meat may prolong gastric emptying time. Additional fasting time (e.g., ≥8 h) may be needed in these cases. Both the amount and type of foods ingested must be considered when determining an appropriate fasting period. Adapted from American Society of Anesthesiologists. Practice guidelines for preoperative fasting and the use of pharmacologic agents to reduce the risk of pulmonary aspiration: application to healthy patients undergoing elective procedures: an updated report by the American Society of Anesthesiologists Task Force on Preoperative Fasting and the Use of Pharmacologic Agents to Reduce the Risk of Pulmonary Aspiration. Anesthesiology. 2017;3:376–393.

increase the risk of pulmonary aspiration in normal healthy individuals.[67] Traditional NPO fasting guidelines did not address the following:

- The time of the procedure
- The time the patient went to bed for the night
- The variability associated with gastric emptying for solids and liquids

Failure to address these critical variables leads to dehydration, hypoglycemia, hypovolemia, increased irritability, enhanced preoperative anxiety, thirst, hunger, and headaches.[68-70] To avoid scheduling delays, patients should be given clear NPO instructions from the health care provider's office or health care facility prior to the procedure.

What are the nursing implications associated with obtaining informed consent prior to the procedure?

An important risk management strategy and legal requirement is to obtain informed consent before the administration of moderate procedural sedation and analgesia. Informed consent requires that the plan, alternatives, and potential complications be explained to the patient in layman's terms. The basis for informed consent stems from the fundamental principle that the patient has the right to exercise control over his or her body and over the treatment plan. Lack of properly obtained informed consent may result in charges of assault and battery. Assault is defined as "the apprehension or anticipation of the application of unauthorized physical force." Battery is defined as "the unconsented, unprivileged touching of another person." A separate area on the consent form, which addresses the procedural risks, reasonable alternatives, and expected benefits associated with procedural sedation, is generally advised. A sample informed consent that can be modified specifically for moderate procedural sedation and analgesia services is identified in Fig. 2.7.

Should sedation providers use the American Society of Anesthesiologist's physical classification system (ASA status classification)?

Incorporation of a physical classification system is a beneficial addition to the presedation assessment form. This physical status classification system was developed in 1940 by a committee of the American Society of Anesthetists, currently the American Society of Anesthesiologists.[71] This system was developed to standardize physical status and assign a potential risk classification. This physical classification system also offers the clinician a numeric summary assessment tool based on the findings of the presedation physical assessment. The ASA Physical Status Classification System is presented in Table 2.17.

What presedation instructions should be given to the patient?

Detailed presedation instructions that must be provided to the patient include the following:

- Fasting guidelines (NPO status)
- Time of arrival
- Estimated procedure time

DIAMONTE HOSPITAL
Diamonte, Arizona

Informed Consent

(example only)

**PATIENT CONSENT TO MEDICAL TREATMENT/SURGICAL PROCEDURE
AND ACKNOWLEDGMENT OF RECEIPT OF MEDICAL INFORMATION**

READ CAREFULLY BEFORE SIGNING

TO THE PATIENT: You have been told that you should consider medical treatment/surgery. State law requires this facility to tell you (1) the nature of your condition, (2) the general nature of the procedure/treatment/surgery, (3) the risks of the proposed treatment/surgery, as defined by the state or as determined by your doctor, and (4) reasonable therapeutic alternatives and risks associated with such alternatives.

You have the right, as a patient, to be informed about your condition and the recommended surgical, medical, or diagnostic procedure to be used so that you may make the decision whether or not to undergo the procedure after knowing the risks and hazards involved.

In keeping with the State law of informed consent, you are being asked to sign a confirmation that we have discussed all these matters. We have already discussed with you the common problems and risks. We wish to inform you as completely as possible. Please read this form carefully. Ask about anything you do not understand, and we will be pleased to explain it.

1. Patient name: _____

2. Treatment/procedure:
    (a) Description, nature of the treatment/procedure: _____
    _____
    Purpose: _____
    _____

3. Patient condition: Patient's diagnosis, description of the nature of the condition or ailment for which the medical treatment, surgical procedure, or other therapy described in Item 2 is indicated and recommended:
    _____
    _____

4. Material risks of treatment procedure:
    (a) All medical or surgical treatment involves risks. Listed below are those risks associated with this procedure that members of this facility believe a reasonable person in your (patient's) position would likely consider significant when deciding whether to have or forego the proposed therapy. Please ask your physician if you would like additional information regarding the nature or consequences of these risks, their likelihood of occurrence, or other associated risks that you might consider significant but may not be listed below.

        - See attachment for risks identified by the State
        - See attachment for risks determined by your doctor

Fig. 2.7 Sample informed consent form. (From Davis N, LaCour M: *Foundations of health information management*, ed 4, St Louis, 2017, Elsevier.)

Continued

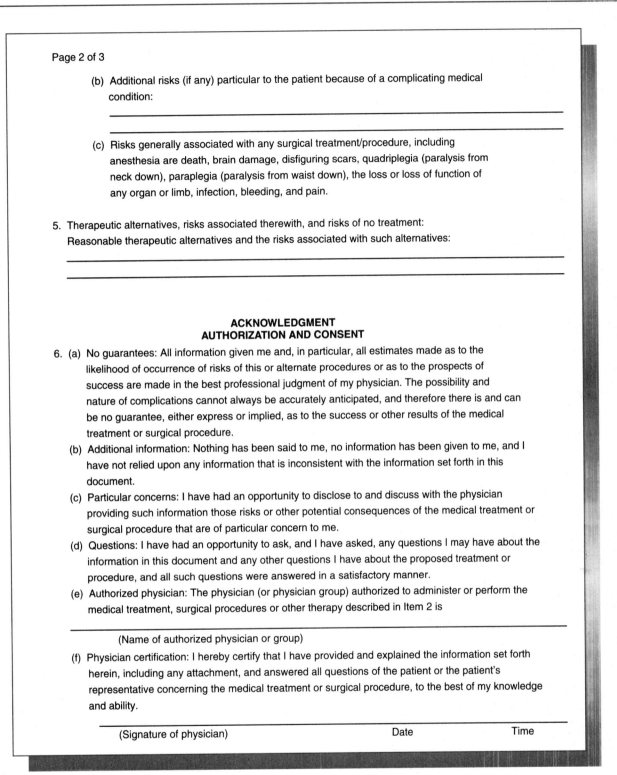

Page 2 of 3

(b) Additional risks (if any) particular to the patient because of a complicating medical condition:

_____

_____

(c) Risks generally associated with any surgical treatment/procedure, including anesthesia are death, brain damage, disfiguring scars, quadriplegia (paralysis from neck down), paraplegia (paralysis from waist down), the loss or loss of function of any organ or limb, infection, bleeding, and pain.

5. Therapeutic alternatives, risks associated therewith, and risks of no treatment:
   Reasonable therapeutic alternatives and the risks associated with such alternatives:

_____

_____

ACKNOWLEDGMENT
AUTHORIZATION AND CONSENT

6. (a) No guarantees: All information given me and, in particular, all estimates made as to the likelihood of occurrence of risks of this or alternate procedures or as to the prospects of success are made in the best professional judgment of my physician. The possibility and nature of complications cannot always be accurately anticipated, and therefore there is and can be no guarantee, either express or implied, as to the success or other results of the medical treatment or surgical procedure.

(b) Additional information: Nothing has been said to me, no information has been given to me, and I have not relied upon any information that is inconsistent with the information set forth in this document.

(c) Particular concerns: I have had an opportunity to disclose to and discuss with the physician providing such information those risks or other potential consequences of the medical treatment or surgical procedure that are of particular concern to me.

(d) Questions: I have had an opportunity to ask, and I have asked, any questions I may have about the information in this document and any other questions I have about the proposed treatment or procedure, and all such questions were answered in a satisfactory manner.

(e) Authorized physician: The physician (or physician group) authorized to administer or perform the medical treatment, surgical procedures or other therapy described in Item 2 is

_____
(Name of authorized physician or group)

(f) Physician certification: I hereby certify that I have provided and explained the information set forth herein, including any attachment, and answered all questions of the patient or the patient's representative concerning the medical treatment or surgical procedure, to the best of my knowledge and ability.

_____
(Signature of physician)   Date   Time

Fig. 2.7 (Continued)

- Presence of a responsible adult for discharge
- Medication instructions
- Procedure-specific guidelines
- Bowel preparation
- Prophylactic antibiotics
- Dye preparations
- Wearing loose-fitting clothing

When instructing patients regarding NPO guidelines, it is important to inform them that they are to have nothing to eat or drink after a specific time. Many patients receiving NPO instructions believe that these instructions pertain only to food, and not to water. Therefore, when instructing patients regarding NPO status, the clinician must specify no ingestion of food, water, juice, coffee, or other drinks. Presedation oral

Page 3 of 3

Consent

I hereby authorize and direct the designated authorized physician/group, together with associates and assistants of his/her choice, to administer or perform the medical treatment or surgical procedure described in Item 2 of this consent form, including any additional procedures or services as they may deem necessary or reasonable, including the administration of any general or regional anesthetic agent, x-ray or other radiological services, laboratory services, and the disposal of any tissue removed during a diagnostic or surgical procedure, and I hereby consent thereto.

I have read and understand all information set forth in this document, and all blanks were filled in prior to my signing. This authorization for and consent to medical treatment or surgical procedure is and shall remain valid until revoked.

I acknowledge that I have had the opportunity to ask any questions about the contemplated medical procedure or surgical procedure described in Item 2 of this consent form, including risks and alternatives, and acknowledge that my questions have been answered to my satisfaction.

_____   _____   _____   _____
Witness   Date/time   Patient or person   Date/time
                                                                                                      authorized to consent

If consent is signed by someone other than patient, indicate relationship: _____

Fig. 2.7 (Continued)

TABLE 2.17   American Society of Anesthesiologists' Physical Status Classification System[a]

ASA Classification	Definition	Examples
ASA I	A normal healthy patient	Healthy, nonsmoking, no or minimal alcohol use
ASA II	A patient with mild systemic disease	Mild diseases, only without substantive functional limitations; examples include (but not limited to) current smoker, social alcohol drinker, pregnancy, obesity (BMI, 30–40), well-controlled DM or HTN, mild lung disease
ASA III	A patient with severe systemic disease	Substantive functional limitations—one or more moderate to severe diseases; examples include (but not limited to) poorly controlled DM or HTN, COPD, morbid obesity (BMI $\geq$ 40), active hepatitis, alcohol dependence or abuse, implanted pacemaker, moderate reduction of ejection fraction, ESRD undergoing regularly scheduled dialysis, premature infant, PCA < 60 wk, history (>3 mo) of MI, CVA, TIA, or CAD/stents.
ASA IV	A patient with severe systemic disease that is a constant threat to life	Examples include (but not limited to) recent (<3 mo) MI, CVA, TIA, or CAD/stents, ongoing cardiac ischemia or severe valve dysfunction, severe reduction of ejection fraction, sepsis, DIC, ARDS, or ESRD not undergoing regularly scheduled dialysis
ASA V	A moribund patient who is not expected to survive without the operation	Examples include (but not limited to) ruptured abdominal or thoracic aneurysm, massive trauma, intracranial bleed with mass effect, ischemic bowel in the face of significant cardiac pathology or multiple organ or system dysfunction
ASA VI	A patient declared brain-dead whose organs are being removed for donor purposes	

ARDS, Acute respiratory distress syndrome; *BMI*, body mass index; *CAD*, coronary artery disease; *COPD*, chronic obstructive pulmonary disease; *CVA*, cerebral vascular accident; *DIC*, disseminated intravascular coagulation; *DM*, diabetes mellitus; *ESRD*, end-stage renal disease; *HTN*, hypertension; *MI*, myocardial infarction; *PCA*, patient-controlled analgesia; *TIA*, transient ischemic attack.

https://www.asahq.org/standards-and-guidelines/asa-physical-status-classification-system.

[a]The addition of E denotes emergency surgery. An emergency is defined as existing when delay in treatment of the patient would lead to a significant increase in the threat to life or body part.

From American Society of Anesthesiologists. ASA physical status classification system.

medications ordered for the morning of the procedure may be taken with a sip of water. It may be necessary to quantify this amount with the patient to avoid ingestion of large amounts of water.

Patients should be instructed to arrive for the procedure at a mutually agreed on time. Sufficient time must be allotted to register the patient properly, obtain baseline vital signs, and prepare the patient for the planned diagnostic examination or procedure. When these presedation duties are performed in an unhurried atmosphere, patient anxiety is decreased through reassurance and timely preparation.

Patients must be instructed to arrange for a competent adult to accompany them home. Early notification of this requirement allows the patient time to make arrangements for transportation and recovery at home. It is not acceptable to discharge a sedation patient to return home by taxi, Uber, Lyft, or any other paid transportation system. A responsible adult who will assume postsedation care and instructions on behalf of the patient should be present during the discharge process.

Procedure-specific guidelines (e.g., bowel preparations, prophylactic antibiotics, dye preparations) must be clearly outlined before the procedure. Written instructions are extremely helpful for many patients and eliminate numerous telephone calls that might request reiteration of the presedation instructions.

SUMMARY

Patients presenting for therapeutic, diagnostic, and minor surgical procedures often have an inherent fear associated with the planned procedure or medications that will be used during the procedure. Common presedation fears include a "bad" diagnosis (e.g., carcinoma), postprocedure nausea, vomiting, pain, and, in some cases, death. During presedation assessment, the clinician must do the following:

- Conduct the interview in an unhurried manner.
- Use an organized interview format.
- Complete a focused physical examination.
- Inform and reassure the patient.

When conducted appropriately, presedation assessment is a useful tool for building a trusting patient-clinician relationship, completed prior to initiating the procedure.

REFERENCES

1. American Society of Anesthesiologists. Practice guidelines for preoperative fasting and use of pharmacologic agents to reduce the risk of pulmonary aspiration: Application to healthy patients undergoing elective procedures. *Anesthesiology*. 2017; 126: 376–393.
2. The Joint Commission. Standards FAQ details: Sedation and anesthesia – pre-induction assessment – time frame. (2018). https://www.jointcommission.org/standards_information/jcfaqdetails.aspx?StandardsFaqId=870&ProgramId=46.
3. Garrow JS, Webster J. Quetelet's index (W/H2) as a measure of fatness. *International Journal of Obesity*. 1985; 9:147–153.
4. Freedman DS, Horlick M, Berenson GS. A comparison of the Slaughter skinfold-thickness equations and BMI in predicting body fatness and cardiovascular disease risk factor levels in children. *American Journal of Clinical Nutrition*. 2013; 98:1417–1424.
5. Wohlfahrt-Veje C, Tinggaard J, Winther K, et al. Body fat throughout childhood in 2647 healthy Danish children: Agreement of BMI, waist circumference, skinfolds with dual x-ray absorptiometry. *European Journal of Clinical Nutrition*. 2014; 68:664–670.
6. Hines RL, Marschall KE. Systemic and Pulmonary Arterial Hypertension. In: Hines RL, Marschall KE, eds. *Stoelting's anesthesia and co-existing disease*. 8th edition Philadelphia, PA: Elsevier; 2018:183–198.
7. Merai R, Siegel C, Rakotz M, et al. CDC grand rounds: A public health approach to detect and control hypertension. *Morbidity and Mortality Weekly Report*. 2016; 65:1261–1264.
8. Centers for Disease Control and Prevention, National Center for Health Statistics. Multiple Cause of Death Data 1999-2015 [data file]. (2016). http://wonder.cdc.gov/mcd-icd10.html; 2016.
9. Hines RL, Marschall KE. Hines RL, Marschall KE, eds. *Stoelting's anesthesia and co-existing disease*. 8th ed. Elsevier: Philadelphia; 2018.
10. Wilson W, Taubert KA, Gewitz M, et al. Prevention of infective endocarditis: guidelines from the American Heart Association: a guideline from the American Heart Association Rheumatic Fever, Endocarditis, and Kawasaki Disease Committee, Council on Cardiovascular Disease in the Young, and the Council on Clinical Cardiology, Council on Cardiovascular Surgery and Anesthesia, and the Quality of Care and Outcomes Research Interdisciplinary Working Group. *Circulation*. 2007; 116: 1736–1754.
11. Schwartzstein RM. Approach to the patient with dyspnea. (2017). https://www.uptodate.com/contents/approach-to-the-patient-with-dyspnea?search=approach%20to%20the%20patient%20with%20dyspnea&source=search_result&selectedTitle=1~150&usage_type=default&display_rank=1; 2017.
12. Mayo Clinic Staff. Shortness of breath (dyspnea). (2018). https://www.mayoclinic.org/symptoms/shortness-of-breath/basics/definition/sym-20050890; 2018.
13. Marx JA, Hockberger R, Walls R. Dyspnea. In: Marx JA, et al. ed. *Rosen's emergency medicine: Concepts and clinical practice*. 8th ed. Philadelphia, PA: Saunders Elsevier; 2013:206–213.
14. Lareau SC, Fahy B, Meek P. Breathlessness. *American Journal of Respiratory Critical Care Medicine*. 2013; 187:3–4.
15. Lechtzin N. Shortness of breath. Merck Manuals. (2018). https://www.merckmanuals.com/home/lung-and-airway-disorders/symptoms-of-lung-disorders/shortness-of-breath; 2018.
16. Quintero DR, Fakhoury K. Assessment of stridor in children. (2017). https://www.uptodate.com/contents/assessment-of-stridor-in-children?search=assessment%20stridor&source=search_result&selectedTitle=1~150&usage_type=default&display_rank=1; 2017.
17. Loftis LL. Emergency evaluation of acute upper airway obstruction in children. (2017). https://www.uptodate.com/contents/emergency-evaluation-of-acute-upper-airway-obstruction-in-children?search=Emergency%20evaluation%20of%20acute%20upper%20airway%20obstruction%20in%20children&source=search_result&selectedTitle=1~150&usage_type=default&display_rank=1; 2017.
18. American Heart Association. Warning signs of heart failure. (2017). http://www.heart.org/HEARTORG/Conditions/HeartFailure/WarningSignsforHeartFailure/Warning-Signs-

for-Heart-Failure_UCM_002045_Article.jsp#.VrTf7fkrJMw; 2017.

19. National Heart, Lung, and Blood Institute (n.d.). COPD. https://www.nhlbi.nih.gov/health-topics/copd. [Accessed 06.01.2019].

20. Gallagher SA, Hackett P, Rosen JM. High altitude illness: Pathophysiology, risk factors, and general prevention. (2017). https://www.uptodate.com/contents/high-altitude-illness-physiology-risk-factors-and-general-prevention?search=high%20altitude%20illness&source =search_result&selectedTitle= 1~32&usage_type=default&display_rank=1; 2017.

21. Olson EJ (expert opinion). Mayo Clinic, Rochester, Minn. Feb. 6, 2016. https://www.mayoclinic.org/symptoms/shortness-of-breath/basics/causes/sym-20050890?p=1. [Accessed 06.01.2019].

22. Global Strategy for the Diagnosis. Management and Prevention of COPD. In: *Global Initiative for Chronic Obstructive Lung Disease (GOLD)*: 2017. (2017). http://goldcopd.org.

23. Centers for Disease Control and Prevention, National Center for Health Statistics. Asthma. (2017). http://www.cdc.gov/nchs/fastats/asthma.htm; 2017.

24. Gupta MK, Gupta R, Khuneteta A, Swarnkar SK. An overview of asthma and its treatment. *Journal of Biomedical and Pharmaceutical Research*. 2017; 6(5):32–36.

25. Farney RJ, Walker BS, Farney RM, et al. The STOP-Bang equivalent model and prediction of severity of obstructive sleep apnea: Relation to polysomnographic measurements of the apnea/hypopnea index. *Journal of Clinical Sleep Medicine*. 2011; 7:459–465.

26. Gross JB, Apfelbaum JL, Connis RT, Nickinovich DG. In reply. *Anesthiology*. 2014; 121:667–668.

27. Chung F, Liao P, Farney R. Correlation between the STOP-Bang score and the severity of obstructive sleep apnea. *Anesthesiology*. 2015; 6:1436–1437.

28. American Society of Anesthesiologists Task Force on the Perioperative Management of Patients with Obstructive Sleep Apnea. Practice guidelines for the perioperative management of patients with obstructive sleep apnea. *Anesthiology*. 2014; 120:268–286.

29. Lautt WW. Overview. In: Granger DN, Granger J, eds. *Hepatic circulation: Physiology and pathophysiology*. San Rafael, CA: Morgan & Claypool Life Sciences; 2009:7–18.

30. Raghunathan K, Shaw A, Nathanson B, et al. Association between the choice of IV crystalloid and in-hospital mortality among critically ill adults with sepsis. *Critical Care Medicine*. 2014; 42:1585–1591.

31. Yunos NM, Bellomo R, Hegarty C, et al. Association between a chloride-liberal vs chloride-restrictive intravenous fluid administration strategy and kidney injury in critically ill adults. *Journal of the American Medical Association*. 2012; 308: 1566–1572.

32. Sharif-Askari FS, Syed Sulaiman SA, Saheb Sharif-Askari N, Al Sayed Hussain A. Development of an adverse drug reaction risk assessment score among hospitalized patients with chronic kidney disease. *PLoS ONE*. 2014; 9. e95991.

33. American Diabetes Association. Classification and diagnosis of diabetes. Sec. 2. In Standards of Medical Care in Diabetes. *Diabetes Care*. 2015; 38:S8–S16. Suppl. 1.

34. Centers for Disease Control and Prevention. Diabetes basics. (2017). https://www.cdc.gov/diabetes/basics/type2.html; 2017.

35. Moghissi ES, Korytkowski MT, DiNardo M, et al. American association of clinical endocrinologists and American diabetes association consensus statement on inpatient glycemic control. *Diabetes Care*. 2009; 32:119–1131.

36. Marley RA, Sheets SA. Preoperative evaluation and preparation of the patient. In: Nagelhout JJ, Elisha S, eds. *Nurse anesthesia (6th ed., pp. 338)*. St. Louis, MO: Elsevier/Saunders; 2018; 338–339.

37. Thompson BM, Stearns JD, Apsey HA, et al. Perioperative management of patients with diabetes and hyperglycemia undergoing elective surgery. *Current Diabetes Reports*. 2016; 16(2).

38. Abdelmalak B, Ibrahim M, Yared JP, et al. Perioperative glycemic management in insulin pump patients undergoing noncardiac surgery. *Current Pharmaceutical Design*. 2012; 18:6204–6214.

39. Connery LE, Coursin DB. Assessment and therapy of selected endocrine disorders. *Anesthesiology Clinics of North America*. 2004; 22:93–123.

40. Loevy HT, Aduss H, Rosenthal IM. Tooth eruption and craniofacial development in congenital hypothyroidism: Report of case. *Journal of the American Dental Association*. 1987; 115:429–431.

41. Hepner DL, Castells MC. Latex allergy: An update. *96: Anesthesia & Analgesia*. 2003. 1219–1229.

42. Benarroch-Gampel J, Sheffield KM, Duncan CB, et al. Preoperative laboratory testing in patients undergoing elective, low-risk ambulatory surgery. *Annals of Surgery*. 2012; 256:518–528.

43. Muntro J, Booth A, Nicholl J. Routine preoperative testing: A systematic review of the evidence. *Health Technology Assessment*. 1997; 1:1–62.

44. National Institute for Health and Care Excellence. *Preoperative tests: the use of routine preoperative tests for elective surgery (NG45)*. (2016). https://www.nice.org.uk/guidance/ng45.

45. Kennedy JM, van Rij AM, Spears GF, et al. Polypharmacy in a general surgical unit and consequences of drug withdrawal. *British Journal of Clinical Pharmacology*. 2000; 49:353–362.

46. Shorrock P, Bakerly N. Effects of smoking on health and anaesthesia. *Anaesthesia and Intensive Care Medicine*. 2016; 17:141–143.

47. Lida H. Preoperative assessment of smoking patient. *Masui*. 2010; 59:838–843.

48. Pearce AC, Jones RM. Smoking and anesthesia: Preoperative abstinence and perioperative morbidity. *Anesthesiology*. 1984; 61:576–584.

49. Lai HK, Hedley AJ, Repace J, et al. Lung function and exposure to workplace second-hand smoke during exemptions from smoking ban legislation: an exposure-response relationship based on indoor PM2.5 and urinary cotinine levels. *Thorax*. 2011; 66:615–623.

50. Treyster Z, Gitterman B. Second-hand smoke exposure in children: Environmental factors, physiological effects, and interventions within pediatrics. *Reviews on Environmental Health*. 2011; 26:187–195.

51. Seyidov TH, Elemen L, Solak M, et al. Passive smoke exposure is associated with perioperative adverse effects in children. *Journal of Clinical Anesthesia*. 2011; 23:47–52.

52. Shapiro B, Coffa D, McCance-Katz EF. A primary care approach to substance misuse. *American Family Physician*. 2013; 88:113–121.

53. Gortney JS, Raub JN, Patel P, et al. Alcohol withdrawal syndrome in medical patients. *Cleveland Clinic Journal of Medicine*. 2016; 83:67–79.

54. Milroy C. Ten years of ecstasy. *Journal of the Royal Society of Medicine.* 1999; 92:68–71.

55. Boot BP, McGregor IS, Hall W. MDMA (Ecstasy) neurotoxicity: Assessing and communicating the risks. *Lancet.* 2000; 355: 1818–1821.

56. Henry JA. Metabolic consequences of drug misuse. *British Journal of Anaesthesia.* 2000; 85:136–142.

57. National Institute on Drug Abuse (NIDA). Cocaine. Retrieved from https://www.drugabuse.gov/drugs-abuse/cocaine on 2019, January 5.

58. American Psychiatric Association. Substance use disorder. In: *Diagnostic and statistical manual of mental disorders.* 5th ed. Washington, DC: Author; 2013.

59. Centers for Disease Control and Prevention. Today's heroin epidemic. (2015). https://www.cdc.gov/vitalsigns/heroin/index.html; 2015.

60. Kester R, Strauss J, Greenlee A, et al. Medical and psychiatric comorbidities associated with opiate use disorder in the geriatric population: A systematic review. *The American Journal of Geriatric Psychiatry.* 2017; 25:S111–S112.

61. Lindstrom A, Ooyen C, Lunch ME, et al. Sales of herbal dietary supplements increase by 7.9% in 2013, marking a decade of rising sales: Turmeric supplements climb to top ranking in natural channel. *HerbalGram.* 2014; 103:52–56.

62. Rosen MA. Anesthesia for the pregnant patient undergoing nonobstetric surgery. In: Rosenblatt MA, Butterworth JFIV, Gross JB, eds. *ASA Refresher Courses in Anesthesiology.* Philadelphia: Lippincott; 2011:134–141.

63. Greene DN, Schmidt RL, Kramer SM, et al. Limitations in qualitative point of care hCG tests for detecting early pregnancy. *Clinica Chimica Acta.* 2013; 415:317–321.

64. Mazze RI, Kallen B. Appendectomy during pregnancy: a Swedish registry study of 778 cases. *Obstetric Gynecology.* 1991; 77:835–840.

65. Mazze RI, Kallen B. Reproductive outcome after anesthesia and operation during pregnancy: A registry study of 5405 cases. *American Journal of Obstetrics & Gynecology.* 1989; 161: 1178–1185.

66. American Society of Anesthesiologists. Practice guidelines for preoperative fasting and the use of pharmacologic agents to reduce the risk of pulmonary aspiration: Application to healthy patients undergoing elective procedures: An updated report by the American Society of Anesthesiologists Task Force on Preoperative Fasting and the Use of Pharmacologic Agents to Reduce the Risk of Pulmonary Aspiration. *Anesthesiology.* 2017; 3:376–393.

67. Stuart PC. The evidence behind modern fasting guidelines. *Best Practice & Research Clinical Anaesthesiology.* 2006; 20:457–469.

68. Smith I, Kranke P, Murat I, et al. Perioperative fasting in adults and children: Guidelines from the European Society of Anaesthesiology. *European Journal of Anaesthesiology.* 2011; 28:556–569.

69. Dose VA, White PF. Effects of fluid therapy on serum glucose levels in fasted outpatients. *Anesthesiology.* 1987; 66:223–226.

70. Splinter WM, Stewart JA, Muir JG. The effect of preoperative apple juice on gastric contents, thirst, and hunger in children. *Canadian Journal of Anaesthesia.* 1989; 36:55–58.

71. Barash P, Calahan M, et al. *Clinical Anesthesia.* 8th ed. Chicago: Wolters Kluwer; 2017.

CHAPTER 2: REVIEW QUESTIONS

1. Which of the following methods of patient weight assessment measures the mass of the body in relation to height and weight?
   A. Basal index
   B. Body mass index
   C. Conversion of pounds into kilograms
   D. Measurement of patient in kilocalories

2. A plan of _____ is frequently indicated when nonanesthesia clinicians are requested to provide administration of moderate procedural sedation and analgesia to the obese patient population.
   A. Deep sedation
   B. Minimal sedation
   C. Mandatory consultation with anesthesia
   D. Moderate procedural sedation and analgesia plan

3. Presedation administration of H_2 blockers and gastrokinetic agents serve to _____
   A. Increase gastric volume and decrease gastric pH.
   B. Decrease gastric volume and increase gastric pH.
   C. Decrease gastric volume and decrease gastric pH.
   D. Increase gastric volume and increase gastric pH.

4. Hypertension is defined by the American Heart Association as a systolic blood pressure greater than _____ and a diastolic blood pressure greater than _____.
   A. 160 mm Hg; 99 mm Hg
   B. 160 mm Hg; 95 mm Hg
   C. 140 mm Hg; 95 mm Hg
   D. 140 mm Hg; 90 mm Hg

5. Current recommendations for managing the hypertensive patient presenting for sedation include the following:
   A. Hold all cardiac medications for 24 hours preprocedure.
   B. Hold all cardiac medications for 12 hours preprocedure.
   C. Administer antihypertensive therapy up to and including the morning of the procedure.
   D. Administer antihypertensive therapy only if the patient has a history of malignant hypertension.

6. Newly diagnosed dysrhythmias or dysrhythmias that impair myocardial performance identified during presedation patient assessment require _____.
   A. Further evaluation and consultation
   B. No further consultation
   C. Administration of presedation digoxin
   D. Administration of presedation lidocaine

7. Diagnosis of sleep apnea is definitively diagnosed with which of the following diagnostic examinations?
   A. MRI
   B. CT scan
   C. Polysomnography
   D. Pulse oximetry

8. The degree of metabolism of pharmacologic compounds is dependent on hepatic blood flow and enzyme activity in the endoplasmic reticulum.
   A. True
   B. False

9. Accentuation of a benzodiazepine effect may be greatly enhanced in patients with renal disease secondary to which of the following physiologic effects?
   A. Increased renal blood flow
   B. Decreased renal blood flow
   C. Ionization of the pharmacologic compounds
   D. Decreased protein binding of the medications

10. Using the CAGE approach of inquiry during social history inquiry is an effective method to identify which of the following substances?
    A. Cigarette smoking
    B. Alcohol ingestion
    C. Marijuana use
    D. Heroin use

11. Diabetic patients presenting for moderate procedural sedation and analgesia should _____.
    A. Withhold all medications on the day of the diagnostic procedure
    B. Eat a full breakfast the morning of the planned procedure
    C. Have their blood sugar checked every 15 minutes in the preprocedure area
    D. Have their procedure scheduled early in the day to prevent a prolonged fast

12. To have diagnostic testing yield beneficial information, it is important to:
    A. Order an ECG, complete blood count (CBC), and electrolytes on all patients.
    B. Order no presedation laboratory testing at any time.
    C. Order presedation laboratory and diagnostic testing based on the patient's past medical history and physical examination.
    D. Only follow hospital policy with regard to presedation testing.

13. A cigarette smoking history should be quantified in _____ and documented on the presedation assessment form.
    A. Carton-years
    B. Pack-years
    C. Individual cigarette years
    D. Cigarettes per day

14. Chronic use of alcohol leads to stimulation of the _____, which may require increased amounts or doses of sedative and analgesic medications.
    A. Cytochrome P-450 system in the liver
    B. Nephrons in the renal tubules
    C. Nephrons in the gray matter
    D. Hepatocytes in the periductal area

15. Current presedation NPO guidelines include the following:
    A. No solids for 3 hours; clear liquids until 1 hour preprocedure
    B. No solids for 6 hours; clear liquids until 2 hours preprocedure
    C. No solids for 8 hours; clear liquid ingestion until the procedure
    D. No solids or clear liquids for 12 hours presedation

Answers can be found in Appendix A.

Basic Pharmacologic Concepts for Sedation Clinical Practice

COMPETENCY STATEMENT

The licensed independent physician prescribing sedative, hypnotic, and analgesic medications, and the health care provider monitoring the moderate procedural sedation and analgesia patient, integrate concepts of pharmacology (pharmacokinetics and pharmacodynamics) when formulating a sedation plan of care.

I already understand the pharmacology of the benzodiazepines and opioids; why do I need to understand pharmacologic concepts further?

As health care providers prepare patients for the administration of moderate procedural sedation and analgesia, a deeper working knowledge of the pharmacology behind the agents used to achieve amnesia, analgesia, and hypnosis is required. Sedation providers must understand and apply basic principles of pharmacology to anticipate the patient care considerations associated with the pharmacokinetics and pharmacodynamics of each medication classification.

This competency module presents an overview of foundational pharmacologic concepts. Specific properties of sedative and analgesic medications are presented in Chapters 4 and 5. It is also critically important for clinicians engaged in the administration of moderate procedural sedation and analgesia to understand the pharmacologic profiles of sedative and analgesic medications so as to anticipate side effects associated with their administration. Pertinent pharmacologic definitions associated with the administration of IV medications are listed in Box 3.1.

What is the definition of pharmacokinetics, and how does it apply to the administration of moderate procedural sedation and analgesic medications?

Pharmacokinetics is the quantitative study of the absorption, distribution, metabolism, and excretion of injected drugs and their metabolites. ADME is the four-letter acronym for the terms *absorption, distribution, metabolism,* and *excretion* that have described pharmacokinetics for over 50 years. These terms were first presented together by Nelson in 1961, rephrasing the terms *resorption, distribution, consumption,* and *elimination* used by Teorell in 1937.[1,2] ADME, as originally used, stood for descriptors quantifying drug: entering the body (A), moving about the body (D), changing within the body (M), and leaving the body (E). Over time, the use of ADME has diversified according to the needs of the user. In particular, it is used to describe mechanisms: crossing the gut wall (A); movement between compartments (D); mechanisms of metabolism (M); and excretion or elimination (E); transport (T) is sometimes added, making the acronym ADME(t).[3]

Pharmacokinetics describes the relationship between the drug dose and drug concentration in plasma or at the site of drug effect over time. In essence, pharmacokinetics is the

---

BOX 3.1   Pharmacologic Definitions

- **Efficacy:** The maximum effect that can be produced by a drug.
- **Half-life:** Half-life is an important pharmacokinetic measurement. The metabolic half-life of a drug is the time taken for its concentration in plasma to decline to half its original level. Half-life refers to the duration of action of a drug and depends on how quickly the drug is eliminated from the plasma. The clearance and distribution of a drug from the plasma are therefore important parameters for the determination of its half-life.
- **Hyperreactive:** Refers to the patient population that requires decreased doses of pharmacologic agents to produce the desired effect.
- **Hyporeactive:** Refers to the patient population that requires increased doses of pharmacologic agents to produce the expected pharmacologic effect.
- **Pharmacodynamics:** A description of what the drug does to the body, including the relationship between drug concentration and pharmacologic effect or, quite simply, what the drug does to the body.
- **Pharmacokinetics:** The relationship between drug dose and drug concentration or, quite simply, what the body does to a drug.
- **Potency:** Pharmacologic dosage required to produce an effect similar to that of another drug.
- **Synergism:** Occurs with use of one medication in conjunction with another. This results in a pharmacologic effect greater than the algebraic sum associated with each of the two individual drugs (e.g., $1 + 1 = 3$).
- **Tachyphylaxis:** Development of an acute tolerance to a drug; it is a rapidly diminishing response to successive doses of a drug, rendering it less effective. The effect is common with drugs acting on the central nervous system.
- **Tolerance:** Development of an increased drug requirement to produce a given effect. It results from chronic exposure to medications or toxins, which results in increased dosages of medications being required to achieve the desired pharmacologic effect.

---

study of what the body does to a drug. The pharmacokinetic profile of a medication considers the following parameters:

- Dose of drug administered
- Drug concentration at the receptor site
- Patient variability

Before the absorption, distribution, metabolism, and excretion of injected medications, transfer of the pharmacologic agent across cell membranes must occur. This transfer is a result of passive diffusion, active transport, or facilitated diffusion.

Passive Diffusion. Passive diffusion requires the presence of a concentration difference on each side of the cell membrane. The degree of pharmacologic transfer is dependent on the magnitude of the concentration gradient across the cell membrane.

Active Transport. Active transport requires energy to move molecules across cell membranes. Energy is required to facilitate the movement of pharmacologic compounds and molecules across cell membranes against a concentration gradient.

Facilitated Diffusion. Facilitated diffusion is a process whereby a specific carrier transport mechanism is used. Facilitated diffusion cannot move compounds and molecules against an electrochemical or concentration gradient.

How do absorption pathways affect pharmacologic bioavailability?

Bioavailability is a pharmacologic term used to indicate the extent to which a drug reaches a site of action or the biologic fluid from which the drug gains access to the site.[4] The absorption of a medication is dependent on the rate at which the pharmacologic compound leaves the site of administration. An important consideration associated with absorption is bioavailability. The mode of absorption is also an important factor for determining the duration and intensity of the pharmacologic effect. Several factors may alter absorption. These include the solubility of the medication, drug form, circulation at the site of absorption,

and protein binding. Generally, highly lipid-soluble drugs are capable of crossing cell membranes with ease. The suspension or drug form also affects absorption. To reach the site of action and exert a pharmacologic effect, all drugs must dissolve in water. Therefore, pharmacologic adjuncts delivered in an aqueous medium are absorbed faster than those delivered in a pill form or suspension. Circulation at the site of absorption also affects bioavailability. An increase in blood flow at the site of absorption increases the rate of absorption. Decreased blood flow at the site of absorption decreases absorption. Factors that decrease blood flow at the site of absorption include hypotension, shock, and utilization of vasoconstrictors.

What is the impact of protein binding on medications used for moderate procedural sedation and analgesia?

Pharmacologic agents bind to plasma proteins to varying degrees. The bound portion of the drug is inactive. The free or unbound portion of a drug is required for pharmacologic effect. Plasma protein binding also contributes to clearance of the drug. The unbound fraction of the drug is also available for metabolism by the hepatic cytochrome P-450 system, renal elimination, or both. Patients with nutritional disorders, carcinoma, recent weight loss, renal disease, or decreased plasma protein levels may demonstrate enhanced or exaggerated effects from pharmacologic adjuncts used to achieve a state of sedation or analgesia.

As always, titration of pharmacologic agents is advised in all situations. Careful assessment of the patient's response is warranted, particularly in patients with altered hepatic or renal function. Patients with decreased plasma protein levels or physical conditions associated with altered plasma protein levels require careful titration of all central nervous system (CNS) depressant medications. Small incremental doses, administered slowly over several minutes, allow the clinician the ability to assess the sedative effects and side effects of the medication fully.

⚡ PATIENT SAFETY SBAR FOCUS

Pharmacokinetic Impact and the Geriatric Patient

Situation

Geriatric patients in our endoscopy center continue to fall into a state of deep sedation as defined by the "Continuum of Sedation."

Background

One of our gastroenterologists follows a specific GI sedation protocol for all patients. At the beginning of the procedure, 2 milligrams of midazolam and 50 micrograms of fentanyl are administrated intravenously. Additional 1-milligram doses of midazolam are administered when the patient moves during the procedure. Patients arrive in the post sedation area with decreased oxygen saturation and depressed levels of consciousness.

Assessment

Older patients frequently demonstrate an increase in sedative response during procedural sedation. Physiologic changes related to the aging process (decreased total body water, increased body fat, decreased plasma proteins, decreased hepatic and renal blood flow) lead to increased drug accumulation. The geriatric patient also demonstrates an increase in the unbound portion of midazolam resulting in higher plasma concentrations, which reduces overall dosing requirements. When the pharmacokinetic changes associated with the geriatric aging process are not appreciated by the prescribing physician, hypotension, apnea, airway obstruction, and oxygen desaturation frequently ensue. Dosage reduction of 30% to 50% may be required when benzodiazepines are administered to the geriatric patient. Considerations with the administration of benzodiazepines include careful titration, decreased total dose, and the use of benzodiazepines with shorter acting half-lives (midazolam).

Recommendation

Sedative and analgesic agents must be appropriately selected based on procedural needs, patient age, and the presence of comorbidities. The geriatric gastroenterology patient is not an appropriate candidate for a *"one size fits all"* pharmacologic approach in the sedation setting. Slow titration to clinical effect technique coupled with ongoing assessment of level of consciousness, spontaneous ventilation, airway, and cardiovascular function is required particularly for the aged patient population. Recommended intravenous administration guidelines for the geriatric patient include slow titration to clinical effect technique. Titration of midazolam in 0.25-mg increments administered slowly over several minutes provides adequate time to pharmacologically assess patient response secondary to the geriatric patient's decreased cardiac output. This prolonged administration and assessment technique (A-A technique) allows careful titration of sedative analgesic agents, reduces total medication requirement, provides for a slow, controlled rise in therapeutic plasma level, and may provide for more rapid patient recovery.

What is the impact of the various routes of administration on medication absorption and distribution?

There are a variety of routes of administration for medication administration. The specific route of administration affects the absorption and distribution of each medication. Routes of medication administration include the following:

Oral Route. Absorption after ingestion of pharmacologic compounds is dependent on the small intestine and stomach. Absorption from the gastrointestinal tract generally occurs in the small intestine, where the epithelial lining is thin and has a large surface area.

First-Pass Effect. As depicted in Fig. 3.1, medications absorbed through the stomach and intestine require passage (first-pass effect) through the liver before they gain entrance to the systemic circulation. During this process, some of the active pharmacologic compound is inactivated by liver metabolism or biliary excretion, resulting in decreased bioavailability. As a result of this hepatic metabolism or biliary excretion, some medications require larger oral doses when compared to the IV route to exert a similar pharmacologic effect (e.g., propranolol [Inderal], oral dose = 40 mg when compared to an IV equivalent dose of 1 mg).

Sublingual Route. Because of the decreased surface area associated with sublingual administration, the sublingual mode of administration is reserved for highly lipid-soluble medications. A common medication given by the sublingual route is nitroglycerin. Because of venous drainage of the sublingual area directly into the superior vena cava, there is no first-pass hepatic effect associated with sublingual administration.

Rectal Route. Pharmacologic agents instilled into the rectum are absorbed via the superior hemorrhoidal veins and transported to the liver.[5] Approximately 50% of rectally administered medications undergo a first-pass hepatic effect. Depending on the site of rectal absorption (proximal or distal), bioavailability varies greatly. Rectal administration is generally reserved for unconscious, uncooperative, or pediatric patients who cannot tolerate oral medication administration. Rectal administration is not popular because of a wide variation in patient response, rectal mucosal irritation, and diarrhea.

Subcutaneous Route. Subcutaneous administration is reserved for nonirritating medications. It offers a more rapid and superior absorption pathway than oral administration. The quantity of medication absorbed depends on the following:

- Surface area
- Local blood flow
- Drug solubility

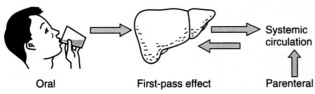

Fig. 3.1 First-pass effect.

Subcutaneous administration of a drug can ensure a steady plasma concentration. This is important for drugs such as insulin that require consistent blood levels to avoid fluctuations in blood sugar.

Intramuscular Route. Intramuscular injections afford sustained release and a more rapid pharmacologic effect. An increased bioavailability is directly proportional to the blood flow of the muscular bed. Pharmacologic suspensions allow prolonged release. However, organic solvents such as propylene glycol used in the suspension of diazepam often result in erratic intramuscular absorption.

Intravenous Route. IV administration of medications results in a rapid rise in the blood plasma level and a more rapid onset of action. Although this rapid onset at the target site of action is desirable, caution must be exercised during the administration of IV medications because side effects can also occur rapidly. Careful titration is required, and adequate time should be allowed to assess an individual patient's response.

Inhalational Route. Medications may be absorbed through the pulmonary tree (e.g., atomized, aerosolized, metered-dose inhaler). Rapid absorption is facilitated by the large pulmonary surface area. Alveolar blood flow closely mimics total cardiac output, with resultant rapid uptake from the pulmonary epithelium. When used properly, metered-dose inhalers and aerosol delivery are efficacious for the delivery of pharmacologic agents to the systemic circulation.

Topical Route. Topically administered medications must be lipid-soluble, and the quantity absorbed is proportional to the body surface area exposed to the medication. Factors affecting delivery of topical medication to the circulation include the following:

- Hydrated skin (more permeable to drug than dry skin)
- Occlusive patch (timed-release patch)
- Blood flow
- Low molecular weight
- Lipid-soluble molecules

Any activity that increases cutaneous blood flow will increase the uptake of topically administered medications. A complete review of the techniques of administration is provided in Table 3.1.

TABLE 3.1 Techniques of Medication Administration

Method	Pattern of Absorption	Advantages	Disadvantages
Oral ingestion	Lower gastrointestinal (GI) tract absorption is dependent on local conditions—blood flow, surface area, physical state of the drug.	Safe, convenient, economical	Emesis secondary to GI upset; drug destruction secondary to digestive enzymes; ineffective in patients with propulsion disorders; requires patient cooperation; requires intact reflexes; first-pass effect
Sublingual	Absorption of highly lipid-soluble, nonionized pharmacologic preparations; sublingual venous return empties into the superior vena cava.	Convenient, elimination of first-pass effect	Decreased surface area; need for highly soluble and potent agents; requires patient cooperation
Rectal	Proximal absorption via the superior hemorrhoidal veins; distal absorption bypasses the hepatic first-pass effect.	Useful in the presence of emesis and nausea	Mucosal irritation; diarrhea; first-pass effect; varied absorption
Subcutaneous	Absorption is dependent on the surface area and absorbing capillary membrane.	May be used for unconscious, uncooperative patients; vasoconstrictors reduce systemic absorption (local anesthetics); sustained release	Pain, necrosis, tissue sloughing; erratic absorption; suitable for only small volumes of injectate; decreased uptake in the presence of decreased blood pressure
Intramuscular	Rapid absorption of the pharmacologic effect is dependent on blood flow to the muscular bed.	May be used in the unconscious, uncooperative patient; sustained release; rapid absorption	Local irritation; erratic absorption; may result in increased laboratory results (creatine phosphokinase)
Intravenous	This bypasses absorption processes, with resultant immediate blood plasma level of the pharmacologic agent.	Rapid blood plasma level; bypasses limiting factors associated with the absorptive process; utilization of large volumes	Requires vascular access; side effects and complications are immediate; requires careful titration
Inhalational	The effect is pulmonary epithelial absorption. Increased alveolar blood flow results in a rapid onset of action.	Drug delivery to specific receptor sites of action (e.g., pulmonary—beta agonists); rapid onset of action	Inability to regulate dose; pulmonary epithelial irritation; improper aerosol delivery
Topical	Highly lipid-soluble medications are absorbed through the epidermis into the systemic circulation.	Slow, timed-release pharmacologic effect; sustained pharmacologic effect; ease of use	Inability to regulate uptake and delivery; may require large body surface contact

How does the pharmacologic distribution process occur after a drug is administered?

Once the absorption process is complete, several phases of pharmacologic distribution occur. The first phase of distribution is a result of cardiac output and regional blood flow. Organs with high blood flow, referred to as vessel-rich organs, receive most of the drug during this initial phase. These organs include the heart, brain, liver, and kidneys. Organ systems that are not considered in the vessel-rich group require minutes to hours to attain equilibrium with pharmacologic agents. These organ systems include muscle, viscera, skin, and fat.

To understand basic pharmacokinetic principles, it is important to envision the body as composed of one or more compartments. Most drugs behave as though they have been distributed within two compartments, one central and the other peripheral. As illustrated in Fig. 3.2, an initial drug dose is injected into the central compartment. After introduction into the central compartment, the drug disseminates to the peripheral compartment. The central compartment consists of intravascular fluid and organs in the vessel-rich group. The peripheral compartment consists of all other fluids and tissues of the body. Eventually, drugs return from the peripheral compartment to the central compartment for elimination from the body.

What is the impact of metabolism on pharmacologic compounds administered to the moderate procedural sedation and analgesia patient?

Metabolism and clearance of drugs from the systemic circulation rely on hepatic, biliary, pulmonary, and renal mechanisms. The goal of metabolic degradation is to transform active compounds into water-soluble, pharmacologically inactive substances. In some cases, the process of metabolism yields pharmacologically active metabolites (e.g., desmethyldiazepam during the metabolism of diazepam) that may prolong the drug's duration of action. Metabolic pathways in the liver responsible for the biodegradation of pharmacologic compounds include oxidation, reduction, hydrolysis, and conjugation. These complex biochemical processes yield inactive pharmacologic compounds.

Two-compartment model

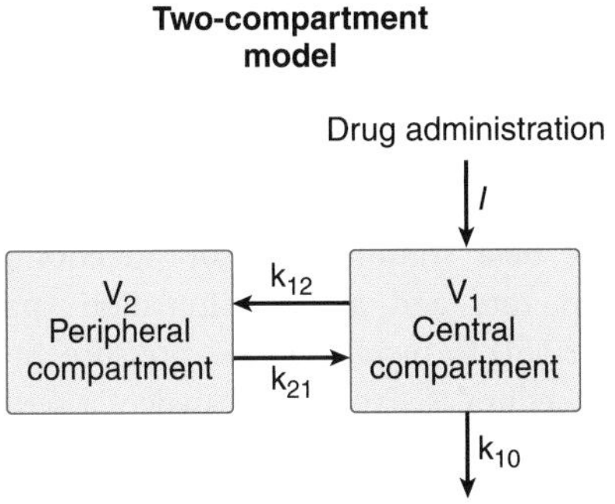

Fig. 3.2 Two compartment pharmacokinetic model. k_{12} and k_{21} are rate constants that signify the intercompartmental transfer of medications. k_{10} is the elimination rate constant for drug elimination. (From Miller RD, ed: *Miller's Anesthesia*. 8th ed. Philadelphia: Saunders; 2015.)

What is the hepatic microsomal enzyme system?

Sites of drug metabolism include plasma, lungs, kidneys, gastrointestinal tract, and liver. The hepatic microsomal enzyme system lies in the smooth endoplasmic reticulum of the liver. The cytochrome P-450 enzyme system is located on hepatic microsomes. The degree of hepatic microsomal enzyme activity is determined genetically. Aside from a genetic predisposition to hepatic microsomal enzyme activity, certain medications may stimulate the cytochrome P-450 system. Prolonged barbiturate, benzodiazepine, or phenytoin use predisposes the patient to an increase in hepatic microsomal enzyme activity. As noted in Chapter 2, it is important to ascertain a thorough patient medication history to assess the use of enzyme-inducing drugs. Enhanced hepatic microsomal enzyme activity generally results in an increased medication requirement for the individual patient.

What is the role of excretion in the pharmacokinetic process?

The kidneys are the major organ system for the excretion of drugs and metabolites. Renal excretion of pharmacologic agents or their metabolites depends on the following:
- Glomerular filtration rate
- Active tubular secretion
- Passive tubular reabsorption

The clearance and excretion of drugs and metabolites require adequate renal function prior to the administration of sedative medications. Patients with suspected renal disease may require nephrology consultation with baseline testing (e.g., creatinine, blood urea nitrogen [BUN]). A summary of the pharmacokinetic and pharmacodynamic process is presented in Fig. 3.3.

What is pharmacodynamics?

Pharmacodynamics is defined as the response of the body to the drug. It refers to the relationship between drug concentration at the site of action and any resulting effects—namely, the intensity and time course of the effect and adverse effects. Pharmacodynamics is affected by receptor binding and sensitivity, postreceptor effects, and chemical interactions. Both pharmacodynamics and pharmacokinetics explain the drug's effects, which is the relationship between the dose and response. The pharmacologic response depends on the drug binding to its target. The concentration of the drug at the receptor site influences the drug's effect. A drug's pharmacodynamics can be affected by physiologic changes due to disease, genetic mutations, aging, or other drugs. These changes occur because of the ability of the disorders to change receptor binding, alter the level of binding proteins, or decrease receptor sensitivity.[6]

In essence, if pharmacokinetics is the study of what the body does to a drug, pharmacodynamics is what the drug does to the body. Pharmacodynamics is the study of the effects of pharmacologic agents on the body and, more specifically, on target sites, which are typically designated as *receptor sites* or *receptors*.

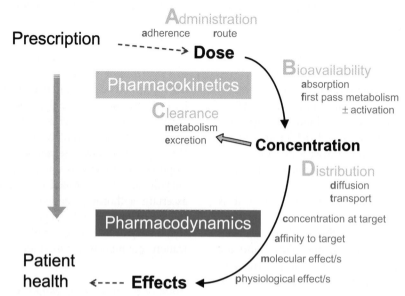

Fig. 3.3 The pharmacokinetic process. (From Doogue MP, Polasek TM: The ABCD of clinical pharmacokinetics. *Ther Adv Drug Saf.* 2013;4(1):5–7.)

What are the pharmacodynamic effects associated with opioids administered during a moderate sedation procedure?

The pharmacodynamic effects associated with opioid use include their clinical and side effects:

Clinical Effects
- Suppression of opioid withdrawal
- Analgesia
- Sedation

Side Effects
- Decreased gastrointestinal motility
- Dysphoria
- Euphoria
- Miosis
- Nausea
- Respiratory depression
- Vomiting

What are the pharmacodynamic effects associated with benzodiazepines administered during a moderate sedation procedure?

The pharmacodynamic effects associated with benzodiazepine use include the following:
- Amnesia
- Anxiolysis
- Muscular relaxation
- Anticonvulsant effects

What is the importance of receptors in the pharmacodynamic process?

Proteins compose one of the most important classes of pharmacologic receptors. Protein macromolecule receptors are present in cell membranes. A signaling process translates information relayed to them by neurotransmitters, hormones, or agonist drugs. Receptors can be triggered by conductance or transmembrane signaling. Receptors are identified and classified based on their agonistic or antagonistic clinical effect.

Examples of receptor activity include the following:
- Alpha
- Beta
- Dopamine
- Gamma-amino butyric acid (GABA)
- Histamine
- Mu
- Serotonin

Pharmacologic agents tend to exert their actions on selective receptors to produce a specific drug response. As noted in Fig. 3.4, pharmacologic agents that bind to physiologic receptors to produce a specific effect are termed *agonists.*[7] The term *pharmacologic antagonists* refers to agents that bind to physiologic receptors but have no pharmacologic effect.[7] Antagonists also inhibit the action of agonists. An example of key agonist and antagonist actions is seen in the autonomic nervous system. Many pharmacologic agents used to control heart rate (e.g., beta blockers) are antagonists. Alpha antagonists (phenoxybenzamine) antagonize alpha receptors and result in peripheral vasodilatation. Pharmacologic antagonists also include reversal agents for benzodiazepines (flumazenil [Romazicon]) and opioids (naloxone [Narcan]) that bind competitively to their respective receptor sites and reverse the benzodiazepine and opioid effects. Examples of agonist stimulation include beta stimulation (isoproterenol [Isuprel]) to increase heart rate and alpha stimulation (phenylephrine [Neo-Synephrine]) to increase blood pressure. Specific to the moderate procedural sedation and analgesia setting, patients who have received flumazenil for the reversal of benzodiazepine effects should be monitored for resedation, respiratory depression, or other residual benzodiazepine effects for an appropriate period (up to 120 minutes) based on the dose and duration of effect of the benzodiazepine used.[8]

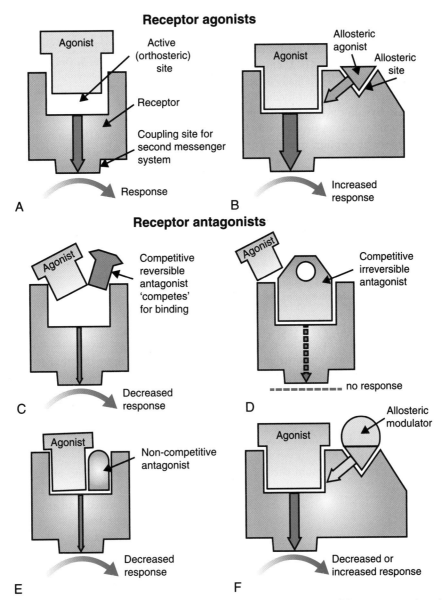

Fig. 3.4 Drug–receptor interactions. A, An agonist drug binds to the active site of the receptor and produces a response; B, An allosteric agonist binds at a site distinct to the active site and in this case increases the response elicited by the agonist; C, A competitive inhibitor 'competes' with the agonist for binding, ultimately causing a decreased response; D, A competitive irreversible antagonist binds to the receptor, irreversibly preventing agonist binding – hence, no response; E, A non-competitive antagonist binds independently, blocking the response to the agonist at some point within the receptor-coupling cascade and causes a decreased response; F, An allosteric modulator binds to the allosteric site producing a change in the protein, either causing reduced affinity of the primary agonist (antagonism) and hence reducing the response or potentiating (facilitating) the effect of the primary agonist and hence increasing the response. (From Bryant B et al: *Pharmacology for health professionals*, ed 5, Chatswood, 2019, Elsevier Australia.)

Many of the medications administered during sedation and analgesia act on individual specific receptor sites (e.g., opioids, benzodiazepines). Concurrent action on these receptor sites can result in a synergism, which causes analgesia and sedation in excess of the effect of either drug alone. When considering pharmacodynamic principles, it is important to consider the individual patient response coupled with the varied drug dosages required during the administration of sedation and analgesia services.

SUMMARY

It is important for the clinician administering sedation and monitoring the patient to realize that the sedative-analgesic medications selected possess specific pharmacokinetic and pharmacodynamic profiles. Pharmacokinetics or dose concentration relationship = drug in syringe (dose) → drug in the bloodstream (plasma concentration). Pharmacodynamics or the concentration-effect relationship is the resulting effect of the pharmacokinetic process of the drug at the target cells → drug interacting with the receptor yielding the pharmacologic effect. Sedation and analgesic medications are generally selected for their pharmacodynamic properties (e.g., amnesia, anxiolysis, analgesia, sedation). However, it is equally important for the clinician to understand that a sedative medication may have an excellent pharmacodynamic action (effect) but a very undesirable pharmacokinetic profile. A prolonged half-life, unpleasant side effects, poor absorption qualities, and cumulative drug effect must all be considered when selecting a medication for sedation.

REFERENCES

1. Nelson E. Kinetics of drug absorption, distribution, metabolism, and excretion. *Journal of Pharmaceutical Scientists.* 1961; 50:181–192.
2. Teorell T. Kinetics of distribution of substances administered to the body (I: The extravascular modes of administration). *Archives Internationales de Pharmacodynamie et de Thérapie.* 1937; 57: 205–225.
3. Doogue M, Polasek TM. The ABCD of clinical pharmacokinetics. *Therapeutic Advances in Drug Safety.* 2013; 4:5–7.
4. Chow S-C. Bioavailability and bioequivalence in drug development. *Wiley Interdiscip Rev Comput Stat.* 2014; 6(4):304–312.
5. Netter FH. *Atlas of Human Anatomy.* 7th ed. Philadelphia, PA: Elsevier; 2019.
6. Campbell JE, Cohall D. Pharmacodynamics—a pharmacognosy perspective. In: McCreath SB, Delgoda R, eds. *Pharmacognosy: Fundamentals, Applications, and Strategy.* Cambridge, MA: Academic Press; 2017:513–525.
7. Neal MJ. *Medical Pharmacology at a Glance.* 8th ed. Hoboken, NJ: Wiley-Blackwell; 2015.
8. U.S. National Library of Medicine. (2013). Flumazenil. https://dailymed.nlm.nih.gov/dailymed/drugInfo.cfm?setid=442ed32b-b508-40cc-9915-ff05674566da#LINK_5811c645-dffe-47c6-bc14-a519a6d0ef7f.

CHAPTER 3: REVIEW QUESTIONS

1. The quantitative study of the absorption, distribution, metabolism, and excretion of injected drugs and their metabolites is defined as _____.
   A. Pharmacodynamics
   B. Synergism
   C. Additive effect
   D. Pharmacokinetics

2. _____ is the maximum effect that can be produced by a drug.
   A. Potency
   B. Efficacy
   C. Tachyphylaxis
   D. Synergism

3. Medications administered via the _____ route must initially undergo a first-pass effect in the liver.
   A. Oral
   B. Intramuscular
   C. Intravenous
   D. Topical

4. The _____ pharmacologic distribution phase is a result of cardiac output and regional blood flow.
   A. First
   B. Final
   C. Delta
   D. Gamma

5. A site of drug metabolism located in the smooth endoplasmic reticulum of the liver is identified as (the) _____.
   A. Golgi apparatus
   B. Hepatic microsomal enzyme system
   C. Mitochondria
   D. Smooth endoplasmic vacuoles

6. Which pharmacokinetic process is dependent on glomerular filtration rate, active tubular secretion, and passive tubular reabsorption?
   A. Absorption
   B. Biotransformation
   C. Metabolism
   D. Excretion

7. Which pharmacologic process quantifies the chemical and physical interactions between the pharmacologic agent administered and the effects on target sites and actions of each drug?
   A. Pharmacodynamics
   B. Pharmacokinetics
   C. Pharmacologic transfer
   D. Active transfer

8. Which pharmacologic agent binds to physiologic receptors to produce a specific effect?
   A. Stereoisomers
   B. Effectors
   C. Agonists
   D. Antagonists

9. Which pharmacologic agents bind to physiologic receptors, but have no pharmacologic effect?
   A. Stereoisomers
   B. Effectors
   C. Agonists
   D. Antagonists

10. The goal of _____ is to transform active compounds into water-soluble, pharmacologically inactive substances.
    A. Absorption
    B. Metabolic degradation
    C. Distribution
    D. Excretion

11. Tachyphylaxis is defined as_____.
    A. The development of an increased drug requirement to produce a given effect
    B. The maximum effect that can be produced by a drug
    C. The effect that occurs when one medication in conjunction with another results in a pharmacologic effect greater than the algebraic summation associated with each of the two individual drugs
    D. The development of an acute tolerance to a drug, demonstrating rapidly diminishing response to successive doses of a drug

12. Which of the following techniques of medication administration bypasses the absorption process, resulting in an immediate rise in blood plasma level of the pharmacologic agent administered?
    A. Sublingual
    B. Subcutaneous
    C. Intravenous
    D. Intramuscular

Answers can be found in Appendix A.

Pharmacology of Moderate Procedural Sedation and Analgesic Agents and Techniques of Administration

At the completion of this chapter, the learner shall:

- Describe the ideal pharmacologic characteristics of sedative, hypnotic, and analgesic medications.
- State end-organ effects and pharmacokinetic and pharmacodynamic considerations associated with benzodiazepines, opioids, sedatives, hypnotics, dissociative anesthetics, and local anesthetics.
- Demonstrate understanding of the techniques of administration for sedative, hypnotic, and analgesic medications to achieve a state of moderate procedural sedation.
- Describe the advantages, disadvantages, and patient care considerations associated with the following techniques of administration:
  - Titration to clinical effect technique
  - Bolus technique
  - Continuous-infusion technique

COMPETENCY STATEMENT

The health care provider will know the recommended dose, recommended dilution, onset, duration, effects, potential adverse reactions, drug compatibility, and contraindications for each moderate procedural sedation and analgesia medication.

What medications are most commonly administered for moderate procedural sedation and analgesia?

There are a number of different medications available for use in the sedation setting. These medications include the following.

Benzodiazepines
- Diazepam
- Midazolam
- Lorazepam

Opioid Agonists
- Meperidine
- Morphine
- Fentanyl

N-Methyl-D-Aspartate (NMDA) Receptor Antagonists
- Ketamine hydrochloride

Alkylphenols (Sedative, Hypnotic)
- Propofol

Reversal Agents
- Flumazenil
- Naloxone

Why are there so many medications available to establish a state of moderate procedural sedation and analgesia?

Ideal characteristics of injected pharmacologic agents used to achieve a sedated state (e.g., anxiolysis, amnesia, analgesia, increased patient cooperation) for therapeutic and diagnostic procedures include the following:

- Rapid onset of action
- Short duration of action
- Lack of cumulative effects
- Rapid recovery
- Minimal side effects
- Rapid metabolism to inactive nontoxic metabolites
- Residual analgesia
- Optimal patient satisfaction

Unfortunately, there is no single pharmacologic agent or technique that satisfies all these requirements. In an attempt to produce an amnestic, pain-free, sedated patient, a combination of medications is required. This combination of medications gives the clinician the ability to manipulate the patient's short-term memory and sense of time.[1-3] Through pharmacologic intervention, the patient's perception of time is altered, and patient cooperation is enhanced. To produce a sedate analgesic state successfully and minimize complications (e.g., respiratory distress, cardiovascular depression, hypoxemia) requires an understanding of the pharmacologic agents used to produce moderate and deep sedation. A complete pharmacologic profile of medications administered in the sedation setting is provided in Chapter 5.

What are the advantages and disadvantages of combining these pharmacologic agents for moderate procedural sedation and analgesia?

The administration of individual pharmacologic agents may produce adequate sedation in some cases. However, there are a number of advantages associated with combining sedative, hypnotic, and analgesic agents to produce a cooperative, sedate patient state. Administering a combination of pharmacologic agents frequently produces a more rapid recovery and decreased overall dosage requirements.

What are the pharmacologic benefits associated with benzodiazepine administration for moderate procedural sedation?

Benzodiazepines are the most commonly administered medications to help achieve a state of moderate sedation. Their anxiolytic, sedative, and hypnotic properties lend themselves to achieving a calm, cooperative, physiologically stable patient for the procedure. Benzodiazepines have a high therapeutic index—the therapeutic index is the ratio between the dosage of a medication that causes a lethal effect and the dosage that causes a therapeutic effect. The ratio between the toxic dose and the therapeutic dose of a drug is used as a measure of the relative safety of the drug. When administered judiciously by the sedation provider, the high therapeutic index associated with the benzodiazepines should achieve the goals of moderate procedural sedation before producing adverse effects (e.g., respiratory depression, cardiovascular compromise).

Pharmacodynamically, how do the benzodiazepines produce a state of sedation and anxiolysis?

Pharmacodynamically, benzodiazepines bind to specific receptor sites in the central nervous system (CNS) within the gamma-amino butyric acid (GABA) receptor complex. This binding does not result in opening of the chloride ion channel, but potentiates opening in response to GABA. GABA therefore triggers a burst of channel openings, and these bursts increase in number if additional receptor sites are concurrently activated by benzodiazepines.[4] GABA receptor site interaction is identified in Fig. 4.1. Benzodiazepine

binding at the GABA site results in a variety of pharmacologic effects, which include the following:
- Anxiolysis
- Sedation
- Hypnosis
- Anticonvulsive effects
- Skeletal muscle relaxation

What are the pharmacokinetic effects associated with benzodiazepines?

Benzodiazepines are administered via the following routes of administration:
- Oral
- Intramuscular
- Intravascular

Benzodiazepines are lipid-soluble and readily penetrate the blood-brain barrier. Metabolism of benzodiazepines occurs by means of hepatic metabolism (hepatic microsomal enzyme activity), with excretion via the renal system.[5] Initially synthesized in 1959, diazepam is the prototype benzodiazepine to which all others are compared. Classified as a long-acting benzodiazepine, diazepam is well absorbed from the gastrointestinal tract, with peak plasma levels achieved in 1 to 2 hours after oral administration and 1 to 2 minutes after intravenous (IV) administration. The initial metabolism of diazepam yields an active metabolite (desmethyldiazepam) and oxazepam. Diazepam has a prolonged half-life (20–50 hours) when compared with its short-acting counterpart, midazolam (1.7–2.6 hours).[6] When compared with midazolam's water-soluble suspension, diazepam's propylene glycol suspension predisposes to venous irritation and phlebitis. The half-life associated with benzodiazepines is secondary to the degree of hepatic extraction and volume of distribution. Older patients may be particularly sensitive to the sedative effects associated with diazepam secondary to the prolonged half-life, active pharmacologic metabolites, and decreased protein binding associated with the aging process

Midazolam is a water-soluble benzodiazepine that was introduced into clinical practice in 1985.[7] Chemical substitutions along the benzene ring structure provide the health care provider administering moderate sedation with an alternative that is superior to diazepam. Midazolam is metabolized to a single metabolite (1-hydroxymidazolam) that has some residual sedative effect, but undergoes further rapid clearance from the body.[8] 1-Hydroxymidazolam does not cause prolonged sedation in patients with normal hepatic and renal function. Because of these distinct pharmacokinetic and pharmacodynamic advantages associated with midazolam, diazepam is rarely selected as the benzodiazepine of choice for moderate procedural sedation.

Remimazolam (CNS-7056; Paion Pharmaceutical, Aachen, Germany) is an ultra–short-acting IV benzodiazepine that has shown positive results in clinical phase III trials. In the human body, remimazolam is rapidly metabolized to an inactive metabolite by tissue esterases and is not metabolized by cytochrome-dependent hepatic pathways. Like other benzodiazepines, remimazolam can be reversed with

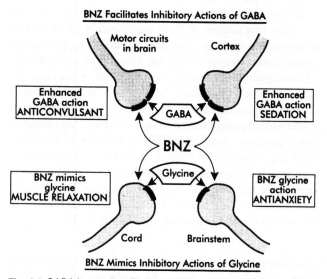

BNZ Facilitates Inhibitory Actions of GABA

Motor circuits in brain — Cortex

Enhanced GABA action **ANTICONVULSANT**

GABA

Enhanced GABA action **SEDATION**

BNZ

BNZ mimics glycine **MUSCLE RELAXATION**

Glycine

BNZ glycine action **ANTIANXIETY**

Cord — Brainstem

BNZ Mimics Inhibitory Actions of Glycine

Fig. 4.1 GABA interaction. Through GABA interaction, enhanced inhibition of neurotransmitters occurs, altering normal neuronal function in the central nervous system. *BNZ*, Benzodiazepine; *GABA*, gamma-amino butyric acid. (From Richter JJ. Neuroleptic drugs. Anesthesiology. 1981;54–56.)

BOX 4.1 Potential Pharmacologic Benefits of Remimazolam[a]

Smaller volume of distribution
Faster clearance
Clearance independent of body weight
Unlikely to yield clinically relevant postprocedure residual sedation
Less prolonged sedation in patients with renal or hepatic disease
Improved patient satisfaction
Improved return to cognitive function post procedure
Pharmacologically reversible (Romazicon [flumazenil])

[a]Subject to final FDA approval in the United States.

---

flumazenil to terminate its sedative effects rapidly. In clinical studies, remimazolam demonstrated efficacy and safety in over 1700 volunteers and patients. Investigative data have indicated that remimazolam has a rapid onset and offset of action, combined with a favorable cardiorespiratory safety profile. Remimazolam is currently in the final stage of clinical development for procedural sedation in the United States. A full clinical development program for general anesthesia was completed in Japan, and a phase II study in general anesthesia was completed in Europe. Based on the positive results of a phase II study, development for intensive care unit (ICU) sedation beyond 24 hours is another attractive indication.[9] Remimazolam use in the United States remains subject to US Food and Drug Administration (FDA) approval with a safety labeling comparable to that of midazolam. Additional potential benefits of remimazolam use per the manufacturer are identified in Box 4.1.

What are the cardiovascular end-organ effects associated with benzodiazepine administration in the moderate procedural sedation patient population?

As a sedation provider, it is important to recognize that the pharmacokinetic properties attributed to the benzodiazepine drug classification are influenced by age, gender, obesity, race, and hepatic and renal status. Specific cardiovascular effects associated with benzodiazepine administration include a slight decrease in arterial blood pressure, cardiac output, and peripheral vascular resistance. The hemodynamic effects associated with midazolam and diazepam are dose-related.[10] Significant hemodynamic changes associated with benzodiazepine use are more likely to develop in the hypovolemic, septic, or catecholamine-depleted patient population.

What are the respiratory system end-organ effects associated with benzodiazepine administration in the moderate procedural sedation patient population?

Benzodiazepines depress the central respiratory system in a dose-dependent fashion. The following respiratory effects are associated with the administration of benzodiazepines[11-13]:
- Reduction of muscular tone, leading to an increased risk of upper airway obstruction

- Flattened response of the respiratory curve of carbon dioxide
- Depressed hypoxic ventilatory response
- Supraadditive respiratory depressant effect
- May result in respiratory arrest when given in conjunction with opioids—use caution when administering to geriatric or debilitated patients

What are the central nervous system end-organ effects associated with benzodiazepine administration in the moderate procedural sedation patient population?

A reduction in cerebral blood flow, cerebral oxygen consumption, and intracranial pressure occurs with the administration of benzodiazepines. In addition to their centrally mediated muscle relaxant properties, all benzodiazepines are effective in treating seizure disorders and increasing the seizure threshold to local anesthetics. The anterograde amnesia, anxiolysis, and hypnosis provided by benzodiazepines are useful adjuncts during the administration of sedation and analgesia.

Is there a reversal agent available to reverse the effects of the benzodiazepines pharmacologically?

The CNS and respiratory depressant effects of benzodiazepines may be reversed with the administration of flumazenil. Flumazenil (Ro 15-1788) is a selective benzodiazepine receptor antagonist administered intravenously or intranasally. It has antagonistic and antidote properties to reverse the effects of benzodiazepines chemically through competitive inhibition. Hoffmann-La Roche Pharmaceuticals (Nutley, NJ) received approval from the FDA to market flumazenil in 1991. Generic formulations of flumazenil are currently available since the original patent expired in 2008. A complete pharmacologic profile of flumazenil is provided in Chapter 5.

Are there any additional precautions associated with benzodiazepine administration?

To avoid respiratory compromise or cardiovascular depression, caution must be exercised when benzodiazepines are administered to patients with the following conditions:
- Chronic obstructive pulmonary disease
- History of sleep apnea
- Cardiopulmonary depression
- Extremes of age
- Alcohol intoxication
- Morbid obesity
- Potential for difficult airway management
- Pathophysiologic disease processes

How has the opioid epidemic in the United States affected the moderate procedural sedation setting?

Pain became recognized as the so-called fifth vital sign in the mid-1990s. As professional organizations mandated managing the patient's pain levels, pain medications, especially opioid prescriptions, increased dramatically.[14] Fig. 4.2 demonstrates the increase in opioid prescriptions that was mirrored by a significant increase in the number of deaths,

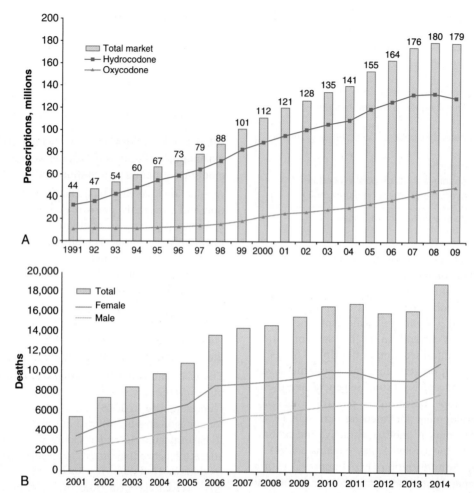

Fig. 4.2 (A) Total number of hydrocodone and oxycodone prescriptions dispensed by US pharmacies, 1991–2009. (B) National overdose deaths—number of deaths from prescription opioid pain relievers, 2001–2014. (A from SDI Vector One. National (VONA), 09-30-10 Hydrocodone and oxycodone, 1991–2009. www.fchealth.org/sites/default/files/pdf_files/OConnor_PPT_052516.pdf; B from Anesthesia Experts. Opioid crisis fueled partly by acute pain management in children. http://anesthesiaexperts.com/uncategorized/opioid-crisis-fueled-partly-acute-pain-management-children.)

which parallels the amount of drug that was dispensed.[15] An additional review of data related to the current opioid crisis has revealed the following[16]:

- Since 1999, the amount of prescription opioids sold in the United States has quadrupled.
- Since 1999, the number of overdose deaths involving opioids has quadrupled.
- In 2012, health care providers wrote 259 million opioid prescriptions.
- From 2000 to 2015, more than 500,000 people died from drug overdoses.

As noted during a presentation at the 2017 meeting of the Society for Pediatric Anesthesia and American Academy of Pediatrics Section on Anesthesiology and Pain Medicine, Dr. Myron Yaster noted that "We're also part of this problem, and we're dispensing much more opioids than these patients need, simply because we have no data to guide prescribers on how much to prescribe. So everybody gets a two-to-three week amount of drugs."[17] University of Pennsylvania's School of Nursing professor, Dr. Peggy Compton, has noted that the

public often misunderstands the role that opioid prescriptions have played in the crisis. The epidemic wasn't caused by people taking pills prescribed by their doctor to treat pain. That idea is a myth. "Simply by giving prescribed opioids to patients with pain, we are not creating addicts. Prescription opioids are easier to obtain in our society than they've ever been in history," Compton stated.[18] Leftover pills and ease of access now allow family members, relatives, and friends immediate access to opioid medications. The current opioid epidemic has led some physicians to prescribe less pain medication.

Pharmacodynamically, what are the benefits of administering opioids for the patient presenting for moderate procedural sedation and analgesia?

The administration of opioids results in binding to specific opiate receptors located in the CNS. Opioids occupy mu (μ), delta (δ), and kappa (κ) receptor subtypes and produce analgesia, drowsiness, and mood alteration. As identified in Table 4.1, the pharmacologic effects of opioids depend on the specific receptor subtypes stimulated. With the pharmacologic effects on the μ, δ, and κ

TABLE 4.1   Summary of Selected Features of Opioid Receptors

Feature	Mu (μ)	Delta (δ)	Kappa (κ)
Tissue bioassay[a]	Guinea pig ileum	Mouse vas deferens	Rabbit vas deferens
Endogenous ligand	β-Endorphin	Leu-enkephalin	Dynorphin
	Endomorphin	Met-enkephalin	
Agonist prototype	Morphine	Deltorphin	Buprenorphine
	Fentanyl		Pentazocine
Antagonist prototype	Naloxone	Naloxone	Naloxone
Supraspinal analgesia	Yes	Yes	Yes
Spinal analgesia	Yes	Yes	Yes
Ventilatory depression	Yes	No	No
Gastrointestinal effects	Yes	No	Yes
Sedation	Yes	No	Yes

From Bailey PL, Egan TD, Stanley TH. Intravenous opioid anesthetics. In Miller RD, ed. *Anesthesia.* 5th ed. New York: Churchill Livingstone; 2000:312.
[a]Traditional experimental method to assess opioid receptor activity in vivo.

receptor subtypes, opioids suppress pain by their action in the brain, spinal cord, and peripheral nervous system. However, the effect on μ receptors is considered to be the most important, with its activation directly linked to both analgesic and euphoric effects.[19] Opioids produce some degree of sedation; however, they are used mainly for their analgesic properties. Increased dosage of narcotics is associated with significant levels of sedation and the potential for severe respiratory depression. Opioids affect multiple organ systems, including the respiratory and cardiovascular systems, and can cause a variety of adverse effects. Proper dosing and monitoring allow these adverse effects to be minimized. Careful titration to clinical effect is required to avoid the development of hypoventilation, airway obstruction, or respiratory insufficiency. See the Patient Safety SBAR box which features an example of how important medication safety checks are when administering moderate procedural sedation and analgesia.

⚡ PATIENT SAFETY SBAR FOCUS

Prevention of Procedural Medication Administration Errors

Situation
Last week, one of our moderate procedural sedation and analgesia patients received 300 micrograms (6 cc's) of fentanyl (Sublimaze) during a routine procedure.

Background
The physician ordering medication for a recent interventional radiology procedure incrementally ordered 0.5-milligram doses of midazolam for patient sedation. The patient continued to demonstrate procedural anxiety and a reduced respiratory rate. Midway through the procedure, the patient's oxygen saturation decreased and end-tidal CO_2 increased dramatically. Root cause analysis revealed that procedural chest wall rigidity resulted from an inadvertent midazolam/fentanyl syringe swap during the procedure.

Assessment
Human error can lead to medication errors that are defined as "any preventable event that may cause or lead to inappropriate medication use or patient harm while the medication is in the control of the health care professional, patient, or consumer. Such events may be related to professional practice, health care products, procedures, and systems, including prescribing, order communication, product labelling, packaging, and nomenclature, compounding, dispensing, distribution, administration, education, monitoring and use." The preventable error associated with the midazolam/fentanyl syringe exchange is referred to as an adverse drug event or ADE. Medication errors can occur during the prescribing, transcribing, dispensing, and administration processes. For more than 35 years, anesthesia providers have been cognizant that drug administration errors are among the most common adverse events in anesthesia, with syringe swap being the most common of these adverse events. Risk factors for drug administration in the moderate procedural sedation setting include inadequate clinical experience in the sedation setting, poor inter-professional communication strategies, distraction, poor labeling technique, apprehension, poor lighting, and production pressure. To compound these factors, many providers simply deny that they could make a drug error. They sincerely believe that they are better than others and too experienced to make such a mistake.

Recommendation
The sedation provider serves as the final safety net in the prevention of medication errors. The six rights of safe medication administration are owed to all patients. These rights include right medication, right dose, right patient, right route, right time, and right documentation. Decreasing adverse drug events will not occur without careful attention to standardization of system processes within the sedation setting. These processes include standardization of drug concentrations, barcode medication identification, use of electronic recording systems for medication documentation, and standardization of the sedation work area. As shown in the figure below, the University of Washington, Department of Anesthesiology created

Continued

⚡ PATIENT SAFETY SBAR FOCUS—cont'd

the Anesthesia Medication Template (AMT) to define a formal way of organizing and identifying medication syringes in the anesthesia workspace. Utilizing input from the visual, interactive, industrial design, and cognitive psychology industries, their team designed a standardized medication organization process as an intuitive, low-cost strategy to improve patient safety and reduce medication errors. Regardless of these system improvement processes, individual providers continue to remain as the final bastion of patient safety. Their responsibility to the patient includes proper administration of the prescribed medication. All health care providers must:

- **Read** the medication label when initially retrieving the medication.

- **Read** the medication label when drawing up the intravenous medication.
- **Read** the medication label AGAIN prior to administering the intravenous medication.

All sedation providers must resist the temptation that allows *normalization of deviance** to creep into their daily clinical. Carrying multiple syringes in scrub pockets and using improperly labeled syringes are classic examples of safe clinical practice deviations that jeopardize patient safety in the sedation setting. Finally, a *Just Culture*** should be utilized within the organization to promote adverse drug event self-reporting, cooperation, and educational opportunities.

Anesthesia Medication Template

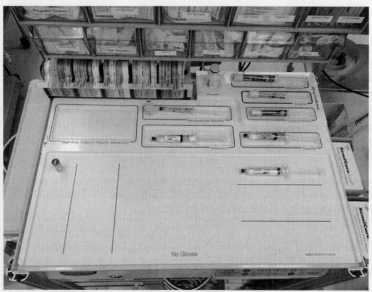

Figure from Grigg EB, et. al. Assessing the impact of the anesthesia medication template on medication errors during anesthesia: a prospective study. *Anesthesia & Analgesia* 124(5): 1617–1625.

(Data from National Coordinating Council for Medication Error Reporting and Prevention. *What is a medication error?* New York, NY: National Coordinating Council for Medication Error Reporting and Prevention; 2015. (http://www.nccmerp.org/about-medication-errors, accessed 15 April 2018); Cooper JB, Newbower RS, Long DC, McPeek B. Preventable anesthesia mishaps: a study of human factors. *Anesthesiology*. 1978;49:399-406; Banja, J. (2010). The normalization of deviance in healthcare delivery. *Business Horizons*, 53(2), 139. https://doi.org/10.1016/j.bushor.2009.10.006; Boysen, P. G. (2013). Just Culture: A Foundation for Balanced Accountability and Patient Safety. *The Ochsner Journal*, 13(3), 400–406; Marx D. *Patient Safety and the Just Culture: A Primer for Health Care Executives.* New York, NY: Trustees of Columbia University; 2001.)
Normalization of deviance: Social normalization of deviance means that people within the organization become so much accustomed to a deviant behavior that they don't consider it as deviant, despite the fact that they far exceed their own rules for elementary safety.
**A just culture balances the need for an open and honest reporting environment with the end of a quality learning environment and culture. While the organization has a duty and responsibility to employees (and ultimately to patients), all employees are held responsible for the quality of their choices. Just culture requires a change in focus from errors and outcomes to system design and management of the behavioral choices of all employees.

What are the pharmacokinetic effects associated with opioid administration?

Intramuscularly, intravenously, and orally administered opioids are readily absorbed to achieve effective plasma levels. Opioid distribution characteristics are presented in Table 4.2. Opioids are metabolized by hepatic biotransformation, with pharmacologic end products excreted through the kidneys. Small fractions of opioids are excreted unchanged in the urine.

How are opioids classified pharmacologically?

Opioids can be categorized as endogenous (e.g., endorphins, enkephalins, dynorphins), opium alkaloids (e.g., morphine,

TABLE 4.2 Opioid Distribution Characteristics

Parameter	OPIOID		
	Morphine	Meperidine (Demerol)	Fentanyl
Potency	1	0.1	75–125 × morphine's
Elimination half-life (min)	102–130	220–265	180–220
Protein binding	30%	64%–82%	85%
Heart rate	↓	↑	↓↓
Mean arterial pressure	a	a	↓
Ventilation	↓↓↓	↓↓↓	↓↓↓
Cerebral blood flow	↓	↓	↓
Cerebral metabolic rate of O_2	↓	↓	↓
Intracranial pressure	↓	↓	↓

aDecrease in mean arterial pressure = degree of histamine release.

BOX 4.2 Classification of Moderate Sedation Opioids by Synthetic Process

Naturally Occurring Opioids
• Morphine

Semisynthetic Opioids
• Codeine
• Oxycodone

Synthetic Opioids
• Meperidine
• Hydromorphone
• Fentanyl
• Alfentanil
• Remifentanil

codeine), semisynthetic (e.g., oxycodone), or synthetic (e.g., methadone, fentanyl). The classes of opioids are phenanthrenes, phenylheptylamines, and phenylpiperidines.[20] Classification of opioids by their synthetic process is outlined in Box 4.2.

What are the cardiovascular end-organ effects associated with opioid administration in the moderate procedural sedation patient population?

Opioids alter the cardiovascular system through a variety of physiologic mechanisms. With the exception of meperidine and the fentanyl derivatives, opioids are devoid of major cardiovascular effects. Meperidine produces tachycardia because of its vagolytic effect. In comparison, fentanyl derivatives (e.g., fentanyl, sufentanil, alfentanil) produce a vagally mediated bradycardia. Blood pressure may decrease secondary to bradycardia, decreased systemic vascular resistance, and alterations in the sympathetic nervous system. Meperidine

and morphine sulfate release histamine, which may significantly decrease systemic vascular resistance and produce bronchoconstriction.

What are the respiratory end-organ effects associated with opioid administration in the moderate procedural sedation patient population?

Binding to the μ receptor results in respiratory depression. The ventilatory response associated with the administration of procedural opioids may lead to the following:
• Increased arterial carbon dioxide levels
• Decreased response to carbon dioxide
• Decreased respiratory rate
• Increased minute ventilation (dose dependent)

The impact of opioids on carbon dioxide levels and minute volume are identified in Fig. 4.3.

An increase in muscle tone may occur with rapid administration of opioids, particularly the fentanyl derivatives. This opioid-induced rigidity results in an increase in muscle tone that may produce chest wall rigidity (wooden chest syndrome) and an inability to ventilate the patient. The exact incidence of rigidity varies. Box 4.3 identifies risk factors for the development of opiate-induced muscle rigidity.[21] The mechanism remains poorly understood but appears to be centrally mediated and is not caused by depression of ventilatory drive. The nucleus raphe pontis in the reticular formation and the caudate nucleus in the basal ganglia have been implicated mechanistically.[22,23] In the presence of opioid-induced muscle rigidity, effective bag-valve-mask ventilation

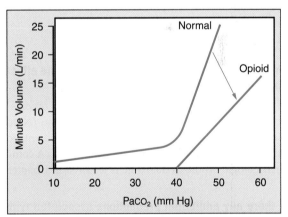

Fig. 4.3 Opioid-induced ventilatory depression. (Adapted from Gross JB. When you breathe IN you inspire, when you DON'T breathe, you . . . expire: new insights regarding opioid-induced ventilatory depression. *Anesthesiology.* 2003;99:767–770.)

BOX 4.3 Risk Factors for Development of Opioid-Induced Rigidity

• Increased dose of opiates
• Speed of injection
• Extremes of age—newborns, geriatric patients
• Critical illness with neurologic or metabolic diseases
• Use of medications that modify dopamine levels

may be extremely difficult. Treatment protocol for chest wall rigidity includes summoning anesthesia personnel to assist with ventilation, administration of naloxone, and muscle relaxants, when required.

What are the central nervous system end-organ effects associated with opioid administration in the moderate procedural sedation patient population?

Opioids increase cerebral blood flow and intracranial pressure through respiratory depression and carbon dioxide retention. Additional CNS effects include the following:

- Analgesia
- Respiratory depression
- Euphoria
- Dysphoria
- Nausea and vomiting

Opioids induce CNS adverse effects that can be divided into three groups.[24]

Group 1: Lower Levels of Consciousness

- Sedation
- Drowsiness
- Sleep disturbances

Group 2: Altered Thinking Process and Ability to React

- Cognitive impairment
- Psychomotor impairment
- Delirium
- Hallucinations
- Dreams
- Nightmares

Group 3: Direct Toxic Effects of Opioids on Neurons

- Myoclonus
- Hyperalgesia
- Tolerance

Is there a reversal agent available to reverse the effects of opioids pharmacologically?

The CNS and respiratory depressant effects of opioids can be reversed with the administration of naloxone (Narcan). As identified in Fig. 4.4, naloxone is a pure opioid antagonist that competitively binds at the opiate receptor site. A complete pharmacologic profile of naloxone is featured in Chapter 5.

Are there any additional precautions associated with opioid administration?

Due to the potential for respiratory depression, airway obstruction, and respiratory arrest, extreme caution must be exercised in the following patient populations receiving IV opioids:

- Chronic obstructive pulmonary disease
- History of sleep apnea
- Cardiopulmonary depression
- Extremes of age
- Acute alcohol intoxication
- Morbid obesity
- Potential for difficult airway management
- Presence of pathophysiologic disease processes

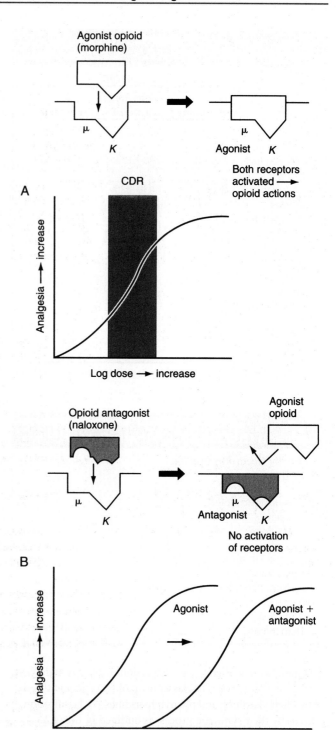

Fig. 4.4 Opioid agonist-antagonist action. (A) An opioid agonist stimulates opioid receptors through a lock and key mechanism to exert a pharmacologic effect. (B) Opioid antagonists reverse the pharmacologic effect of opioids by binding at the opioid receptor but do not exert any pharmacologic response.

Are there any opioid alternatives currently available for the moderate procedural sedation patient?

Given the current opioid crisis, drug manufacturers are increasing their efforts to develop alternative pain medications for procedural patient care. The current opioid market is valued at over 4 billion dollars, but opioids have cost the country significantly through the following:

- Addiction
- Overdoses
- Fatalities

As a result of regulatory scrutiny associated with the overuse of opioids in the United States, the pharmaceutical industry is currently exploring nonopioid alternatives. One alternative currently being investigated is synthetic capsaicin, the active ingredient in chili peppers. In midstate testing, a single injection delivered up to 6 months of substantial relief to arthritic participants by reducing the ultrasensitive nerve endings in the knee. Additional options include nerve growth factor inhibitors, which work by blocking pain signals in nerve cells in the skin, muscle, and other parts of the body besides the brain. Some drug manufacturers are focusing on experimental treatments that channel the pain-modifying properties of cannabis. Nav 1.7 ion channel blockers are also under investigation. These ion channel blockers modulate a newly discovered pathway in the body that affects pain. Another experimental option includes the use for IV administration of a toxin that is found in cone snails.[25] Marine cone snail venom contains a variety of peptides (conotoxins), many of which could act as painkillers in humans. Continued research in this area may eventually lead to the development of synthetic forms of these peptides to manage specific types of neuropathic pain.

What are the pharmacologic benefits associated with administering propofol for moderate procedural sedation?

Propofol has been available in the United States since November 1989. It is now the most widely administered IV hypnotic medication; it is chemically classified as an alkylphenol. Originally marketed with a Cremophor base (a drug additive, because medications are rarely administered in their pure chemical state), it was withdrawn from the market secondary to the high incidence of anaphylactic reactions.[26] It is currently marketed as a 1% aqueous solution (10 mg/mL) for IV use. Its current formulation consists of the following:

- 1% propofol
- 10% soybean oil
- 1.2% purified egg phospholipid (emulsifier)
- 2.25% glycerol (tonicity-adjusting agent)

As a sedative-hypnotic, propofol produces rapid hypnosis, with minimal excitation. It produces nonspecific cortical depression and is characterized by a rapid awakening and recovery phase.

Can propofol be administered to a patient with soy or egg allergies?

Approximately 0.4% of children are allergic to soy. Studies have shown that an allergy to soy usually occurs early in childhood and often is outgrown by the age of 3 years. Most children with soy allergy will outgrow the allergy by age 10.[27] Egg allergies affect 1/1000 of the patient population.[28] Because of its physiochemical formulation, propofol has been contraindicated in individuals with soy and egg allergies. However, recent research has demonstrated convincing evidence that propofol is safe in patients who are allergic to peanut, soy, and egg.[29] In addition, the American Academy of Asthma, Allergy & Immunology (AAAA) recently commented on the safety of asthma inhalers in patients allergic to soy and peanuts, despite some concern based on misperceptions regarding ingredients in the inhalers.[30] A similar concern has been raised regarding possible food allergens in IV medications used for anesthesia.

Propofol is an IV medication used for anesthesia prior to some surgical and other medical procedures and for some patients on ventilators. The propofol is mixed in a liquid containing soybean oil and a substance called *egg lecithin*. Lecithin is a fatty substance found in some plant and animal tissues. Patients who are allergic to certain foods, including soy and egg, are allergic to proteins in the foods but are not allergic to the oils or fats in the foods. Soybean oil and egg lecithin may contain trace amounts of residual protein; however, no allergic reactions have resulted. Although peanuts and soybeans are both in the legume family, the overwhelming majority of peanut-allergic patients are not clinically allergic to soy and, even if they were, would not be expected to react to soybean oil.

There are reports of reactions to propofol involving hives or other symptoms of systemic allergic reactions (anaphylaxis). However, most reports of anaphylaxis to propofol have occurred in patients without egg allergy, and the vast majority of patients with egg allergy can receive propofol without reaction. Some patients may be allergic to the propofol itself. Also, most patients who react after receiving propofol have received other drugs at the same time that can cause or worsen anaphylaxis, including antibiotics, muscle relaxants, and narcotic pain medications. Although it is clear that propofol can cause anaphylactic reactions, the exact cause of these reactions is unclear and appears not to be related to soy or egg allergy. The latest recommendation from the AAAA indicates that patients with soy allergy or egg allergy can receive propofol without any special precautions.[30]

Pharmacodynamically, what are the benefits of administering propofol to the patient presenting for moderate procedural sedation and analgesia procedures?

Propofol exerts its pharmacologic effect at the GABA receptor complex. Through an interaction at this GABA receptor complex, opening of the chloride ion channel results in hyperpolarization of cell membranes. Neuroinhibition in the CNS is produced, resulting in sedation, hypnosis, and unconsciousness. Additional pharmacodynamic research on propofol has revealed that it produces widespread inhibition of the *N*-methyl-D-aspartate (NMDA) subtype of glutamate receptor through modulation of sodium channel gating, an action that also may contribute to the drug's CNS effects.[31,32] Additional pharmacodynamic effects associated with propofol use include the following[33-35]:

- Direct depressant effect on neurons of the spinal cord
- Increase in dopamine concentrations in the nucleus accumbens
- Decreased serotonin levels in the area postrema, resulting in antiemetic effect

What are the pharmacokinetic effects associated with propofol administration?

The high degree of lipid solubility of propofol results in a rapid onset of action, with rapid awakening after a general anesthesia induction dose (half-life, 2–8 minutes). Plasma clearance of propofol exceeds hepatic blood flow. Inactive water-soluble metabolites are excreted by the kidneys. The hemodynamic depression associated with propofol administration may result in decreased drug metabolism secondary to reduced hepatic blood flow. Reduced hepatic blood flow may decrease the clearance of other drugs metabolized by the liver.

What are the cardiovascular end-organ effects associated with propofol administration in the moderate procedural sedation patient population?

IV administration of propofol can result in decreased systemic vascular resistance associated with inhibition of sympathetic vasoconstrictor activity and cardiac contractility, which can lead to decreased arterial blood pressure, cardiac output, and cardiac index. Clinically, the myocardial depressant effect and the degree of vasodilation are dependent on the dose and resultant plasma concentration.[36] Changes in heart rate are generally insignificant in the healthy patient; however, cardiac output and contractility manifestations in the older patient population may lead to significant hypotension and cardiac dysrhythmias. Large medication doses, rapid injection, and/or administration to older adults or patients with multisystemic disease states results in an exacerbation of cardiovascular effects.

What are the respiratory system end-organ effects associated with propofol administration in the moderate procedural sedation patient population?

Even small doses of propofol (sedative dosage range) can cause respiratory depression, airway obstruction, and respiratory insufficiency. Propofol inhibits the hypoxic ventilatory drive and depresses the normal response to hypercarbia. The ventilatory depression is enhanced with the simultaneous administration of other CNS depressant medications (e.g., benzodiazepines, opioids). Propofol induces bronchodilation in patients with chronic obstructive pulmonary disease. Because of the significant respiratory depressant effects associated with propofol, it should only be administered by health care practitioners who demonstrate clinical competency in advanced cardiorespiratory management.

What are the central nervous system end-organ effects associated with propofol administration in the moderate procedural sedation patient population?

The cerebral metabolic rate of oxygen consumption, cerebral blood flow, and intracranial pressure are decreased with the administration of propofol. Additionally, propofol demonstrates significant antipruritic and antiemetic effects. In a small percentage of patients, an excitatory phenomenon may be seen (e.g., muscle twitching, spontaneous movement, hiccoughs). The excitatory phenomenon may be secondary to subcortical glycine antagonism.

Is there a reversal agent available to reverse propofol pharmacologically?

There is no pharmacologic reversal agent available for propofol. In the event of an overdose, cardiovascular and ventilatory support are required.

As a nonanesthesia provider, is it safe for me to push propofol in the moderate procedural sedation setting?

Chapter 1 outlines the patient care considerations, clinical competency requirements, and professional nursing organization guidelines for the health care provider to consider prior to administering propofol in the moderate procedural sedation setting.

Are there any additional precautions associated with propofol administration?

Propofol formulations support bacterial growth. Strict aseptic technique must always be maintained during handling. Propofol is a single-access parenteral product (single-patient infusion vial), which contains 0.005% disodium edetate (EDTA) to inhibit the rate of growth of microorganisms for up to 12 hours, in the event of accidental extrinsic contamination. However, propofol can still support the growth of microorganisms, because it is not an antimicrobially preserved product under US Pharmacopeia (USP) standards. It should not be used if contamination is suspected. Discard any unused drug product as directed, within the required time limits. There have been reports in which failure to use aseptic technique when handling propofol was associated with microbial contamination of the product and with fever, infection, sepsis, other life-threatening illness, and/or death.

There have been reports, in the literature and other public sources, of the transmission of bloodborne pathogens (e.g., hepatitis B, hepatitis C, and human immunodeficiency virus [HIV]) from unsafe injection practices and the use of propofol vials intended for single use on multiple persons. Propofol vials are never to be accessed more than once or used on more than one person.[37]

Propofol infusion syndrome (PRIS) is a rare but extremely dangerous complication of propofol administration that is generally associated with prolonged administration (>48 hours) of propofol or dosages in excess of 4 mg/kg per hour. Certain risk factors for the development of propofol infusion syndrome include the following:

- Total propofol dose
- Duration of administration
- Carbohydrate depletion
- Severe illness
- Concomitant administration of catecholamines and glucocorticosteroids

The pathophysiology of PRIS includes impairment of mitochondrial beta oxidation of fatty acids, disruption of the electron transport chain, and blockage of beta-adrenoreceptors and cardiac calcium channels. The complications commonly present as an otherwise unexplained high anion gap metabolic acidosis, rhabdomyolysis, hyperkalemia, acute kidney injury, elevated liver enzyme levels, and cardiac dysfunction. Management of PRIS includes the following[38]:

- Immediately discontinuing the propofol infusion
- Supportive management
- Hemodynamic support
- Extracorporeal membrane oxygenation in refractory cases

One of the physicians I work with has stated that they administered fospropofol when a resident. What is fospropofol?

Lusedra (fospropofol disodium) was approved by the FDA in 2008 and is a water-soluble prodrug of propofol. Prodrugs are medications or compounds that after administration are metabolized into a pharmacologically active drug. This method of administration increases the safety profile and effectiveness during the procedure. Additional benefits associated with fospropofol administration are noteworthy:

- Fospropofol is manufactured without the need for lecithin, soy bean extract, or glycerol diluents.
- Water solubility decreases the risk of contamination.
- There is no risk of hypertriglyceridemia, which is associated with propofol.
- Pain on injection is comparatively less.

In 2010, original studies on the pharmacology of fospropofol were retracted as a result of an analytic assay inaccuracy that was discovered after publication of these studies.[39,40] Although fospropofol remains available, many health care facilities continue to provide propofol for use in the moderate procedural sedation setting.

Pharmacodynamically, how does ketamine produce analgesia and a dissociative state of sedation?

Ketamine (Ketalar, Ketaject) is a derivative of phencyclidine that produces a dissociative state. In subanesthetic doses, ketamine provides profound analgesia. Ketamine yields dissociative anesthetic effects secondary to antagonistic actions at the phencyclidine site of the NMDA receptor (NMDAR), which is a glutamate receptor and ion channel protein found in nerve cells. The characteristic appearance of the dissociative state includes the following:

- Intense analgesia
- Cataleptic state
- Nystagmus
- Open-eyed gaze
- Noncommunicative patient
- Skeletal muscle movement

What are the pharmacokinetic effects associated with ketamine administration?

After IV administration, ketamine has a rapid onset and a short duration of action. Its distribution half-life is approximately 10 to 15 minutes. Redistribution to the vessel-poor group (e.g., fat, skeletal muscle, bone) and biotransformation

by the hepatic microsomal enzyme system in the liver result in awakening. Biotransformation results in pharmacologically active metabolites (norketamine) that are excreted in the urine.

What are the cardiovascular end-organ effects associated with ketamine administration in the moderate procedural sedation patient population?

Stimulation of the sympathetic nervous system increases heart rate, cardiac output, and arterial blood pressure. Increased myocardial oxygen consumption occurs in conjunction with these changes. Ketamine is contraindicated in patients with coronary artery disease, hypertension, congestive heart failure, or impaired myocardial performance.

What are the respiratory system end-organ effects associated with ketamine administration in the moderate procedural sedation patient population?

Ketamine produces bronchodilation and minimal reduction of the ventilatory drive. Upper airway muscle tone is maintained, and airway reflexes remain intact. Salivary and mucous secretions are enhanced with ketamine administration. These effects may be counteracted with the administration of an antisialogogue (atropine, glycopyrrolate [Robinul]).

What are the central nervous system end-organ effects associated with ketamine administration in the moderate procedural sedation patient population?

Increased cerebral blood flow, cerebral oxygen consumption, and intracranial pressure occur as a result of cerebral vasodilation. Therefore, ketamine use is contraindicated in patients with intracranial disease. Myoclonic activity is characteristic of ketamine administration. Emergence delirium and undesirable CNS side effects include visual and auditory illusions, dreams, and combativeness and may persist for 24 hours. Emergence delirium generally occurs as the patient is recovering from the pharmacologic effects of ketamine administration. The administration of benzodiazepines has been shown to decrease the incidence of postprocedure ketamine delirium.[41]

Is there a reversal agent available to reverse ketamine pharmacologically?

There is no pharmacologic reversal agent for ketamine. Cardiorespiratory support is required in the event of ketamine overdose.

What role do local anesthetics have in the moderate procedural sedation setting?

Local anesthetics may be used to anesthetize specific anatomic areas (e.g., esophagus, line insertion sites) to complete therapeutic, diagnostic, or minor surgical procedures. It is important for the clinician administering moderate procedural sedation to be cognizant of the pharmacodynamics and pharmacokinetics of the local anesthetic used.

What are the pharmacodynamic effects associated with local anesthetic administration?

Local anesthetics provide temporary loss of motor, sensory, and autonomic nervous system function. Local anesthetic chemical structures generally consist of the following:

- A lipophilic group (benzene ring)
- A hydrophylic group (tertiary amine)
- An intermediate chain (ester or amide linkage)

Local anesthetics are classified as amides or esters. Amide local anesthetics include the following:

- Bupivacaine (Marcaine, Sensorcaine)
- Etidocaine (Duranest)
- Lidocaine (Xylocaine)
- Mepivicaine (Carbocaine, Polocaine)
- Ropivacaine (Naropin)

Ester local anesthetics include the following:

- Chloroprocaine (Nesacaine)
- Cocaine
- Procaine (Novocain)
- Tetracaine (Pontocaine)

Local anesthetics differ specifically with regard to the following:

- Potency
- Time of onset
- Duration of pharmacologic effect
- Toxicity

Local anesthetics prevent the development of the action potential required for depolarization of nerve cells by blocking sodium channels. For transmission of impulses to occur, movement of sodium and potassium ions via these channels is required. Depolarization occurs when sodium ions move from extracellular fluid to the intracellular space. Repolarization occurs when potassium ions move from the intracellular to the extracellular space. Fig. 4.5 depicts channel entry positions under normal physiologic function and after local anesthetic solution is administered, preventing the development of an action potential, thereby impairing nerve conduction.

What are the pharmacokinetic effects associated with local anesthetic administration?

Local anesthetic absorption is dependent on a variety of factors:

- Increased vascularity at the injection site results in increased local anesthetic uptake
- Vasoconstrictors decrease the rate of absorption
- Increased protein binding increases the duration of action
- Increased lipid solubility increases potency

Ester local anesthetics are derived from para-aminobenzoic acid (PABA). Ester local anesthetics are metabolized by ester hydrolysis via pseudocholinesterase, which is found in the plasma.[42] Amide local anesthetics are metabolized by dealkylation and hydrolysis in the liver.[42] Local anesthetic potency is determined by lipid solubility. Protein binding determines the duration of effect because the highly bound local anesthetic remains in the lipoprotein of the nerve membrane for a longer duration. The chemical configurations of commonly administered local anesthetics used for therapeutic, diagnostic, and minor surgical procedures are listed in Fig. 4.6. At times, combinations of local anesthetics are used. This admixture of local anesthetics offers the clinician the beneficial pharmacologic effects of each local anesthetic selected.

Is epinephrine added to all local anesthetic solutions?

Epinephrine may be added to local anesthetics to promote local vasoconstriction. This vasoconstriction limits uptake into the tissue and prolongs the local anesthetic effect. The

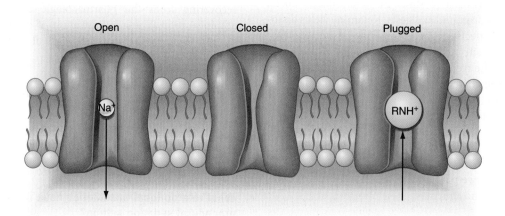

Fig. 4.5 Local anesthetic agents and nerve conduction. On the left is an open channel, inward-permeant to sodium ions (Na+). The center channel is in the resting closed configuration; although impermeant to sodium ions here, the channel remains voltage-responsive. The channel on the right, although in open configuration, is impermeant because it has a local anesthetic cation (RNH+) bound to the gating receptor site. Note that local anesthetic enters the channel from the axoplasmic (lower) side; the channel filter precludes direct entry via the external mouth. Local anesthetic renders the membrane impermeant to sodium ions—hence, inexcitable by local action currents. (Redrawn from De Jong RH: *Local Anesthetics*. St. Louis: Mosby; 1994.)

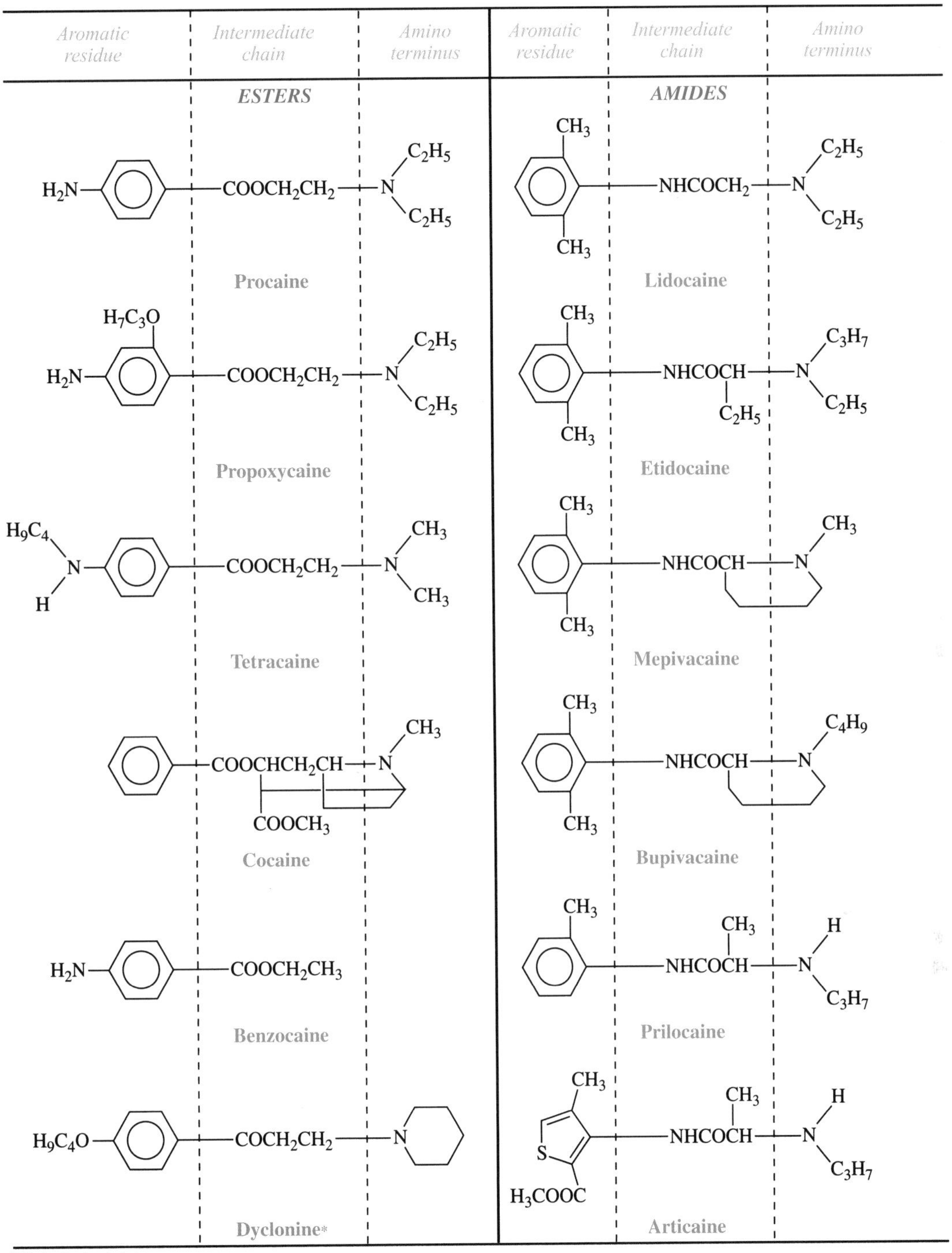

Aromatic residue	Intermediate chain	Amino terminus	Aromatic residue	Intermediate chain	Amino terminus

Fig. 4.6 Chemical configurations of commonly administered local anesthetic solutions. (From Yagiela JA, Neidle EA, Dowd FJ: *Pharmacology and Therapeutics for Dentistry.* 6th ed. St. Louis: Mosby; 2010.)

addition of epinephrine to the local anesthetic solution is contraindicated in the following patient populations:
- Patients with unstable angina
- Patients with cardiac dysrhythmias
- Infiltration into areas without adequate collateral blood flow (e.g., fingers, toes, ears)
- Hyperthyroid patients
- Patients with uteroplacental insufficiency
- Patients with increased sympathetic nervous system activity

What are the cardiovascular end-organ effects associated with local anesthetic administration in the moderate procedural sedation patient population?

All local anesthetics depress the automaticity of the myocardium.[43] Myocardial contractility is also reduced as the local anesthetic concentration increases. Decreased contractility occurs secondary to cardiac membrane changes and alterations in the response of the autonomic nervous system.

What cardiovascular effects are seen when a large a dose of local anesthetic is administered?

Toxic manifestations associated with local anesthetic overdose that affect the cardiovascular system include the following:

- Bradycardia
- Heart block
- Hypotension
- Cardiac arrest
- Circulatory collapse

What are the respiratory end-organ effects associated with local anesthetic administration in the moderate procedural sedation patient population?

Apnea after the administration of local anesthetics may occur following specific nerve paralysis (phrenic, intercostal) or medullary center depression (retrobulbar block). Treatment of local anesthetic–induced respiratory center depression includes administration of oxygen, ventilation, and advanced airway management.

What are the central nervous system end-organ effects associated with local anesthetic administration in the moderate procedural sedation patient population?

The CNS is extremely sensitive to the effects of local anesthetic agents. Neurologic signs and symptoms of local anesthetic-induced toxicity include the following:

- Agitation
- Numbness of the tongue and mouth
- Dizziness
- Visual disturbance
- Tinnitus
- Restlessness
- Slurred speech
- Irrational behavior
- Muscle twitching
- Apnea
- Convulsions

CNS symptoms may range from mild complaints to life-threatening complications. As symptoms progress, tonic-clonic seizures, respiratory arrest, vomiting with aspiration, and loss of consciousness may ensue. The signs and symptoms of local anesthesia toxicity are not limited to the cardiovascular or central nervous system. Box 4.4 outlines multiple signs and symptoms associated with an overdose of local anesthetic solution.

What are the maximum recommended doses of local anesthetics for administration?

The maximum dosages of local anesthetic medications (with and without epinephrine) are highlighted in Table 4.3.

When should the total dose of a local anesthetic solution be reduced in the moderate procedural sedation setting?

A variety of factors must be considered to avoid signs and symptoms of local anesthesia toxicity. These factors include the following:

BOX 4.4 Central Nervous & Cardiovascular Effects of Increased Local Anesthetic Blood Levels

Signs
Talkativeness
Apprehension
Excitability
Slurred speech
Generalized stutter, leading to muscular twitching and tremor in the face and distal extremities
Euphoria
Dysarthria
Nystagmus
Sweating
Vomiting
Failure to follow commands or be reasoned with
Elevated blood pressure
Elevated heart rate
Elevated respiratory rate

Symptoms (progressive with increasing blood levels)
Nervousness
Sensation of twitching before actual twitching is observed (see "Generalized stutter," above)
Metallic taste
Visual disturbances (inability to focus)
Auditory disturbances (tinnitus)
Drowsiness and disorientation
Loss of consciousness

Moderate to High Overdose Levels
Tonic-clonic seizure activity followed by:
- Generalized central nervous system depression
- Depressed blood pressure, heart rate, and respiratory rate

From Malamed SF: *Medical Emergencies in the Dental Office.* 6th ed. St. Louis: Mosby; 2007.

TABLE 4.3 Maximum Recommended Dose (MRD) of Local Anesthetics

Drug	Formulation	MRD	DOSAGE	
			mg/lb	mg/kg
Articaine	With epinephrine	None listed[a]	3.2	7.0
Lidocaine	Plain	300[b]	2.0	4.4[b]
	With epinephrine	500[b]	3.3	7.0[b]
Mepivacaine	Plain	400[b]	2.6	5.7[b]
	With levonordefrin	400[b]	2.6	5.7[b]
Prilocaine	Plain	600[b]	4.0	8.8[b]
	With epinephrine	600[b]	4.0	8.8[b]

From Malamed SF: *Handbook of Local Anesthesia.* 6th ed. St. Louis: Elsevier; 2013.
[a]Manufacturer's recommendation: Prescribing information, New Castle, DE, 2000.
[b]Manufacturer's recommendation: Prescribing information, dental, Westborough, MA, 1990, Astra Pharmaceutical Products.

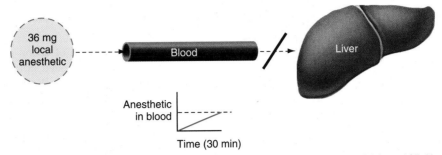

Fig. 4.7 Removal of local anesthetic in a patient with significant liver dysfunction. (From Malamed SF: *Handbook of Local Anesthesia*. 6th ed. St. Louis: Elsevier; 2013.)

- Patient age—decreased dosage should be considered for patients at both ends of the age spectrum.
  - Pediatric patients
  - Geriatric patients
- Presence of concomitant disease processes
  - Reduced dosage of local anesthetic solution should be considered for medically comprised patients.
  - In patients with significant liver dysfunction, removal of a local anesthetic from the blood may be slower than its absorption in the blood, leading to a slow but steady rise in the blood anesthetic level (Fig. 4.7).
- Patient weight
  - Heavier patients generally have a larger volume of distribution; therefore, slightly larger doses of local anesthetic solution can be administered.

However, this generally accepted rule has its limits, and the patient must be carefully assessed for any signs or symptoms of impending local anesthetic toxicity.

What is the treatment protocol in the event of a local anesthetic toxicity reaction?

A reaction to the administration of local anesthesia can occur for a variety of reasons. Table 4.4 offers a comparison of forms of local anesthetic overdose. Use of the PABCD acronym (*p*osition, *a*irway, *b*reathing, *c*irculation, *d*efinitive care) used for the treatment of local anesthetic reactions is highlighted in Box 4.5. In addition to treatment protocols outlined in Box 4.5, anticonvulsant medications (midazolam, 1 mg/min IV slowly) may be ordered by the attending physician when CNS stimulation appears to be intensifying.[44]

We recently had a department in-service and the speaker mentioned that lipids have been administered to rescue patients successfully from local anesthesia toxicity reactions. What role do lipids play in the treatment of the patient exhibiting signs and symptoms of local anesthesia toxicity?

In addition to providing immediate care to the patient experiencing local anesthesia toxicity signs and symptoms using the PABCD acronym, increasing evidence has suggested that the IV infusion of lipid emulsions can reverse the cardiac and neurologic effects of local anesthetic toxicity. Although no blinded studies have been conducted in humans, studies in animal models and multiple case reports in human patients have shown favorable results. Case reports have supported the early use of lipid emulsion at the first sign of

TABLE 4.4 Comparison of Forms of Local Anesthetic Overdose

Parameter	Rapid Intravascular	Too Large a Total Dose	Rapid Absorption	Slow Biotransformation	Slow Elimination
Likelihood of occurrence	Common	Most common	Likely with high-normal doses if no vasoconstrictors are used	Uncommon	Least common
Onset of signs and symptoms	Most rapid (seconds); intraarterial faster than IV	3–5 min	3–5 min	10–30 min	10 min–several hours
Intensity of signs and symptoms	Usually most intense	Gradual onset with increased intensity; may prove quite severe		Gradual onset, with slow increase in intensity of symptoms	
Duration of signs and symptoms	1–2 min	Usually 5–30 min; depends on dose and ability to metabolize or excrete		Potentially longest duration because of inability to metabolize or excrete agents	
Primary prevention	Aspirate, slow injection	Administer minimal doses.	Use vasoconstrictor; limit topical anesthetic use or use nonabsorbed type (base).	Adequate pretreatment physical evaluation of patient	
Drug groups	Amides and esters	Amides; esters only, rarely	Amides; esters only, rarely	Amides and esters	Amides and esters

From Malamed SF: *Handbook of Local Anesthesia*. 6th ed. St. Louis: Elsevier; 2013.

BOX 4.5   Basic Emergency Management for Local Anesthesia Reactions

P—Position
- ↓ Unconscious—supine, with feet elevated slightly
- Conscious—based on patient comfort

A—Airway
- ↓ Unconscious—assess and maintain airway.
- Conscious—assess airway.

B—Breathing
- ↓ Unconscious—assess and ventilate if necessary.
- Conscious—assess breathing.

C—Circulation
- ↓ Unconscious—assess and provide external cardiac compression if necessary.
- Conscious—assess circulation.

D—Definitive care
- Diagnosis, management—emergency drugs and/or assistance (emergency medical services, dial 911)

Adapted from Malamed SF: *Handbook of Local Anesthesia*. 6th ed. St. Louis: Elsevier; 2013.

arrhythmia, prolonged seizure activity, or rapid progression of toxic manifestations in patients with suspected local anesthetic toxicity.[45–51]

IV infusion of a 20% lipid emulsion (eg, Intralipid 20%) has become an accepted part of treatment for systemic toxicity from local anesthetics, particularly for cardiac arrest that is unresponsive to standard therapy. The American Society of Regional Anesthesia and Pain Management (ASRA) checklist for treatment of local anesthesia systemic toxicity (LAST) guidelines identified in Table 4.5 recommend considering the use of lipid emulsion therapy at the first signs of systemic toxicity from local anesthetics, after airway management.[52]

TABLE 4.5   Checklist for Treatment of Local Anesthesia Systemic Toxicity (LAST) Guidelines[a]

>70-kg Patient	<70-kg Patient
Bolus 100-mL lipid emulsion 20%, rapidly over 2–3 minutes	Bolus 1.5-mL/kg lipid emulsion 20%, rapidly over 2–3 minutes
• Lipid emulsion infusion 200–250 mL over 15–20 min	• Lipid emulsion infusion 0.25 mL/kg/min (ideal body weight)
• If patient remains unstable, rebolus once or twice at the same dose and double infusion rate; be aware of dosing limit (12 mL/kg).	
• Total volume of lipid emulsion can approach 1 L in a prolonged resuscitation (e.g., >30 min).	

From https://www.asra.com/advisory-guidelines/article/3/checklist-for-treatment-of-local-anesthetic-systemic-toxicity.
[a]Precise volume and flow rate are not crucial.

How do lipids reverse the effects of the local anesthetic solutions?

The proposed mechanism of action occurs when the lipids administered create a so-called lipid sink that extracts the lipid-soluble local anesthetic solution from the plasma. This theory is referred to as the *lipid sink hypothesis*, first described in 1998.[53] The well-documented, experimentally tested lipid sink theory suggests that the lipid emulsion absorbs the local anesthetic from several tissues (e.g., myocardium, brain, vascular smooth muscle), which increases the metabolic capacity of the liver and, consequently, the catabolism of the local anesthetic.[53–55]

A case report related to decreased oxygen saturation and upper airway benzocaine administration was presented at a recent conference I attended; how does benzocaine administration affect oxygen saturation levels?

Benzocaine is a topical anesthetic that is used by a wide variety of sedation practitioners to anesthetize the upper airway prior to instrumentation (e.g., upper endoscopy, transesophageal echocardiography, bronchoscopy). Physicians and health care providers using topical anesthetic solutions (e.g., Americaine, HurriCaine, Cetacaine) containing benzocaine should be familiar with the potential complication of benzocaine-induced methemoglobinemia. Prompt recognition of this complication and its prescribed treatment protocol is required by the sedation practitioner to avoid the development of neurologic hypoxia or death.

The FDA notified health care professionals and patients that it has continued to receive reports of methemoglobinemia associated with the use of benzocaine products. In 2006, the FDA issued a Public Health Advisory warning about methemoglobinemia with the use of benzocaine sprays during medical procedures. Since then, the FDA has received reports of 72 new cases of methemoglobinemia associated with the use of benzocaine sprays, including 3 resulting in death, bringing the total to 319 cases. Symptoms of methemoglobinemia may appear within minutes to 1 or 2 hours after using benzocaine.[56] Methemoglobinemia is a condition characterized by the oxidation of iron within the hemoglobin molecule from the ferrous form (Fe^{2+}) to the ferric state (Fe^{3+}). This results in an elevated circulating fraction of methemoglobinemia in the erythrocyte. The results of this oxidation of iron in the hemoglobin molecule include the following:
- A significant decrease in the oxygen-carrying capacity of red blood cells
- Central and peripheral cyanosis
- Metabolic acidosis secondary to the cells' inability to carry out aerobic metabolism
- Coma
- Death

The clinical presentation of methemoglobinemia generally would be seen after the administration of an oxidizing toxin that has been metabolized by the cytochrome P-450 system, with resultant free oxygen radicals. The increased levels of methemoglobinemia cause changes in pulse oximetry and oxygen saturation. Oxygen saturation reveals a decreased SpO_2 due to the small difference in light absorption by methemoglobin to hemoglobin. Pulse oximetry yields information based on the differential light absorption of oxyhemoglobin and reduced hemoglobin. Oxyhemoglobin absorbs more light at 940 nm, and reduced hemoglobin absorbs more light at 660 nm. Methemoglobin absorbs light equally at both of these wavelengths, with pulse oximetry displaying an SpO_2 of 85%. The higher the methemoglobin concentration, the closer the SpO_2 value is to 85%. However, the actual percentage of the arterial oxyhemoglobin concentration can be underestimated or overestimated in the SpO_2 value.[57,58]

The diagnosis of methemoglobinemia may be difficult. Clinical symptoms generally occur when methemoglobin production exceeds rates of reduction. Patients frequently do not display initial symptoms of respiratory distress. However, as methemoglobin levels begin to rise (normal methemoglobin levels <1%–2% in erythrocytes), the following symptoms may occur:
- Fatigue
- Headache
- Syncope
- Dysrhythmia
- Dyspnea
- Lethargy
- Dizziness
- Metabolic acidosis
- Stupor
- Coma
- Death

The symptoms outlined may occur within 20 to 60 minutes of drug administration. Initial symptoms may occur when the methemoglobin concentration exceeds 20%—anxiety, fatigue, dyspnea, dizziness, tachycardia, headache, syncope. As methemoglobin levels increase (>50%), oxygen delivery decreases, and marked dyspnea may occur in conjunction with metabolic acidosis, dysrhythmias, and lethargy. These symptoms may progress to stupor and death. Death has been reported from levels greater than 70% and may be attributed to dysrhythmias, circulatory collapse, or neurologic compromise.[59,60] Older, pediatric, and hypoxic patients are also more sensitive to methemoglobin formation.[61,62]

What is the treatment protocol for methemoglobinemia?

Methemoglobinemia is a medical emergency that requires prompt treatment. Diagnosis should be considered when oxygen saturation levels fall significantly and remain unresponsive to increased oxygen administration. Treatment protocol includes the following:
- Identify and discontinue the offending agent immediately.
- Administer supplemental oxygen with high flow rates.
- Administer IV methylene blue, 1–2 mg/kg as a 1% solution over 5 to 10 minutes.
  - Methylene blue acts by providing an artificial electron acceptor for nicotinamide adenine dinucleotide phosphate (NADPH) methemoglobin reductase.

- The dose should be repeated within 60 minutes for an inadequate response, marked by sustained elevation in methemoglobin levels. However, it should be noted that excessive methylene blue can actually promote increased methemoglobin levels.
- Monitor arterial blood gases (ABGs) to assess response to therapy.
- In severe cases, exchange blood transfusion may be necessary.[63,64]

Methylene blue should be available in all sedation settings in which benzocaine topical spray is administered. Although rare, methemoglobin is a fatal complication associated with benzocaine topical anesthetic solutions. Initial symptoms mimic other clinical syndromes that may occur during moderate procedural sedation.

How can the risk of methemoglobinemia be minimized for the patient presenting for moderate procedural sedation?

There are a number of ways to decrease the risk of methemoglobinemia in the procedural sedation setting. These methods include the following[65]:
- Affix labels to topical anesthetic spray bottles warning staff of danger of excessive patient use.
- Identify risk factors while obtaining the patient's medical history.
- Document the amount of drug administered, including measuring and recording the number of sprays applied. The use of a reference chart with maximum recommended doses of anesthetics may be helpful.
- Supplemental oxygen and methylene blue should be kept readily available whenever topical anesthetics are administered.
- Use delivery devices that provide more precision in drug administration, such as atomizers.

What is the best technique to administer sedative, hypnotic, and analgesic medications?

When administered properly, the use of sedatives and analgesics provides a sedate patient with minimal side effects. The variety of sedative medications and modes of administration offer the clinician a wide range of options to achieve the goals and objectives of sedation and analgesia. Medication selection and administration by a particular technique are dependent on the patient's presedation physical status, presence of pathophysiologic disease states, age, and planned procedure. Understanding the technique of administration is equally important to understanding the pharmacokinetics and pharmacodynamics of selected sedative or analgesic medication. Therefore, a variety of techniques of medication administration are available to the clinician administering sedation to avoid the development of deep sedative states or severe respiratory depression.

What is titration to clinical effect technique?

Medications used for therapeutic, diagnostic, and minor surgical procedures may be administered in a variety of ways. As depicted in Fig. 4.8, the titration to clinical effect

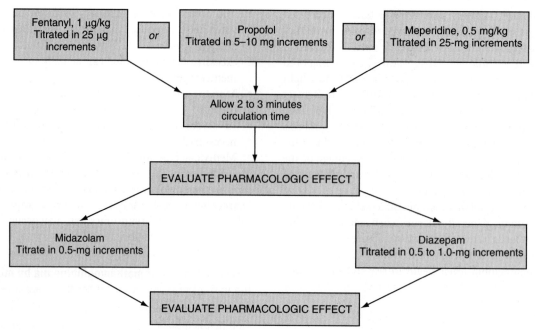

Fig. 4.8 Titration to clinical effect technique.

technique uses individual medications titrated slowly to clinical effect. To establish an analgesic base, opioids are frequently administered before benzodiazepines. Two to 3 minutes prior to the procedure, IV fentanyl, 1 µg/kg (titrated in 25-µg increments), may be slowly administered to establish analgesia.

Combining medications (narcotics and benzodiazepines) reduces total dosage through their synergistic action, assists the clinician in the maintenance of the sedate state, and promotes rapid patient recovery. However, respiratory depression is frequently associated with the pharmacologic synergism achieved through concurrent administration of medications. Overdose, rapid administration (not allowing adequate circulation time), and failure to appreciate patient pathophysiologic disease processes frequently result in the development of airway obstruction, hypoxia, and respiratory insufficiency.

In conjunction with the preexisting analgesia established with opioids, the addition of benzodiazepines (midazolam in 0.5-mg increments, or propofol, 5- to 10-mg increments) titrated to a clinical end point of nystagmus or slurred speech may result in a sedate patient. To avoid cardiopulmonary depression, it is important to titrate medications slowly to the clinical end points outlined earlier. At times, barbiturates or sedative-hypnotics have been advocated in the literature to provide an increase in the depth of sedation. A complete pharmacologic profile for narcotics, benzodiazepines, and sedative hypnotic agents is outlined in Chapter 5.

Note that propofol administration is permitted provided that it is approved by agencies or guidelines such as the state board of nursing, hospital policy and procedure, and clinical competencies achieved.

What is the bolus technique?

A popular technique used for procedures of short duration (e.g., oral surgery, gastroenterologic procedures) is the bolus technique. Based on a predetermined dosage (in mg/kg), the entire dose or a large percentage is administered in one single injection. This technique is particularly popular for the administration of benzodiazepines. One advantage of this technique is its ability to provide a rapid medication plasma level immediately before the procedure.

BOX 4.6   Continuous Infusion Technique Sedation Approach[a]

- Initiate IV line with carrier solution (e.g., normal saline, lactated Ringer's).
- Establish narcotic medication base:
  - Fentanyl, 1 µg/kg (titrated in 25-µg increments)
  or
  - Meperidine, 0.5 mg/kg (titrated in 25-mg increments)
- Sedation can be initiated slowly with a continuous infusion technique to achieve the desired level of sedation and avoid cardiorespiratory depression.
- Begin administration of propofol, 5 µg/kg/min.
- Infusion rate may be increased at 5-µg/kg/min intervals.

If a continuous infusion sedation technique with propofol is selected, it is imperative to ensure that the prescribing clinician understands the pharmacokinetics and pharmacodynamics associated with this agent. The prescribing clinician and health care provider administering the medication (or monitoring the patient) should possess advanced airway management skills, demonstrate proficiency in managing cardiovascular complications, and recognize that propofol (Diprivan) can induce deep sedative states and/or general anesthesia. Propofol is not pharmacologically reversible.

[a]Most patients exhibit clinical end points associated with sedation and analgesia (e.g., nystagmus, slurred speech) at dosage ranges of 5–40 µg/kg/min. Dosage and rate of administration must be established slowly. Clinically relevant factors that decrease total dosage of medication administered include presedation patient status, age, presence of pathophysiologic disease, and desired level of sedation.

Disadvantages of bolus injection include oversedation leading to respiratory insufficiency, unconsciousness, chest wall rigidity, and cardiovascular depression. The bolus technique eliminates the safety features of slow titration, which assesses for individual patient response and clinical sedation end points (e.g., nystagmus, slurred speech). Despite the speed with which a desired plasma concentration can be achieved, the risks associated with the bolus technique often outweigh its potential benefits. Small incremental boluses offer the ability to produce therapeutic plasma levels slowly while potentially using less medication to produce the same pharmacologic end point.

What are continuous infusion techniques?

Continuous infusion techniques permit a constant plasma level to be attained through a continuous infusion of medication. The continuous infusion technique avoids the fluctuations in plasma levels associated with bolus techniques. Additional potential benefits include decreased recovery time, less total drug administered, and minimized side effects.

Careful titration based on predetermined clinical end points (e.g., nystagmus, slurred speech, sedation) allows the infusion to be discontinued at the conclusion of the procedure, with a rapid return to an alert state.

Continuous infusion techniques are popular with propofol administered at a microgram/kilogram per minute administration rate (Box 4.6). Continuous infusion techniques require a carrier IV solution, with the continuous infusion piggybacked into the carrier solution. Extreme care must be exercised to avoid running the carrier solution at a keep vein open or slow rate, thereby allowing a buildup of the infusion within the Venoset tubing. Once the carrier fluid is opened, the patient then receives a large bolus of medications and may experience a relative overdose and concurrent side effects. Regardless of the technique of administration, clinicians must appreciate the pharmacokinetics, pharmacodynamics, and clinical effects associated with sedative and analgesic agents.

Careful titration is warranted in all situations to prevent the development of deep sedation states, respiratory

TABLE 4.6 Techniques of Administration

Technique	Advantages	Disadvantages	Oversedation
Titration to clinical effect technique	1. Allows careful titration of sedative and analgesic medications 2. Reduces total medication requirement via synergistic action 3. Provides for a slow controlled rise in therapeutic plasma level 4. May provide for more rapid patient recovery	1. May be time-consuming	
Bolus technique	1. Provides a rapid rise in therapeutic plasma level for short procedures 2. Provides a sedate and/or analgesic state rapidly based on predetermined dosage (in mg/kg)	1. Rapid administration of sedative or analgesic medications may result in excess therapeutic plasma level. 2. Respiratory obstruction, ventilatory depression, respiratory insufficiency, hypotension, bradycardia, and cardiovascular instability frequentiy occur with excess plasma levels of medication.	
Continuous infusion technique	1. Permits constant plasma level through a continuous infusion of medication 2. Once a therapeutic plasma level is achieved, continuous infusion technique avoids fluctuations in plasma levels. 3. May decrease recovery time secondary to reduction in total dose of medication administered	1. Difficult for nonanesthesia practitioners to master technique in nonintubated patients 2. Initial attempts to reach a therapeutic plasma level may result in oversedation. 3. May be difficult to adjust initial continuous infusion rate based on the patient's level of consciousness	

insufficiency, airway obstruction, hypoxia, and cardiovascular depression. Clinician compliance with hospital policy, manufacturer's recommendations, The Joint Commission, professional practice guidelines, and specialty organization position statements is required to provide quality pharmacologic intervention for patients receiving sedation and analgesia.

SUMMARY

When administered properly, the use of sedatives, analgesics, hypnotics, and tranquilizers can sedate a patient, with minimal side effects. The variety of sedative medications and modes of administration offer the prescribing physician and health care provider managing the patient a wide range of options to achieve the goals and objectives of moderate sedation. Selection of any medication or administration by a particular technique is dependent on the patient's presedation physical status, presence of pathophysiologic disease states, age, and planned procedure. Table 4.6 identifies specific advantages and disadvantages associated with various techniques of medication administration.

REFERENCES

1. Spires G. The Big Mac. In: *Conscious vs. Unconscious Sedation. Early Bird Symposium, 63rd AANA National Meeting*; August, 1996.
2. Lister RG. The amnesic action of benzodiazepines in man. *Neuroscience & Biobehavioral Reviews*. 1985; 9:87–94.
3. Veselis RA, Reinsel RA, Feshchenko VA, Johnson Jr. R. Information loss over time defines the memory defect of propofol: A comparative response with thiopental and dexmedetomidine. *Anesthesiology*. 2004; 101:831–841.
4. Mihic SJ, Harris RA. Hypnotics and sedatives. In: Brunton LL, Chabner BA, Knollman BC, eds. *Goodman and Gilman's The Pharmacologic Basis of Therapeutics*. 13th ed New York: McGraw-Hill; 2017.
5. Stoelting R. Pharmacology and Physiology in Anesthetic Practice. In: *Alphen aan den Rijn*. 5th ed The Netherlands: Wolters Kluwer Health; 2015.
6. Saari TI, Uusi-Oukari M, Ahonen J, Olikkola KT. Enhancement of GABAergic activity: neuropharmacological effects of benzodiazepines and therapeutic use in anesthesiology. *Pharmacol Rev*. 2011; 63:243–267.
7. Ariano RE, Kassum DA, Aronson KJ. Comparison of sedative recovery time after midazolam versus diazepam administration. *Crit Care Med*. 1994; 22:1492–1496.
8. Vuyk J, Sitsen E, Reekers M. Intravenous anesthetics. In: Miller RD, ed. *Miller's Anesthesia*. 8th ed Philadelphia: Elsevier; 2015:821–863.
9. Sohngen, W. Paion Pharmaceuticals. Remimazolam. http://www.paion.com/remimazolam/product-information/about-remimazolam/.
10. Vuyk J, Sitsen E, Reekers M. Intravenous anesthetics. In: Miller RD, ed. *Miller's Anesthesia*. 8th ed. Philadelphia: Elsevier; 2015:840.
11. Norton JR, Ward DS, Karan S, et al. Differences between midazolam and propofol sedation on upper airway collapsibility using dynamic negative airway pressure. *Anesthesiology*. 2006; 104:1155–1164.
12. Sunzel M, Paalzow L, Berggren L, Eriksson I. Respiratory and cardiovascular effects in relation to plasma levels of midazolam and diazepam. *Br J Clin Pharmacol*. 1988; 25:561–569.
13. Tverskoy M, Fleyshman G, Ezry J, et al. Midazolam-morphine sedative interaction in patients. *Anesth Analg*. 1989; 68:282–285.
14. Anesthesia Experts. Opioid crisis fueled partly by acute pain management in children. http://anesthesiaexperts.com/uncategorized/opioid-crisis-fueled-partly-acute-pain-management-children.
15. Vector One SDI. National (VONA), 09-30-10 Hydrocodone and oxycodone. (1991-2009). www.fchealth.org/sites/default/files/pdf_files/OConnor_PPT_052516.pdf; 1991-2009.
16. Centers for Disease Control and Prevention (CDC). Understanding the epidemic. https://www.cdc.gov/drugoverdose/epidemic.
17. Yaster M. The opioid problem; how clinical research leads to discovery. In: *Presented at the Pediatric Anesthesia (SPA)/American Academy of Pediatrics Section on Anesthesiology and Pain Medicine (AAP) Pediatric Anesthesiology 2017 meeting, Austin Texas*; March 4, 2017.
18. Wolfram J. Leftover painkillers driving opioid crisis. http://www.wesa.fm/post/leftover-painkillers-driving-opioid-crisis-penn-researcher-says#stream/0.
19. Schumacher M, Basbaum AI, Naidu RK, et al. Opioid analgesics and antagonists. In: *Katzung Basic and Clinical Pharmacology*. 11th ed. New York, NY: McGraw Hill; 2009:531–550.
20. Chan HCS, McCarthy D, Li J, et al. Designing safer analgesics via μ-opioid receptor pathways. *Trends Pharmacol Sci*. 2017; 38 (11):1016–1037.
21. Coruh B, Tonelli M, Park D. Fentanyl-induced chest rigidity. *Chest*. 2013; 143(4):1145–1146.
22. Sokoll MD, Hoyt JL, Gergis SD. Studies in muscle rigidity, nitrous oxide, and narcotic analgesic agents. *Anesth Analg*. 1972; 51:16–20.
23. Freye F, Kuschtusky K. Effects of fentanyl and droperidol on the dopamine metabolism of the rat striatum. *Pharmacology*. 1976; 14(1):1–7.
24. Brincat J, Macleod M. Adverse effects of opioids on the central nervous systems of palliative care patients. *Journal of Pain & Palliative Care Pharmacotherapy*. 2007; 21(1):15–25.
25. Chen, C. Drug makers are racing to find alternatives to opioids. https://www.bloomberg.com/news/articles/2017-06-28/life-after-opioids-drugmakers-scramble-to-concoct-alternatives.
26. Glen J, Hunter S. Pharmacology of an emulsion formula. *Br J Anaesth*. 1984; 56:617–626.
27. Savage JH, Kaeding AJ, Matsui EC, Wood RA. The natural history of soy allergy. *J Allergy Clin Immunol*. 2010; 125:683–686.
28. Clark T, Skypala I, Leech SC, et al. British Society for Allergy and Clinical Immunology guidelines for the management of egg allergy. *Clinical & Experimental Allergy*. 2010; 40:1116–1129.
29. Harper NJN. Propofol and food allergy. *British Journal of Anaesthesia*. 2016; 116(1):11–13.
30. Thanai P. Soy allergic and egg allergic patients can safely receive anesthetic. https://www.aaaai.org/conditions-and-treatments/library/allergy-library/soy-egg-anesthesia.
31. Zorumski CF, Izumi Y, Mennerick S. Ketamine: NMDA Receptors and Beyond. *The Journal of Neuroscience: The Official Journal of the Society for Neuroscience*. 2016; 36(44):11158–11164.
32. Essential drugs in anesthetic practice. In Evers A, Maze M, & Kharasch E, eds, *Anesthetic Pharmacology: Basic Principles and Clinical Practice*. Cambridge: Cambridge University Press; 2013:359–384. https://doi.org/10.1017/CBO9780511781933.025.

33. Folino TB, Parks LJ. Propofol. In: StatPearls [Internet]. Treasure Island (FL): StatPearls Publishing; 2018. Available from: https://www.ncbi.nlm.nih.gov/books/NBK430884/.

34. Sahinovic MM, Struys MMRF, Absalom AR. Clinical Pharmacokinetics and Pharmacodynamics of Propofol. *Clinical Pharmacokinetics*. 2018; 57(12):1539–1558. https://doi.org/10.1007/s40262-018-0672-3.

35. Sahinovic MM, Struys MMRF, Absalom AR. Clinical Pharmacokinetics and Pharmacodynamics of Propofol. *Clinical Pharmacokinetics*. 2018; 57(12):1539–1558.

36. Pagel PS, Wartlier DC. Negative inotropic effects of propofol as evaluated by the regional preload recruitable stroke work relationship in chronically instrumented dogs. *Anesthesiology*. 1993; 78(1):100–108.

37. Propofol injection emulsion, USP. Package insert. Fresenius-Kabi, Lake Zurich, IL.

38. Mirrakhimov AE, Voore P1, Halytskyy O, et al. Propofol infusion syndrome in adults: a clinical update. *Crit Care Res Pract*. 2015; 2015:260385.

39. Michel M, Struys J, Fechner J, et al. Requested retraction of six studies the PK/PD and tolerability of fospropofol. *Eur J Anaesthesiol*. 2010; 27:395–396.

40. Struys MJ, Fechner J, Schüttler H. Erroneously published fospropofol pharma- cokinetic–pharmacodynamic data and retraction of the affected publications. *Anesthesiology*. 2011; 112:1056–1058.

41. Sener S, Eken C, Schultz CH, et al. Ketamine with and without midazolam for emergency department sedation in adults: a randomized controlled trial. *Ann Emerg Med*. 2011; 57:109–114.

42. Yazdi CA. Local anesthetics. In: Aglio L, Urman R, eds. *Anesthesiology*. Cham: Springer International Publication; 2017:347–358.

43. Butterworth J, Wasnick J, Mackey D. *Morgan and Mikhail's Clinical Anesthesiology*. 6th ed. New York: McGraw Hill Education; 2018.

44. Malamed S. *Handbook of Local Anesthesia*. 6th ed. St. Louis: Elsevier-Mosby; 2014323.

45. Neal JM, Mulroy MF, Weinberg GL. American Society of Regional Anesthesia and Pain Medicine checklist for managing local anesthetic systemic toxicity: 2012 version. *Reg Anesth Pain Med*. 2012; 37(1):16–18.

46. Litz RJ, Roessel T, Heller AR, Stehr SN. Reversal of central nervous system and cardiac toxicity after local anesthetic intoxication by lipid emulsion injection. *Anesth Analg*. 2008; 106 (5):1575–1577.

47. Litz RJ, Popp M, Stehr SN, Koch T. Successful resuscitation of a patient with ropivacaine-induced asystole after axillary plexus block using lipid infusion. *Anaesthesia*. 2006 Aug.; 61(8):800–801.

48. Foxall G, McCahon R, Lamb J, et al. Levobupivacaine-induced seizures and cardiovascular collapse treated with Intralipid. *Anaesthesia*. 2007; 62(5):516–518.

49. Zimmer C, Piepenbrink K, Riest G, Peters J. Cardiotoxic and neurotoxic effects after accidental intravascular bupivacaine administration. Therapy with lidocaine propofol and lipid emulsion. *Anaesthetist*. 2007; 56(5):449–453.

50. Ludot H, Tharin JY, Belouadah M, et al. Successful resuscitation after ropivacaine and lidocaine-induced ventricular arrhythmia following posterior lumbar plexus block in a child. *Anesth Analg*. 2008; 106(5):1572–1574.

51. Warren JA, Thoma RB, Georgescu A, Shah SJ. Intravenous lipid infusion in the successful resuscitation of local anesthetic-induced cardiovascular collapse after supraclavicular brachial plexus block. *Anesth Analg*. 2008; 106(5):1578–1580.

52. Neal JM, Barrington MJ, Fettiplace MR, et al. The Third American Society of Regional Anesthesia and Pain Medicine Practice Advisory on Local Anesthetic Systemic Toxicity. *Executive Summary 2017 Reg Anesth Pain Med*. 2018; 43:113–123.

53. Weinberg GL, VadeBoncouer T, Ramaraju GA, et al. Pretreatment or resuscitation with a lipid infusion shifts the dose-response to bupivacaine-induced asystole in rats. *Anesthesiology*. 1998; 88:1071–1075.

54. Weinberg GL. Lipid emulsion infusion: resuscitation for local anesthetic and other drug overdose. *Anesthesiology*. 2012; 117:180–187.

55. Shi K, Xia Y, Wang Q, et al. The effect of lipid emulsion on pharmacokinetics and tissue distribution of bupivacaine in rats. *Anesth Analg*. 2013; 116:804–809.

56. FDA warns of methemoglobinemia with benzocaine topical products. https://www.empr.com/safety-alerts-and-recalls/fda-warns-of-methemoglobinemia-with-benzocaine-topical-products/article/200164.

57. Sandza Jr. JG, Roberts RW, Shaw RC, et al. Symptomatic methemoglobinemia with a commonly used topical anesthetic, cetacaine. *Ann Thorac Surg*. 1980; 30:187–190.

58. Gupta P, Deepa L, Edward I, et al. Benzocaine-induced methemoglobinemia. *South Med J*. 2000; 93(1):83–86.

59. Bunn HF. Disorders of hemoglobin. In: Wilson JD, Braunwald E, Isselbacher KJ, et al. *Harrison's Principles of Medicine*. 12th ed. New York: McGraw-Hill; 1991:1543–1552.

60. Douglas WW, Fairbanks VF. Methemoglobinemia-induced topical anesthetic spray (cetacaine). *Chest*. 1977; 71:587–591.

61. Scott EM, Hoskins DD. Hereditary methemoglobinemia in Alaskan Eskimos and Indians. *Blood*. 1958; 12:795–802.

62. Muchmoree EA, Dahl BJ. One blue man with mucositis [letter]. *N Engl J Med*. 1992; 327:133.

63. Grauer SE, Giraud GD. Toxic methemoglobinemia after topical anesthesia for transesophageal echocardiography. *J Am Soc Echocardiogr*. 1996; 9:874–876.

64. Clary B, Skaryak L, Tedder M, et al. Methemoglobinemia complicating topical anesthesia during bronchoscopic procedures. *J Thorac Cardiovasc Surg*. 1997; 114:293–295.

65. Anesthesia Experts. Use of topical anesthetics to support intubation. http://anesthesiaexperts.com/uncategorized/topical-anesthetics-support-intubation/Pharm.

CHAPTER 4: REVIEW QUESTIONS

1. Benzodiazepines bind to specific receptors in the central nervous system and enhance the transmission of _____ in the brain.
   A. Norepinephrine
   B. Gamma-amino butyric acid (GABA)
   C. Dopamine
   D. Epinephrine

2. Which of the following is not a pharmacodynamic effect associated with the administration of benzodiazepines?
   A. Anxiolysis
   B. Sedation
   C. Hypnosis
   D. Analgesia

3. Which of the following sedative medications possesses a long half-life and yields an active metabolite?
   A. Diazepam
   B. Midazolam
   C. Morphine
   D. Fentanyl

4. Reversal of pharmacologic effect with benzodiazepines can be achieved with which of the following medications?
   A. Naloxone
   B. Flumazenil
   C. Compazine
   D. Flumazenil

5. Opioids exert pharmacologic action secondary to their pharmacodynamic effects, including which of the following?
   A. Occupation of the GABA receptor
   B. Functional dissociation between the reticular activating system and the thalamus
   C. Occupation of the mu, kappa, delta, and sigma receptors
   D. Stimulation of dopamine release

6. Chest wall rigidity can occur with which of the following medications?
   A. Morphine
   B. Meperidine
   C. Hydromorphone
   D. Fentanyl

7. Which narcotic analgesic elicits a tachycardia secondary to its vagolytic properties?
   A. Morphine
   B. Meperidine
   C. Hydromorphone
   D. Fentanyl

8. Benzocaine-induced methemoglobinemia may be treated with which pharmacologic agent?
   A. Indigo carmine
   B. Methylene blue
   C. Atropine sulfate
   D. Lidocaine hydrochloride

9. A derivative of phencyclidine, which produces a dissociative state and has been used in subanesthetic doses to produce profound analgesia during sedation procedures, is identified as which of the following?
   A. Inapsine
   B. Lorazepam
   C. Propofol
   D. Ketamine

10. The incidence of emergence delirium associated with dissociative anesthetics may be decreased with the administration of which of the following medications?
    A. Opioids
    B. Phenothiazines
    C. Benzodiazepines
    D. Barbiturates

11. Which of the following drugs is a prodrug of propofol?
    A. Midazolam
    B. Fentanyl
    C. Ketamine
    D. Fospropofol

12. Respiratory depression, hypotension, and hypercarbia are frequent complications associated with which of the following techniques of medication administration?
    A. Titration technique
    B. Bolus technique
    C. Continuous infusion technique
    D. Liberal flow technique

Answers can be found in Appendix A.

Sedation-Analgesia Pharmacologic Profile

LEARNING OUTCOMES

At the completion of this chapter, the learner shall:
- Identify the pharmacokinetic profile associated with sedative, analgesic, and hypnotic medications used in the sedation setting.
- Identify the pharmacodynamic profile associated with sedative, analgesic, and hypnotic medications used in the sedation setting.
- List medications used in the sedation setting that are contraindicated in the presence of specific disease states.
- Identify the indications, side effects, and clinical pharmacology associated with sedative, hypnotic, and analgesic medications.
- State the cardiovascular, respiratory, and central nervous system effects associated with sedative, hypnotic, and analgesic medications used for diagnostic, therapeutic, and minor surgical procedures.

COMPETENCY STATEMENT

The health care provider will know the recommended dose, recommended dilution, onset, duration, effects, potential adverse reactions, drug compatibility, and contraindications for each moderate procedural sedation and analgesia medication.

What pharmacologic competencies are required for the health care practitioner ordering moderate procedural sedation medications?

Health care providers administering moderate procedural sedation and analgesia medications must follow proper monitoring procedures and clinical assessment strategies. It is critical that every licensed independent practitioner prescribing medications and, ultimately, each health care provider administering sedation or monitoring the patient receiving sedation, have a clear and definitive understanding of the pharmacodynamics and pharmacokinetics associated with each medication administered. A failure to appreciate the clinical effects of each medication administered, particularly when combinations are used, may result in an increase in patient morbidity and mortality.

Before the administration of any medication, it is imperative that each health care professional be well versed in the pharmacology of the specific medication. A comprehensive understanding of the clinical pharmacology, onset, duration, indications, contraindications, drug interaction, central nervous system and cardiorespiratory effects, metabolism, excretion, and management of an overdose is essential in providing quality patient care.

What does it mean when a drug is listed as Schedule I, II, III, IV, or V?

The Controlled Substances Act (CSA) places all substances that were in some manner regulated under existing federal law into one of five schedules. This is based on the substance's medical use, potential for abuse, and safety or dependence liability. Additional information related to the Controlled Substancs Act can be found at https://www.dea.gov/druginfo/csa.shtml. In determining into which schedule a drug or other substance should be placed, or whether a substance should be decontrolled or rescheduled, certain factors must be considered. These factors of the CSA include the following:
- Its actual or relative potential for abuse
- Scientific evidence of its pharmacologic effect
- The state of current scientific knowledge regarding the drug or other substance
- Its history and current pattern of abuse
- The scope, duration, and significance of abuse
- What, if any, risk there is to the public health
- Its psychic or physiologic dependence liability
- Whether the substance is an immediate precursor of a substance already controlled

Box 5.1 identifies the schedule of controlled substances as defined by the US Drug Enforcement Agency (DEA). A detailed summary of moderate procedural sedation and analgesia medications is presented in this chapter.

BOX 5.1 Schedule of Controlled Substances

Drugs that come under the jurisdiction of the Controlled Substances Act are divided into five schedules. Adherence to federal and state guidelines regarding administration, dispensing, distribution, and accountability is imperative. Copies of the Controlled Substances Act may be obtained from the Superintendent of Documents, US Government Printing Office, Washington, DC, 20402.

Schedule I

The substances in this schedule are those that have no accepted medical use in the United States but have a high abuse potential. Some examples are heroin, lysergic acid diethylamide (LSD), peyote, and methaqualone.

Schedule II

The substances in this schedule have a high abuse potential, with severe psychic, psychological, and/or physical dependence. Schedule II substances consist of specific narcotics, stimulants, and depressant medications. Examples include opium, morphine, codeine, fentanyl, sufentanil, hydromorphone, meperidine, and oxycodone. Additional Schedule II medications are amphetamines, methylphenidate (Ritalin), pentobarbital, and secobarbital.

Schedule III

Schedule III substances have an abuse potential less than those in Schedules I and II and include compounds containing limited quantities of certain narcotic and non-narcotic medications. Examples of Schedule III drugs include derivatives of barbituric acid (except those identified in earlier schedules), phentermine, paregoric, and any compound, mixture, preparation, or suppository dosage form containing amobarbital, secobarbital, or pentobarbital.

Schedule IV

The substances in this schedule have an abuse potential less than those listed in Schedules I, II, and III. Examples of Schedule IV medications include chloral hydrate, meprobamate, paraldehyde, methohexital, diazepam, midazolam, lorazepam, and pentazocine.

Schedule V

The substances in this schedule have an abuse potential less than those listed in Schedules I, II, III, and IV. These substances consist primarily of medications containing limited quantities of narcotics and stimulant drugs used for their antitussive, antidiarrheal, and analgesic effects. Examples include buprenorphine and propylhexedrine.

SEDATIVE, ANALGESIC, AND HYPNOTIC MEDICATIONS

These are classified as follows (trade name followed by the generic name):
- Opioid agonists
  - Alfenta—alfentanil hydrochloride
  - Demerol—meperidine hydrochloride
  - Dilaudid—hydromorphone hydrochloride
  - Morphine—morphine sulfate
  - Sublimaze—fentanyl citrate
- Benzodiazepine agonists
  - Valium—diazepam
  - Versed—midazolam
- Hypnotics
  - Diprivan—propofol[a]

- Dissociative anesthetic
  - Ketamine—ketamine hydrochloride[a]
- Resuscitative medications
- Opiate receptor antagonist
  - Narcan—naloxone hydrochloride
- Benzodiazepine receptor antagonist
  - Romazicon—flumazenil
- Cardiovascular stimulants
  - Atropine sulfate
  - Ephedrine
  - Adrenalin—epinephrine

Sedation-analgesia is an ever-changing field. The medications outlined in this chapter are provided as a guide for the sedation clinician. A variety of dosing protocols have been proposed in the literature and are outlined in Tables 5.1 through 5.4. Licensed independent practitioners are advised to check the product information currently provided by the manufacturer of each drug to be administered to verify the recommended dose associated with the specific procedure, patient's physiologic status, and level of sedation desired. It is the responsibility of the treating physician relying on experience and knowledge of the patient to determine dosages and the best treatment for the patient. Neither the publisher nor the author assumes any responsibility for any injury and/or damage to persons or property.

---

[a]It is the author's opinion that these medications should only be administered by anesthesia providers (physician anesthesiologist or certified registered nurse anesthetist) unless extensive didactic and clinical education is completed. Licensed independent clinicians and health care professionals who are nonanesthesia providers should not under any circumstance administer these drugs unless they have received comprehensive education and are credentialed accordingly. If these medications are used by nonanesthesia providers, it is imperative to ensure that the prescribing clinician understands the pharmacokinetics and pharmacodynamics associated with each agent. The prescribing clinician and health care provider administering the medication (or monitoring the patient) should possess advanced airway management skills, demonstrate proficiency in managing cardiovascular complications, and recognize that each medication can induce deep sedative states and/or general anesthesia. These medications are not pharmacologically reversible.

⚡ PATIENT SAFETY SBAR FOCUS

Moderate Procedural Sedation and Analgesia Medications

Situation

During administration of moderate procedural sedation in our radiology suite, our last patient of the day suddenly stopped breathing. Immediately prior to the respiratory arrest, 100 micrograms of Sublimaze (fentanyl) was administered.

Background

Several minutes after the administration of fentanyl, the chest and abdominal wall became very rigid. It became difficult to ventilate the patient with a bag-valve-mask device. The oxygen saturation dropped very rapidly, and an airway could not be maintained for the patient. Application of a chin lift and jaw thrust did help to restore airflow. The patient continued to become more hypoxic, and ST segment depression was noted on the EKG monitor. Ultimately, a rapid response was called.

Assessment

Opioid-induced muscle rigidity generally occurs with the infusion of large doses of opioids administered rapidly. However, relatively small doses of opioids may also induce muscle rigidity in sedation patients. Opioids capable of inducing this phenomenon include:

- Alfenta (alfentanil)
- Demerol (meperidine)
- Morphine
- Sublimaze (fentanyl citrate)
- Sufenta (sufentanil)
- Ultiva (remifentanil)

First described in 1953, opioid-induced muscle rigidity has also been referred to as "wooden chest syndrome" characterized primarily by abdominal and chest wall rigidity. However, the rigidity can affect other muscle groups including the muscles of the neck, masseter, and jaw. Untreated, opioid-induced muscle rigidity is a life-threatening respiratory complication. Left untreated chest wall rigidity results in decreased chest wall compliance, increased resistance to ventilation, an immediate rise in right atrial pressure, and decreased venous return and cardiac output with a resultant increase in systemic arterial blood pressure.

The exact physiology associated with the development of muscle rigidity is not fully understood; however, inhibition of striatal release of GABA and increased dopamine production are cited as a potential etiologic factor. Additionally, vocal cord closure may occur as low doses of fentanyl act on vagal postinspiratory (laryngeal adductor) motoneurons, whereas in vagal laryngeal adductor and pharyngeal constrictor motoneurons, depression of depolarizing synaptic drive potentials led to sparse, very low frequency discharges. Such effects on three types of vagal motoneurons may explain the tonic vocal fold closure and pharyngeal obstruction of airflow.

Recommendations

It is important for the sedation provider to be knowledgeable regarding risk factors associated with opioid-induced muscle rigidity. Risk factors include:

- Dose and rapidity of injection of opiates
- Extremes of age (e.g, newborns, older adult patients)
- Critical illness with neurologic or metabolic diseases
- Use of medications that modify dopamine levels

Opioid-induced muscle rigidity is not responsive to traditional bag-valve-mask ventilation; however, there are several options for its clinical treatment.

Low-dose intravenous Narcan (naloxone) administration is effective in reversing the effects of opioid-induced muscle rigidity. In addition to reversing the effects of rigidity, naloxone can cause increased heart rate and cardiac index with resultant increased myocardial oxygen concentration. The lowest dose of pharmacologic reversal agent should always be used, particularly in patients with ischemic cardiovascular disease. Intravenous administration of muscle relaxants (depolarizing or non-depolarizing) may also assist in relieving rigidity. Depolarizing muscle relaxants (succinylcholine [Anectine]) or non-depolarizing muscle relaxants (vecuronium [Norcuron]), (rocuronium [Zemuron]), administered by an anesthesia provider, can ultimately lead to successful ventilation and endotracheal intubation in most patients. Although there are no true prevention strategies to eliminate opioid-induced muscle rigidity, the following precautions have been shown to reduce the incidence:

- Administration of opioid
  - Slow injection
  - Avoiding large doses
- Pretreatment with midazolam (0.1 mg/kg)
  - Has been shown to reduce myoclonus
- Clonidine administration
  - Reverses muscle rigidity through inhibition of sympatho-adrenal outflow

TABLE 5.1 Sedation Dosing Protocols

Agent	Suggested Dosing	Onset and Duration	Clinical Considerations
Analgesics			
Morphine sulfate	1-mg increments; peak clinical effects not apparent for up to 20 min	Onset: 5–10 min, peak CNS effect delayed up to 20 min Duration: 2–4 h	Respiratory: potent respiratory depressant in presence of other sedatives; in absence of pain, may produce excessive sedation and dysphoria; respiratory monitoring (pulse oximetry, respiratory rate and depth) essential Cardiovascular: hypotension may follow administration to hypovolemic patient.

Continued

TABLE 5.1 Sedation Dosing Protocols—cont'd

Agent	Suggested Dosing	Onset and Duration	Clinical Considerations
Meperidine (Demerol), 10% as potent as morphine (8–10 mg equivalent to 1 mg morphine)	Dilute and titrate 5- to 10-mg increments, evaluating patient response within onset time.	Onset: 3–5 min Duration: 1–3 h	Gastrointestinal: nausea and vomiting; excessive sedation may lead to aspiration. Genitourinary: urinary retention In equal analgesic doses produces same sedation, respiratory depression, and incidence of nausea and vomiting as morphine.
Fentanyl (Sublimaze), 100 times more potent than morphine	50–100 times more potent than morphine	Onset of analgesia: 3–5 min Duration of analgesia: 30- to 60-min period of respiratory depression longer than analgesic duration (3–5 h) Onset of sedation: almost immediate, dependent on concomitant drug administration Duration of sedation: highly variable but generally 15–90 min	Respiratory: potent respiratory depressant alone and when combined with benzodiazepines; skeletal muscle (chest wall) rigidity with rapid administration; rigidity may be so pronounced that ventilation is difficult or impossible. Cardiovascular: vagotonic producing bradycardia; hypotension in hypovolemic patient
Benzodiazepines Diazepam (Valium)	Titrated in 2-mg increments; large interpatient variability in response to titrated doses	Onset: 1–2 min Duration: in hours equal to patient age (20-year-old = 20 h; 70-year-old = 70 h)	Respiratory: minimal respiratory depression unless large doses or concomitant opioid administration Cardiovascular: minimal depressant effects, although the occasional patient may experience hypotension. Other: pain on injection may cause phlebitis, local irritation, and venous thrombosis.
Midazolam (Versed); four times as potent as diazepam	Titrate 0.5- to 1-mg doses and never exceed 2.5 mg; most rapid-acting benzodiazepine; allow a minimum of 2 min between doses to assess patient effect; like diazepam, large interpatient variability to titrated doses; following established sedation, decrease subsequent doses 20%–40%.	Onset: 3–5 min Duration: 1–5 h in healthy patients; duration doubled in older and obese patients	Respiratory: central respiratory depressant, may produce apnea with rapid administration; effects are pronounced with concomitant opioid administration; observant respiratory monitoring critical to avert potential problems Cardiovascular: hypotension in hypovolemic patient; incidence of hypotension increased with concomitant opioid administration
Antagonist Agents Naloxone (Narcan)	0.1-mg increments titrated to obtain respiratory rate of 12 breaths/min	Onset: 1–2 min Duration: 30–45 min; opioid may outlast expected opioid duration; repeat doses are often necessary.	Opioid antagonist; titrate to achieve an acceptable respiratory rate; continued evaluation of respiratory function essential; will reverse previously established analgesia following painful procedure
Flumazenil (Romazicon)	0.2 mg administered over 10–15 s; additional 0.2 mg after 45 s, repeating at 60-s intervals up to 1 mg; no more than 3 mg is recommended in any 1-h period.	Onset: 1–2 min Duration: 30–60 min	Specific benzodiazepine antagonist; titrated to reverse respiratory depression and sedation; duration of benzodiazepines exceeds duration of flumazenil; continued ventilatory assessment required

From Biddle C, Aker J. Conscious sedation: between Scylla and Charybdis. Quality of Life—A Nursing Challenge. 1995;4(4):107.

TABLE 5.2   Sedation Dosing Protocols

Drug	Onset of Action	Usual Dosage	Duration
Benzodiazepines			
Midazolam	1–5 min	0.5–2.0 mg IV over 2 min; may repeat at 5-min intervals with 0.5 mg to a maximum of 5 mg	60–90 min
Diazepam	3–10 min IV 15–30 min PO	2–5 mg IV over 5 min; may repeat at 5-min intervals, with 2 mg to a maximum of 10 mg	2–8 h
Lorazepam	5–10 min	0.5–2.0 mg IV, slow, to a maximum of 4 mg	4–6 hr
Opioids			
Morphine	2–5 min	2–5 mg IV over 5 min; may repeat at 5-min intervals in increments of 2–5 mg to a maximum of 20 mg	2–7 h
Meperidine	1–3 min	25–50 mg IV over 2 min; may repeat at 5-min intervals in increments of 10–15 mg to a maximum of 150 mg (use with caution in patients with renal disease)	2–4 h
Fentanyl	1–2 min	25–50 µg IV over 2 min; may repeat at 5-min intervals in increments of 25 µg to a maximum of 500 µg/4 h	30–60 min
Reversal Agents			
Flumazenil (for benzodiazepines)	1–2 min	0.2 mg IV over 15 s; may repeat in 1-min intervals to a maximum of 1 mg	1–2 h
Naloxone (for opioids)	1–2 min	0.02–0.04 mg IV over 30 s; may repeat at 1-min intervals to a maximum of 10 mg (dilute 0.4 mg naloxone in 10 mL to make 0.04 mg/mL)	1–4 h

From Messinger J, Hoffman L, O'Donnell J, Dunworth B. Getting conscious sedation right. Am J Nurs. 1999;99(12):44–49.

TABLE 5.3   Sedation Dosing Protocols

Class	Drug	Dosage and Administration[a]	Advantages	Cautions[b]
Opioids	Fentanyl	0.5–1 µg/kg IV over 2 min until appropriate analgesia reached	Short-acting analgesic; reversal agent (naloxone) available	May cause apnea, respiratory depression, bradycardia, dysphoria, muscle rigidity, nausea, and vomiting; hypotension is described but is uncommon when used as a single agent; use lower aliquots and/or longer dosing intervals for older people or those with renal or hepatic dysfunction.
	Morphine	50–100 µg/kg IV then 0.8–1 mg/h IV as needed	Reversal agent (naloxone) available; prolonged analgesic properties (longer duration of action than fentanyl, alfentanil, sufentanil, and remifentanil)	Uncommon first-line agent for procedural analgesia; slow onset and peak effect time and less reliable than fentanyl, alfentanil, sufentanil, and remifentanil
	Remifentanil	0.025–0.1 µg/kg per minute IV	Ultra–short-acting; no solid organ involved in metabolic clearance	Difficult to use without an infusion pump
Benzodiazepines	Midazolam	Small IV doses of 0.02–0.03 mg/kg until clinical effect ("sleepy," ptosis, dizziness, slurred speech) achieved; repeat dosing of 0.5–1 mg for 3–5 min, with total dose < 5 mg	Familiar emergency drug; minimal effect on respiration; reversal agent (flumazenil) available	No analgesic effect; may cause hypotension, particularly when given rapidly or combined with opioids (may need to decrease midazolam dose); paradoxic excitation can occur (uncommon).

Continued

TABLE 5.3 Sedation Dosing Protocols—cont'd

Class	Drug	Dosage and Administration	Advantages	Cautions
Volatile agents	Nitrous oxide	50% nitrous oxide-50% oxygen mixture delivered by physician or patient holding mask over mouth and nose	Rapid onset and recovery; cardiovascular and respiratory stability; few contraindications	Acute tolerance may develop; specialized equipment needed; for prolonged use, requires a well-ventilated space, possibly with scavenging system of waste gases
Propofol	Propofol	Intermittent bolus of 0.1–0.3 mg/kg IV over 1–5 min or continuous infusion of 100 µg/kg/min for 3–5 min then reduce to ~50 µg/kg/min titrated to effect	Rapid onset; short-acting; anticonvulsant properties	May cause rapidly deepening sedation, airway obstruction, apnea, hypotension secondary to myocardial depression; consider reducing the dosage (by 50% or more) in older patients or those with reduced physiologic reserve.
Phencyclidines	Ketamine	0.2–0.5 mg/kg IV over 2–3 min; 2–4 mg/kg IM	Rapid onset; short-acting; potent analgesic, even at low doses; cardiovascular stability; bronchodilator; synergy with propofol; few contraindications	Avoid in patients with a history of psychosis because it may activate (or reactivate) psychiatric disease; may cause nausea and vomiting; emergence reactions common,[c] but midazolam, 0.03 mg/kg IV, may attenuate or eliminate these reactions, and quiet spaces for recovery may also help; consider adding an antisialagogue, such as glycopyrrolate.
Etomidate	Etomidate	0.1–0.15 mg/kg, slow (30–60 s) IV injection; may readminister every 3–5 min	Rapid onset; short-acting; cardiovascular stability in nonhypovolemic patients; respiratory depression rare	May cause myoclonus, pain on injection, nausea, vomiting, lower seizure threshold (caution when using in patients with seizure disorders, epilepsy—may induce seizures), and adrenal suppression (importance unclear in trauma); recommended IV dose lasts 5–15 min.

[a]Dosing regimens and protocols should be verified for each individual institution before starting any procedural sedation technique. The doses given are suggestions only, and doses and injection intervals may need to be adjusted on the basis of individual clinical presentation and comorbidities.
[b]Combinations of sedatives and analgesic drugs—synergistic combinations of these agents can augment their depressive effects on respiration and slow the patient's return to consciousness compared with the use of each drug alone. Dosages should therefore be appropriately reduced when multiple agents are used. Certain combinations have better safety profiles. For example, before propofol-induced deep sedation, low-dose ketamine (at subdissociative levels) seems to be a safer analgesic than fentanyl; a small prospective trial for this indication has shown that ketamine is associated with fewer significant intrasedative adverse events (47% [95% confidence interval (CI), 31% to 64%] vs. 34% [CI, 67% to 93%]).
[c]Emergence reactions are undesirable psychological reactions that can occur during recovery from sedative regimens when ketamine is a key component. They can vary in severity and composition but commonly involve vivid dreaming, a sensation of floating or leaving one's body, and misinterpretations of true sensory stimuli (illusions). These are often associated with excitement, confusion, euphoria, and fear.
Adapted from Atkinson P, French J, Nice A. Procedural sedation and analgesia for adults in the emergency department. BMJ 2014;348:g2965.

TABLE 5.4 Sedation Dosing Protocols

Drug	Sedation	Anxiolysis	Analgesia	Route, Dose	Onset (min)	Peak (min)	Duration (min)	Comments
Sedative-Hypnotics[a]								
Midazolam	Yes	Yes	No	IV: 0.5 mg (titrate to effect, up to max of 5 mg)	1–2	3–5	10–30	Minimal cardiorespiratory depression
				IM: 0.08 mg/kg	10–15	20–45	60–120	Reduce dose when used in combination with opioids.
				PO: 0.5 mg/kg	15–50	35–45	60–90	

TABLE 5.4 Sedation Dosing Protocols—cont'd

Drug	Sedation	Anxiolysis	Analgesia	Route, Dose	Onset (min)	Peak (min)	Duration (min)	Comments
Diazepam	Yes	Yes	No	IV: 2–3 mg (titrate to effect, up to 15 mg) PO: 5–10 mg	1–2	8–15	15–45	Midazolam is the benzodiazepine of choice for short procedures.
					30–60	45–60	60–100	Antagonist—flumazenil
Opioids								
Fentanyl	No	No	Yes	IV: 25–50 µg intermittent boluses	1–2	5	30–40	Respiratory depression; decreased response to hypercarbia and hypoxia. Synergistic sedative and respiratory depressant effects (reduce dose with sedatives). Nausea, vomiting. Meperidine—histamine release. Antagonist—naloxone
Reversal Agents (Antagonists)								
Flumazenil	No	No	No	IV: 0.1–0.2 mg (titrate to effect to max of 5 mg)	1–2	5–10	45–90	Short-acting; repeat doses may be required. Avoid in patients receiving benzodiazepines for seizure control. Caution with chronic benzodiazepine therapy (withdrawal effect) or with tricyclic antidepressants.
Naloxone	No	No	No	IV: 0.02–0.04 mg (titrate to effect)	1–2	2–3	30–60	Short-acting, repeat doses may be required. May cause hypertension and tachycardia. Pulmonary edema reported
Anesthetics								
Ketamine	Yes	No	Yes	IV: 0.2–0.5 mg/kg (titrate to effect)	1	1–2	10–20	Dissociative anesthetic
				IM: 2–5 mg/kg	5	15	15–30	Emergence reactions blunted with midazolam. Minimal respiratory depression, bronchodilator. Hypersalivation, laryngospasm. Cardiac stimulant—increase in blood pressure and heart rate. Increase in intracranial pressure and intraocular pressure
Propofol	Yes	Yes	No	IV: 0.5 mg/kg (intermittent boluses) Infusion: 25–75 µg/kg per minute	<1	1–2	5–8	Cardiorespiratory depression. Pain on injection. Antiemetic properties

Max, Maximum.

[a]Alterations in dosing may be indicated based on the clinical situation and the practitioner's experience with these agents. Individual dosages may vary depending on age and coexistent diseases. Doses should be reduced for sicker patients and older adults. When using drug combinations, the potential for significant respiratory impairment and airway obstruction is increased. Drugs should be titrated to achieve optimal effect, and sufficient time for dose effect should be allowed before administering an additional dose or another medication.

From Metzner J, Domino KB. Moderate sedation: a primer for perioperative nurses. AORN J. 2015;102:526–535.

ALFENTANIL HYDROCHLORIDE (ALFENTA)

Class	Opioid agonist
Schedule	Alfentanil is subject to Schedule II control under the Controlled Substances Act of 1970.
Clinical	Alfentanil is an opioid analgesic with a rapid onset of action.
Pharmacology	Alfentanil is 10% to 20% as potent as fentanyl and has one-third the duration of action of fentanyl. Lower doses provide analgesia, whereas higher doses promote hypnosis and attenuate catecholamine response. Opioids bind to opiate receptors located throughout the central nervous system (CNS). Opioid receptors that have been identified include mu, kappa, delta, and sigma. The pharmacodynamic properties of each opioid is dependent on which specific opioid receptor is occupied.
Onset	IV = immediate, produces analgesia in 1 minute
Peak effect	IV = 1–2 minutes
Duration	IV = 5–15 minutes
Indications	Analgesic adjunct given in incremental doses in the maintenance of anesthesia with sedative hypnotic, nitrous oxide or oxygen; analgesic administered by continuous infusion with nitrous oxide or oxygen in the maintenance of general anesthesia; as a primary anesthetic agent for the induction of anesthesia in patients undergoing general surgery in which endotracheal intubation and mechanical ventilation are required; as the analgesic component for monitored anesthesia care (MAC).
Contraindications	Known hypersensitivity to alfentanil. Depressed ventilatory function, increased intracranial pressure.
Protein binding	92%
Half-life	90–111 minutes
Considerations	Individualize dose. Titrate medication to effect. Reduction of dosage (30–50%) in older and debilitated patients. Calculate drug dose based on lean body weight in obese patients (>20% above ideal body weight.). Crosses placental barrier, excreted in breast milk.
Drug interactions	Pronounced synergism and respiratory depression occur when used in conjunction with CNS depressants (e.g., barbiturates, benzodiazepines, sedatives, hypnotics).
Respiratory effects	Apnea, respiratory depression, hypoxia, bronchospasm, as well as diminished respiratory reserve. Extreme caution must be used in patients with pulmonary disease, decreased respiratory reserve, or compromised respiratory status. Dose-related muscle rigidity, (particularly truncal rigidity) may occur. Facilities must be fully equipped to monitor and treat respiratory depression. Respiratory depressant effects outlast its analgesic effect.
Cardiovascular (CV) effects	Dysrhythmias, bradycardia, tachycardia, hypotension. Bradycardia may be treated with atropine. Use with caution in patients with bradyarrhythmias.
CNS effects	The magnitude and duration of CNS effects are enhanced when alfentanil is used with other CNS depressant drugs. Dosages of alfentanil and other CNS depressant drugs should be reduced when used in combination. Caution should be exercised in patients with increased intracranial pressure or head injury. Increased intracranial pressure is associated with the development of hypercapnia and the respiratory depressant effects associated with opioid use. Additional neurologic effects include confusion or euphoria.
Metabolism	Alfentanil is metabolized to inactive metabolites via hepatic mechanisms. Erythromycin can inhibit alfentanil metabolism.
Elimination	Excretion via urine.
Overdose	Signs and symptoms of narcotic overdose include decreased respiratory rate and volume, extreme somnolence, cold clammy skin, bradycardia, and hypotension. In the event of an overdose, maintenance of a patent airway, coupled with cardiac and respiratory support, is required. Ventilation and oxygenation must be maintained until the respiratory depressant effects have dissipated.
	Naloxone (Narcan), a narcotic antagonist, will reverse the respiratory and cardiovascular depressant effects associated with alfentanil overdose. Naloxone may also reverse additional side effects associated with narcotic administration. These side effects include urinary retention, pruritis, respiratory depression, nausea, and vomiting. Careful titration is required to avoid full reversal of analgesia.
	Patients treated with naloxone must remain adequately monitored and reassessed postsedation for a minimum of 120 minutes to avoid the development of renarcotization and respiratory depression.
Dosage	3–8 μg/kg based on lean body weight, titrated in 125-μg increments. Dosage should be individualized and reduced in older adults, debilitated patients, renal or hepatic disease patients, or patients with hypothyroidism. Titration to individual patient response is required. If used for conscious sedation, slow IV injection is required.
Supplied	500 μg/mL

MEPERIDINE HYDROCHLORIDE (DEMEROL)

Class	Opioid agonist
Schedule	Meperidine is subject to Schedule II control under the Controlled Substances Act of 1970.
Clinical pharmacology	Meperidine is a synthetic opioid analgesic similar to morphine sulfate, but less potent. Meperidine is 10% as potent as morphine (8–10 mg is equivalent to 1 mg morphine). Its principal therapeutic actions are analgesia and sedation. Pain threshold is elevated, and the CNS is depressed. May cause less spasm of smooth muscle, constipation, and suppression of the cough reflex than morphine. Opioids bind to opioid receptors located throughout the CNS. The pharmacodynamic properties of each opioid are dependent on which specific opioid receptor is occupied.
Onset	IV = 1–5 minutes IM = 10–15 minutes Oral = 15–45 minutes
Peak	IV = 5–7 minutes IM = 30–50 minutes Oral = 60–90 minutes
Duration	2–4 hours
Indications	Meperidine is indicated for the short-term relief of moderate to severe pain.
Contraindications	Known hypersensitivity to meperidine. Depressed ventilatory function, acute asthma, increased intracranial pressure. It has been reported that patients receiving monoamine oxidase (MAO) inhibitors have had fatal reactions when treated with meperidine, although the exact mechanism is unclear. Reactions include severe respiratory depression, cyanosis, hypotension, hyperexcitability, convulsions, tachycardia, and hypertension. When narcotics are required in this patient population, meperidine is contraindicated. Monitoring and follow-up are required if narcotics are used in the presence of MAO inhibitors.
Protein binding	60%–80%
Half-life	3–5 hours
Considerations	The administration of IV meperidine must be titrated to effect and injected slowly. Rapid injection increases the incidence of adverse reactions, which include severe respiratory depression, apnea, hypotension, circulatory collapse, and cardiac arrest. Pharmacologic breakdown results in toxic metabolite (normeperidine); therefore long-term use is not recommended in older adults. Meperidine (pethidine) offers little therapeutic advantage over other opioids and produces a neurotoxic metabolite with a long half-life. The ISMP issued warnings in 2004 and 2005 suggesting that meperidine be avoided. When used, it should be in limited doses (<600 mg/24 h in <48 h).
Drug interactions	Dry mouth, constipation, spasm of the sphincter of Oddi (biliary spasm), flushing, urinary retention, pruritis, urticaria, rash, skin wheals, local irritation at the injection site, and antidiuretic effect. Drug effects are potentiated by antacids, anticholinergics, cimetidine, tricyclic antidepressants, oral contraceptives, phenothiazines, and CNS depressant medications.
Respiratory effects	Severe respiratory depression and arrest may occur with the IV administration of meperidine. Extreme caution should be exercised in patients with asthma, chronic obstructive pulmonary disease (COPD), cor pulmonale, decreased respiratory reserve, hypoxia, or hypercapnia. Facilities must be fully equipped to monitor and treat respiratory depression.
CV effects	Tachycardia, bradycardia, shock, cardiac arrest, palpitations, syncope, orthostatic hypotension. Hypotension may be severe in hypovolemic, critically ill patients.
CNS effects	Euphoria, dysphoria, weakness, headache, sedation, convulsions, agitation, tremor, uncoordinated muscle movements, transient hallucinations, disorientation, and visual disturbances. Extreme caution should be exercised with the use of any narcotic in patients with increased intracranial pressure or head injury. Increased intracranial pressure is associated with the development of hypercapnia and the respiratory depressant effects of opioids.
Metabolism	Meperidine undergoes extensive metabolism in the liver to normeperidine. Normeperidine's extended half-life of 15 to 30 hours may lead to cumulative effects. See considerations identified above.
Excretion	Urinary excretion is pH-dependent. Secreted in breast milk.
Overdose	Signs and symptoms of overdose include decreased respiratory rate and volume, extreme somnolence, cold clammy skin, bradycardia, and hypotension. In the event of an overdose, maintenance of a patent airway, coupled with cardiac and respiratory support, is required. Ventilation and oxygenation must be maintained until the respiratory depressant effects have dissipated.
Reversal	Naloxone (Narcan), an opioid receptor antagonist, will reverse the respiratory and cardiovascular depressant effects associated with meperidine overdose. Naloxone may also reverse additional side effects associated with opioid administration. These side effects include urinary retention, pruritis, respiratory depression, nausea, and vomiting. Careful titration is required to avoid full reversal of analgesia.

Continued

MEPERIDINE HYDROCHLORIDE (DEMEROL)—cont'd

	Patients treated with naloxone must remain adequately monitored and reassessed postsedation for a minimum of 120 minutes to avoid the development of renarcotization and respiratory depression.
Dosage	Should be individualized and reduced in older adults, debilitated patients, presence of renal/hepatic disease, or patients with hypothyroidism. Titration to individual patient response is required. If used IV for moderate sedation, slow IV injection is required.
	IV: 0.25–1 mg/kg slowly in 5- to 10-mg increments titrated to patient effect.
Supplied	Ampules = 50 mg/mL, 100 mg/mL
	Vials = 50 mg/mL, 100 mg/mL
	Carpujects and Tubex dispensers also available.

HYDROMORPHONE HYDROCHLORIDE (DILAUDID)

Class	Opioid agonist
Schedule	Hydromorphone is subject to Schedule II control under the Controlled Substances Act of 1970.
Clinical pharmacology	Hydromorphone is a semisynthetic opioid agonist (derivative of morphine). It is six times as potent as morphine, with a shorter duration of action and a more rapid onset. It produces potent analgesia, more sedation, and less euphoria than morphine.
Onset	IV = 1 minute
Peak	IV = 15–30 minutes
Duration	IV = 2–3 hours
Indications	Analgesic agonist for the relief of moderate to severe pain.
Contraindications	Known hypersensitivity to hydromorphone; patients who are not already receiving increased doses of parenteral narcotics, increased intracranial pressure, depressed ventilatory function, acute asthma.
Protein binding	<30%
Half-life	2–3 hours
Considerations	Respiratory depression is dose-related. Hydromorphone must be given slowly when used for IV administration (over 3 minutes). Rapid administration of hydromorphone increases narcotic-related side effects.
Drug interactions	Hypotension, bradycardia, urinary retention, dysphoria, constipation, nausea, vomiting, pruritis, urticaria. Patients taking other CNS depressants may have synergistic effects when hydromorphone is used. Decreased doses of hydromorphone are required when used in the presence of other CNS depressant drugs.
Respiratory effects	Respiratory depression, decreased respiratory rate and tidal volume, with resultant cyanosis and hypoxemia. Facilities must be fully equipped to monitor and treat respiratory depression.
CV effects	Orthostatic hypotension, syncope, circulatory depression, bradycardia, hypotension.
CNS effects	Sedation, drowsiness, lethargy, mental and/or physical impairment, anxiety, fear, dysphoria, dizziness, mood alterations, psychological dependence.
Metabolism	Conjugation in the liver.
Excretion	Excreted as glucuronidated conjugate via the kidney. May be excreted in breast milk.
Overdose	Naloxone (Narcan), a narcotic antagonist, will reverse the respiratory and cardiovascular depressant effects associated with hydromorphone overdose. Naloxone may also reverse additional side effects associated with narcotic administration. These side effects include urinary retention, pruritis, respiratory depression, nausea, and vomiting. Careful titration is required to avoid full reversal of analgesia.
	Patients treated with naloxone must remain adequately monitored and reassessed postsedation for a minimum of 120 minutes to avoid the development of renarcotization and respiratory depression.
Dosage	Slow IV administration, 0.5-mg increments, titrated to patient response.
	Should be individualized and reduced (30%–50%) in older adults, debilitated patients, presence of renal or hepatic disease, or patients with hypothyroidism. Titration to individual patient response is required.
Supplied	Injection: 1 mg/mL, 2 mg/mL, 3 mg/mL, 4 mg/mL

MORPHINE SULFATE (MORPHINE)

Class	Opioid agonist
Schedule	Morphine sulfate is subject to Schedule II control under the Controlled Substances Act of 1970.
Clinical pharmacology	Morphine is an alkaloid derivative of opium that produces analgesia, sedation, euphoria, and dose-related respiratory depression. Hypotension and decreased systemic vascular resistance are related to the degree of histamine release. Nausea and vomiting associated with morphine sulfate administration are a result of stimulation of the chemoreceptor trigger zone. It induces sleep and inhibits perception of pain by binding to

MORPHINE SULFATE (MORPHINE)—cont'd

	opiate receptors, decreasing sodium permeability, and inhibiting transmission of pain impulses. Opioids bind to opiate receptors located throughout the CNS. Opioid receptors that have been identified include mu, kappa, and delta. The pharmacodynamic profile of each opioid is dependent on which specific opioid receptor is occupied.
Onset	IM = 10–30 minutes IV = 5–10 minutes; CNS effect delayed up to 20 minutes
Peak	IM = 30–60 minutes IV = 20 minutes
Duration	IM = 4–5 hours IV = 4–5 hours
Indications	Morphine is a systemic opioid receptor agonist that may be administered through a variety of routes, which include oral, intramuscular, and IV. Morphine may be used as a narcotic analgesic for the relief of moderate to severe pain. Analgesic of choice associated with myocardial infarction. Treatment of acute pulmonary edema associated with left ventricular failure.
Contraindications	Known hypersensitivity to morphine or natural opioids, bronchial asthma, decreased respiratory reserve, and increased intracranial pressure.
Protein binding	33%
Half-life	2–4 hours
Considerations	As with all opioid adjuncts, individualized dosing is required, with titration to patient effect.
Drug interactions	Histamine release (urticaria, skin wheals, local tissue irritation), constipation, headache, anxiety, depression, convulsions, bradycardia, dysphoria, pruritis, nausea, vomiting, urinary retention, and biliary colic, as well as interference with thermal regulation.
Respiratory effects	Caution must be used in patients with decreased respiratory reserve and increased intracranial pressure. Acute respiratory failure and bronchospasm may occur in patients with COPD, acute asthma, or signs of respiratory embarrassment. The degree of bronchoconstriction is dependent on the magnitude of histamine release associated with the administration of morphine sulfate. Facilities must be fully equipped to monitor and treat respiratory depression.
CV effects	Hypotension, bradycardia, and chest wall rigidity. Extreme caution must be exercised in patients with decreased circulating blood volume or impaired myocardial function. Hypotension may occur after IV injection secondary to histamine-mediated vasodilation.
CNS effects	Euphoria, somnolence. The use of CNS depressant drugs, sedatives, and hypnotics potentiate morphine sulfate's central nervous system depressant effects.
Metabolism	The principal site of metabolism is the liver.
Excretion	90% of urinary excretion occurs within 24 hours; 7%–10% of morphine is excreted in the feces.
Overdose	Signs and symptoms of opioid overdose include decreased respiratory rate and volume, extreme somnolence, cold clammy skin, bradycardia, and hypotension. In the event of an overdose, maintenance of a patent airway coupled with cardiac and respiratory support is required. Ventilation and oxygenation must be maintained until the respiratory depressant effects have dissipated. Narcan (naloxone), an opioid antagonist, will reverse the respiratory and cardiovascular depressant effects associated with morphine overdose. Naloxone may also reverse additional side effects associated with narcotic administration. These side effects include urinary retention, pruritis, respiratory depression, nausea, and vomiting. Careful titration is required to avoid full reversal of analgesia. Patients treated with naloxone must remain adequately monitored and reassessed postsedation for a minimum of 120 minutes to avoid the development of renarcotization and respiratory depression.
Dosage	0.03–0.1 mg/kg in 1-mg incremental IV, titrated to patient response. Dosage should be individualized and reduced in older adults, debilitated patients, or patients with hypothyroidism or renal or hepatic disease.
Supplied	Injection = 1 mg/mL, 2 mg/mL, 4 mg/mL, 8 mg/mL, 20 mg/mL, 15 mg/mL

FENTANYL CITRATE (SUBLIMAZE)

Class	Opioid agonist
Schedule	Fentanyl is subject to Schedule II control under the Controlled Substances Act of 1970.
Clinical pharmacology	Fentanyl is a phenylpiperidine derivative, which is a potent opioid agonist and descending CNS depressant. The analgesic activity of 100 μg (2 mL) of fentanyl is equivalent to 10 mg of morphine, or 75 mg of meperidine. It is approximately 75 to 125 times more potent than morphine, milligram for milligram. It has a rapid onset and relatively short duration of action. Its use is associated with little hypnotic activity, and histamine release rarely occurs. Opioids bind to opiate receptors located throughout the CNS. Opioid receptors that have been identified include mu, kappa, delta, and sigma. The pharmacodynamic properties of each opioid is dependent on which specific opioid receptor is occupied. Fentanyl's principal actions are analgesia and sedation.

Continued

FENTANYL CITRATE (SUBLIMAZE)—cont'd

Onset	IV = 3–5 minutes
	Transmucosal = 5–15 minutes
Peak effect	IV = 5–15 minutes
	Transmucosal = 20–40 minutes
Duration	IV = 30–60 minutes
	Transmucosal: 1–3 hours
Indications	Analgesic action of short duration during anesthetic periods, premedication, induction, and maintenance of anesthesia. As a narcotic analgesic supplement in general or regional anesthesia. Useful in short-duration minor surgery in outpatients and in diagnostic procedures or treatments that require the patient to be awake or lightly sedated.
Contraindications	Known hypersensitivity to fentanyl. Depressed ventilatory function, presence of airway obstruction, acute or severe bronchial asthma, increased intracranial pressure. Contraindicated in patients taking MAO inhibitors
Protein binding	80% protein-bound.
Half-life	1.5–6 hours
Considerations	Titration to effect is required. Dosage reduction and extreme caution must be used when administering to older adults, debilitated patients, and patients susceptible to respiratory depression. When administered in large doses or injected rapidly, chest wall rigidity may result in inability to ventilate the patient. Chest wall rigidity may be treated with a narcotic antagonist and/or paralysis by muscle relaxant.
Drug interactions	Circulatory and respiratory depression. Profound synergism occurs when used with sedatives and CNS depressants. Concurrent use with diazepam (Valium) with higher doses of fentanyl may produce vasodilation and prolonged hypotension and result in delayed recovery.
Respiratory effects	Duration of respiratory depression may last longer than analgesic effects. As the dose of narcotic is increased, the degree of pulmonary exchange is decreased. Apnea, respiratory depression, and chest wall rigidity may occur. Extreme caution must be exercised when administering to patients with COPD, decreased respiratory reserve, and compromised respiratory status. Facilities must be fully equipped to monitor and treat respiratory depression. In healthy individuals, respiratory rate returns to normal more quickly than with other opiates.
CV effects	Vagally mediated bradycardia, shock, cardiac arrest, palpitations, syncope, hypotension.
CNS effects	Euphoria, dysphoria, weakness, sedation, agitation, tremor. Extreme caution should be exercised with patients with intracranial hypertension. CNS depressant drugs produce a synergistic effect and potentiate the effects of CNS depressant drugs.
Metabolism	Hepatic biotransformation.
Elimination	Renal excretion. Caution should be exercised in older patients due to decreased clearance rates and those with liver and kidney disease. Fentanyl is excreted in breast milk.
Overdose	Signs and symptoms of narcotic overdose include decreased respiratory rate and volume, extreme somnolence, cold clammy skin, bradycardia, and hypotension. In the event of an overdose, maintenance of a patent airway coupled with cardiac and respiratory support is required. Ventilation and oxygenation must be maintained until the respiratory depressant effects have dissipated.
	Naloxone (Narcan), a narcotic antagonist, will reverse the respiratory and cardiovascular depressant effects associated with fentanyl overdose. Naloxone may also reverse additional side effects associated with narcotic administration. These side effects include urinary retention, pruritis, respiratory depression, nausea, and vomiting. Careful titration is required to avoid full reversal of analgesia.
	Patients treated with naloxone must remain adequately monitored and reassessed postsedation for a minimum of 120 minutes to avoid the development of renarcotization and respiratory depression.
Dosage	0.5–2 µg/kg or 25–100 µg titrated in 25-µg increments to patient response.
	Dosage should be individualized and reduced in older adults, debilitated patients, patients with renal or hepatic disease, or patients with hypothyroidism. Titration to individual patient response is required. If used for sedation/analgesia, slow IV (over 3–5 minutes) injection is required.
Supplied	50 µg/mL

DIAZEPAM (VALIUM)

Class	Benzodiazepine agonist, sedative-hypnotic, anxiolytic, anticonvulsant, amnestic
Schedule	Diazepam is subject to Schedule IV control under the Controlled Substances Act of 1970.
Clinical pharmacology	Diazepam is a benzodiazepine that depresses the central, autonomic, and peripheral nervous systems to produce amnesia, anxiolysis, muscle relaxation, and a calming effect. The pharmacologic effects of benzodiazepines are primarily exerted via facilitated action of the inhibitory neurotransmitter gamma-amino butyric acid (GABA). This

DIAZEPAM (VALIUM)—cont'd

GABA interaction enhances the inhibitory effects of various neurotransmitters. Benzodiazepines affect the limbic system, thalamus, and hypothalamus producing a calm, sedate state. The effects of diazepam on the central nervous system are based on the dose administered, route of administration, presence of other premedications and concurrent medications administered (opioids).

Diazepam is the benzodiazepine to which all other benzodiazepines are compared. It possesses a long half-life, active metabolites, and a propylene glycol suspension that causes pain on injection.

Onset	IV = 2–5 minutes
Peak	IV = 3–5 minutes
Duration	IV = 15–60 minutes
	PO = 3–8 hours
Indications	Anxiety, acute alcohol withdrawal, skeletal muscle spasm, sedation, sedation-analgesia procedures, preoperative sedation, status epilepticus, severe recurrent seizures.
Contraindications	Known hypersensitivity to diazepam. Acute narrow-angle glaucoma, untreated open angle glaucoma, shock, coma, acute alcohol intoxication; children younger than 6 months of age.
Protein binding	98%
Half-life	30–50 hours
	or
	IV in hours equal to the patient's age (20-year-old = 20 hours; 70-year-old = 70 hours)
Considerations	When used IV, diazepam must be injected slowly. A large vein must be used to prevent venous irritation and possible thrombophlebitis. Use of hand and wrist veins may result in increased incidence of venous irritation. Extreme caution must be used to avoid extravasation or intraarterial administration. Hypoalbuminemia may increase the incidence of side effects. A new formulation as a lipid emulsion has decreased the incidence of pain on injection.
Drug interactions	Drug effect is accentuated (synergism) by the concomitant use of sedatives, hypnotics, or narcotic analgesics. Drug dosage should be decreased based on the type, amount, and time that adjunct medications are administered.
	Complications associated with IV diazepam include venous thrombosis, phlebitis, local irritation, swelling, and vascular impairment. It is recommended not to mix or dilute the medication once it is withdrawn into the syringe.
Respiratory effects	IV diazepam may cause respiratory depression and apnea. Respiratory depression is generally minimal unless large doses are given with concomitant opioid administration. Extreme caution should be used in patients with decreased respiratory reserve. Coughing and laryngospasm have been reported with the administration of diazepam during endoscopic procedures.
CV effects	Decreased systemic vascular resistance and cardiac output. Vagotonic action may lead to bradycardia and hypotension particularly in hypovolemic and debilitated patients. Extreme caution should be used in critically ill or hypovolemic patients.
CNS effects	Drowsiness, confusion, depression, dysarthria, headache, hypoactivity, slurred speech, syncope, vertigo, tremor, ataxia, restlessness, anterograde amnesia, venous irritation, blurred vision, diplopia, rash, urticaria, hiccoughs. May also cause increased CNS depression with concomitant administration of other CNS depressant medications. Physical and psychological dependence have been reported, as well as acute withdrawal after sudden discontinuation in addicted patients.
Metabolism	Hepatic metabolism yields metabolite (desmethyldiazepam), with active pharmacologic effect.
Excretion	Urine
Overdose	In the event of an overdose (respiratory depression, apnea, cardiovascular collapse), maintenance of a patent airway and respiratory and cardiovascular support are required. Reversal with flumazenil, which is a specific benzodiazepine antagonist, generally restores the patient to a clear-headed state. Patients who have responded to flumazenil should be carefully monitored (up to 120 minutes) for signs of resedation, respiratory depression, and residual depressant effects of benzodiazepines.
Dosage	0.05–0.15 mg/kg titrated in 1- to 2-mg increments; large interpatient variability in response to titrated doses. Prior to the planned procedure, 1–2 mg of IV diazepam titrated over 2 minutes may be administered. Additional 1-mg increments administered over several minutes provide sedation for the planned procedure. Additional time must be allowed to evaluate pharmacologic effects in geriatric patients, debilitated patients, or patients with decreased cardiac output. Do not administer by rapid or single bolus injection. Titration to effect includes administration of drug until somnolence, slurring of speech, or nystagmus occurs. Extreme care must be exercised when administering diazepam in the presence of concurrent opioid administration.
Supplied	Diazepam rectal gel (Diastat): 1 mL/5 mg
	Diazepam oral solution: 1 mL, 5 mg, 5 mL
	Diazepam (Dizac/Valium Intramuscular Injectable Solution): 1 mL, 5 mg
	Diazepam (Dizac/Valium Intramuscular Solution): 1 mL, 5 mg
	Diazepam (Dizac/Valium Intravenous Injectable Solution): 1 mL, 5 mg
	Diazepam (Dizac/Valium Intravenous Solution): 1 mL, 5 mg
	Diazepam (Valium Oral Tablets): 2 mg, 5 mg, 10 mg

MIDAZOLAM (VERSED)

Class	Benzodiazepine agonist, sedative-hypnotic, anesthetic adjunct, amnestic
Schedule	Midazolam is subject to Schedule IV control under the Controlled Substances Act of 1970; US Food and Drug Administration (FDA)–approved, 1986.
Clinical pharmacology	Midazolam is a water-soluble benzodiazepine. It is classified as a short-acting benzodiazepine CNS depressant with potent amnestic activity. It is three to four times more potent than diazepam. Depressant effects are dependent on dose, route of administration, and the presence or absence of other CNS depressant drugs. The pharmacologic effect of benzodiazepines is primarily exerted via facilitated action of the inhibitory neurotransmitter GABA. This GABA interaction enhances the inhibitory effects of various neurotransmitters. Benzodiazepines affect the limbic system, thalamus, and hypothalamus, producing a calm, sedate state. The effects of midazolam on the CNS are based on the dose administered, route of administration, presence of other premedications, and concurrent medications administered (opioids).
	Specific advantages of midazolam use include a short half-life, superior sedation, amnesia, and anxiolysis when compared to other benzodiazepines. Midazolam is a water-soluble benzodiazepine. Diazepam and lorazepam use a propylene glycol suspension, which causes pain on injection, venous irritation, and phlebitis.
Onset	IV = 1–5 minutes
	IM = 5–15 minutes
	Intranasal ≤ 5 minutes
Peak	IV = immediate
	IM = 15–60 minutes
	Intranasal = 10 minutes
Duration	2–6 hours
Indications	Preoperative medication, sedation, anxiolysis, and IV induction agent for general anesthesia.
Contraindications	Known hypersensitivity to midazolam, acute narrow-angle glaucoma, dosage reduction in debilitated patients, shock, coma, or acute alcohol intoxication.
Protein binding	97%
Half-life	1–4 hours
Considerations	Individualized dosage. Reduce dose in older patients. Titrate medication to effect. Midazolam must never be used without individualization of dose. Bolus administration is not recommended for sedation-analgesia procedures.
Drug interactions	Drug effect is accentuated (synergism) by concomitant use of sedatives, hypnotics, or narcotic analgesics. Drug dosage should be decreased based on the type, amount, and time adjunct medications are administered. Patients receiving erythromycin and cimetidine may have a decrease in the plasma clearance of midazolam.
Respiratory effects	Potent respiratory depressant. Decrease in respiratory rate and tidal volume. Apnea, respiratory depression, and cardiac arrest. Can depress the ventilatory response to carbon dioxide stimulation. May produce apnea with rapid administration; effects are pronounced with concomitant opioid administration. Patients with COPD are extremely sensitive to the respiratory depressant effects associated with midazolam.
CV effects	Mean arterial pressure, cardiac output, stroke volume, and systemic vascular resistance may be slightly decreased. Hypotension and bradycardia occur more frequently in patients premedicated with a narcotic. Patients with congestive heart failure eliminate midazolam more slowly.
CNS effects	Anxiolytic, hypnotic, sedative effects. Agitation, involuntary movement, hyperactivity, and combativeness. These reactions may be due to excessive dosing, inadequate dosing, hypoxia.
	Use of other CNS depressant medications accentuates the respiratory depressant effects of midazolam.
Metabolism	Midazolam undergoes hepatic microsomal metabolism (hydroxymidazolam). There are no active metabolites. Hepatic clearance may be decreased the with use of enzyme-inhibiting drugs.
Elimination	Metabolites are excreted in the urine.
Overdose	In the event of an overdose (respiratory depression, apnea, cardiovascular collapse), maintenance of a patent airway and respiratory and cardiovascular support are required. Reversal with flumazenil, which is a specific benzodiazepine antagonist, generally restores the patient to a clear-headed state. Patients must be continuously monitored postsedation to assess for resedation, respiratory depression, and residual depressant effects of benzodiazepines
Dosage	Sedation: 0.025–0.1 mg/kg titrated to clinical effect. Do not administer by rapid or single bolus injection. Titration to effect includes administration of drug until somnolence, nystagmus, or slurring of speech occur.
	or
	Per package insert: Initial—usually 0.5–1.0 mg given over 2 minutes (not to exceed 2.5 mg/dose); wait 2 to 3 minutes to evaluate sedative effect after each dose adjustment; total dose > 5 mg usually not necessary to reach desired sedation; use 30% less midazolam if patient premedicated with narcotics or other CNS depressants.
	Debilitated or chronically ill patients—1.5 mg IV initially; may repeat with 1 mg/dose IV q2–3 minutes PRN; not to exceed cumulative dose of 3.5 mg; peak effect may be delayed in older adults, so increments should be smaller and rate of injection slower.

MIDAZOLAM (VERSED)—cont'd

Precautions	IV midazolam should only be used where appropriate equipment and personnel are available for continuous monitoring of cardiorespiratory function and for resuscitation procedures. Midazolam must never be used without individualization of dosage. Midazolam should not be administered by rapid or single bolus IV administration (see dosage, above). Extravasation should also be avoided. The hazards of intraarterial injection of midazolam into humans are unknown. Precautions against unintended intraarterial injection should be taken.
	• Patients should be continuously monitored for early signs of underventilation or apnea. Vital signs should continue to be monitored during the recovery period. During IV application of midazolam, respiratory depression, apnea, respiratory, and/or cardiac arrest have occurred. In some cases where this was not recognized promptly and treated, hypoxic encephalopathy or death has resulted. These life-threatening incidents may occur especially in older patients or patients with preexisting respiratory insufficiency, especially if the injection is given too rapidly or with excessive doses. Particular care must be taken when administering the drug by IV route to older adults, very ill patients, high-risk surgical patients, and those with significant hepatic impairment, chronic renal insufficiency, congestive heart failure, or limited pulmonary reserve because of the possibility of apnea or respiratory depression. These patients require lower doses, whether premedicated or not.

PROPOFOL (DIPRIVAN)

Class	Sedative-hypnotic
Schedule	Not currently a controlled substance. On October 27, 2010, the DEA proposed a rule in the Federal Register to add it as a Schedule IV controlled substance. Although a public comment period followed, it has not been added as a scheduled drug. However, Alabama has made propofol a controlled substance in its state.
Clinical pharmacology	Propofol is a sedative-hypnotic for IV use.
	Produces rapid hypnosis with minimal excitation. It produces nonspecific cortical depression and a more complete and rapid awakening. Rapid awakening is associated with extensive redistribution from the CNS to other tissues and high metabolic clearance. It possesses intrinsic antiemetic effects and has no analgesic properties. Action is dose- and rate-dependent.
Onset	40 seconds
Peak effect	1 minute
Duration	5–10 minutes
Indications	For the induction and maintenance of general anesthesia and as an adjunct to MAC anesthesia.
Contraindications	Known hypersensitivity to propofol.
Protein binding	97%–99%
Considerations	Individualized dose and titration to effect. Reduce dose in older, hypovolemic, and high-risk patients. Potentiation occurs when combined with narcotic analgesics and CNS depressants. Pain on injection has been reported.
	For general anesthesia or care (MAC) sedation, propofol should be administered only by persons trained in the administration of general anesthesia and not involved in the conduct of the surgical or diagnostic procedure. Sedated patients should be continuously monitored, and facilities for maintenance of a patent airway, providing artificial ventilation, administering supplemental oxygen, and instituting cardiovascular resuscitation must be immediately available. Patients should be continuously monitored for early signs of hypotension, apnea, airway obstruction, and/or oxygen desaturation. These cardiorespiratory effects are more likely to occur following rapid bolus administration, especially in older adults, debilitated patients, or American Society of Anesthesiologists (ASA) physical status (ASA-PS) III or IV patients.
Special handling	Shake well before use. Do not use if there is evidence of excessive creaming or aggregation, if large droplets are visible, or if there are other forms of phase separation indicating that the stability of the product has been compromised. Slight creaming, which should disappear after shaking, may be visible on prolonged standing.
	Parenteral drug products should be inspected visually for particulate matter and discoloration prior to administration whenever solution and container permit. Clinical experience with the use of inline filters and propofol during anesthesia or ICU MAC sedation is limited. Propofol should only be administered through a filter with a pore size of 5 µm or greater unless it has been demonstrated that the filter does not restrict the flow of propofol and/or cause the breakdown of the emulsion. Filters should be used with caution and where clinically appropriate. Continuous monitoring is necessary due to the potential for restricted flow and/or breakdown of the emulsion. Do not use if there is evidence of separation of the phases of the emulsion.
	NOTE: Strict aseptic technique must always be maintained during handling. Propofol is a single-access parenteral product (single-patient infusion vial) that contains 0.005% disodium edetate to inhibit the rate of growth of microorganisms, up to 12 hours, in the event of accidental extrinsic contamination. However, propofol can still

Continued

PROPOFOL (DIPRIVAN)—cont'd

support the growth of microorganisms because it is not an antimicrobially preserved product under US Pharmacopeia (USP) standards. Do not use if contamination is suspected. Discard unused drug product as directed within the required time limits. There have been reports in which failure to use aseptic technique when handling propofol was associated with microbial contamination of the product and with fever, infection or sepsis, other life-threatening illness, and/or death. There have been reports in the literature and other public sources of the transmission of bloodborne pathogenic infections (e.g., hepatitis B, hepatitis C, and human immunodeficiency virus [HIV]) from unsafe injection practices, and use of propofol vials intended for single use on multiple persons. Propofol vials are never to be accessed more than once or used on more than one person.

Propofol with ethylenediaminetetraacetic acid (EDTA) inhibits microbial growth for up to 12 hours, as demonstrated by test data for representative USP microorganisms.

Guidelines for aseptic technique for general anesthesia and MAC sedation

Propofol must be prepared for use just prior to initiation of each individual anesthetic or sedative procedure. The vial rubber stopper should be disinfected using 70% isopropyl alcohol. Propofol should be drawn into a sterile syringe immediately after a vial is opened. When withdrawing propofol from vials, a sterile vent spike should be used. The syringe should be labeled with appropriate information, including the date and time the vial was opened. Administration should commence promptly and be completed within 12 hours after the vial has been opened. Propofol must be prepared for single-patient use only. Any unused propofol drug product, reservoirs, dedicated administration tubing, and/or solutions containing propofol must be discarded at the end of the anesthetic procedure or at 12 hours, whichever occurs sooner. The IV line should be flushed every 12 hours and at the end of the anesthetic procedure to remove residual propofol.

Guidelines for aseptic technique for ICU sedation

Propofol must be prepared for single-patient use only. Strict aseptic techniques must be followed. The vial rubber stopper should be disinfected using 70% isopropyl alcohol. A sterile vent spike and sterile tubing must be used for administration of propofol. As with other lipid emulsions, the number of IV line manipulations should be minimized. Administration should commence promptly and must be completed within 12 hours after the vial has been spiked. The tubing and any unused propofol drug product must be discarded after 12 hours.

If propofol is transferred to a syringe prior to administration, it should be drawn into a sterile syringe immediately after a vial is opened. When withdrawing from a vial, a sterile vent spike should be used. The syringe should be labeled with appropriate information, including the date and time the vial was opened. Administration should commence promptly and be completed within 12 hours after the vial has been opened. Propofol should be discarded and administration lines changed after 12 hours.

Respiratory effects	Dose-dependent respiratory depression, apnea, hiccoughs, laryngospasm, bronchospasm, wheezing, and coughing.
CV effects	Hypotension associated with a decrease in cardiac output, cardiac contractility and preload, arrhythmias, tachycardia, bradycardia, decreased cardiac output.
CNS effects	Headache, dizziness, confusion, euphoria, myoclonic or clonic movement, seizures, sexual illusions, and possible additive effect with other CNS drugs, sedatives, and opioids.
Metabolism	Hepatic conjugation to inactive metabolites.
Elimination	Inactive metabolites are eliminated via urine.
Overdose	In the event of an overdose, maintenance of a patent airway and respiratory and cardiovascular support are required. There is no pharmacologic reversal agent for overdose.
Dosage	Indication, dosage, and administration

Induction of general anesthesia: healthy adults < 55 years of age: 40 mg every 10 seconds until induction onset (2–2.5 mg/kg)

Older, debilitated, or ASA-PS III or IV patients: 20 mg every 10 seconds until induction onset (1–1.5 mg/kg)

Cardiac anesthesia: 20 mg every 10 seconds until induction onset (0.5–1.5 mg/kg)

Neurosurgical patients: 20 mg every 10 seconds until induction onset (1–2 mg/kg)

MAINTENANCE OF GENERAL ANESTHESIA: INFUSION

Healthy adults < 55 years of age: 100–200 μg/kg per minute (6–12 mg/kg per hour)

Older, debilitated, ASA-PS III or IV patients: 50–100 μg/kg per minute (3–6 mg/kg per hour)

Cardiac anesthesia—most patients require the following:

Primary propofol with secondary opioid—100–150 μg/kg per minute

Low-dose propofol with primary opioid—50–100 μg/kg per minute

Neurosurgical patients: 100–200 μg/kg per minute (6–12 mg/kg per hour)

MAINTENANCE OF GENERAL ANESTHESIA: INTERMITTENT BOLUS

Healthy adults < 55 years of age: increments of 20–50 mg as needed

PROPOFOL (DIPRIVAN)—cont'd

Initiation of MAC sedation: healthy adults < 55 years of age—slow infusion or slow injection techniques are recommended to avoid apnea or hypotension. Most patients require an infusion of 100–150 µg/kg per minute (6–9 mg/kg per hout) for 3–5 minutes or a slow infusion 3–5 minutes followed immediately by a maintenance infusion.

Older, debilitated, neurosurgical, or ASA-PS III or IV patients: most patients require dosages similar to healthy adults. Rapid boluses are to be avoided.

MAINTENANCE OF MAC SEDATION

Healthy adults < 55 years of age: variable rate infusion technique is preferable over an intermittent bolus technique. Most patients require an infusion of 25–75 µg/kg per minute (1.5–4.5 mg/kg per hour) or incremental bolus doses of 10 mg.

Older, debilitated, neurosurgical, or ASA-PS III or IV patients: most patients require 80% of the usual adult dose. A rapid (single or repeated) bolus dose should not be used. Some physicians prescribe outside of the manufacturer's recommended guidelines listed above for moderate procedural sedation procedures:

Incremental bolus

Propofol in 10-mg (bolus) increments to augment the effects of benzodiazepines and opioids. To avoid deep sedation states or general anesthesia, extreme caution must be used when administering supplemental propofol. Incremental doses must be given slowly over several minutes and adequate circulation time allowed to assess the full pharmacologic effect.

When propofol is used by nonanesthesia providers, it is imperative to ensure that the prescribing clinician understands the pharmacokinetics and pharmacodynamics associated with this pharmacologic agent. Additionally, the prescribing clinician and health care provider administering the sedation and monitoring the patient should possess advanced airway management skills, demonstrate proficiency in managing cardiovascular complications, and recognize that propofol can induce deep sedative states and/or general anesthesia. Propofol is not pharmacologically reversible.

Supplied	200 mg/20 mL (10 mg/mL), 500 mg/50 mL (10 mg/mL), 1000 mg/100 mL (10 mg/mL)

KETAMINE

Class	Dissociative anesthetic
Clinical pharmacology	A phencyclidine derivative that produces rapid dissociative anesthesia, which causes the patient to appear conscious (eyes open, swallowing, enhanced laryngeal-pharyngeal reflexes, muscle contractures, respiratory stimulation). However, the patient loses the ability to process or respond to sensory input. Ketamine has been demonstrated to be an N-methyl-D-aspartate (NMDA) receptor (a subtype of the glutamate receptor) antagonist. Through selective disorganization of nonspecific pathways in the midbrain and thalamic areas, it produces analgesia, amnesia and unconsciousness. Central sympathetic stimulation occurs with systemic, pulmonary arterial pressure, heart rate, and cardiac output increases. Ketamine also produces significant bronchodilation.
Onset	IV = <60 seconds IM = 3–8 minutes
Peak	IV = 5–10 minutes IM = 5–20 minutes
Duration	IV = 5–15 minutes IM = 12–25 minutes
Indications	IV, IM anesthetic induction agent; used as a sedation-analgesia agent for therapeutic and diagnostic procedures.
Contraindications	Patients with increased intracranial pressure, open eye injury, or psychiatric illness. Caution must be exercised in patients with ischemic heart disease, hypertension, and dysrhythmias. Contraindicated for procedures of the pharynx, larynx, and bronchial secondary to increased secretions.
Protein binding	12%
Half-life	3 hours
Considerations	Due to ketamine's ability to produce hypertension and tachycardia, increased myocardial oxygen consumption occurs. Psychological reactions (illusions, dreams, fear, anxiety, excitement, out of body experiences), termed *emergence delirium*, occur in approximately 40% of patients. Emergence reactions generally manifest within the first several hours of recovery and are diminished with the administration of small doses of benzodiazepines. Ketamine should be administered by qualified personnel specially trained in the administration of anesthesia and in the management of the airway and cardiovascular system.
Drug interactions	A combination of theophylline and ketamine may produce seizures. Diazepam and lithium prolong the elimination half-life of ketamine.

Continued

KETAMINE—cont'd

Respiratory effects	Minimal decrease in ventilatory drive. Potent bronchodilator. Increased upper airway secretions are exhibited, particularly in children.
CV effects	Hypertension, tachycardia, increased cardiac output.
CNS effects	Euphoria, unconsciousness, disassociation, and production of a cataleptic state. Increase in intracranial pressure, cerebral oxygen consumption, and cerebral blood flow.
Metabolism	Biotransformation to active and inactive metabolites.
Elimination	Excretion via the kidney.
Overdose	In the event of overdose, maintenance of a patent airway and respiratory and cardiovascular support are required.
Dosage	Sedation and analgesia: IV = 0.2–1 mg/kg IM = 1–2.5 mg/kg If ketamine is used by nonanesthesia providers, it is imperative to ensure that the prescribing clinician understands the pharmacokinetics and pharmacodynamics associated with this agent. In addition, the clinician should also possess advanced airway management skills, demonstrate proficiency in managing cardiovascular complications, and recognize that ketamine can induce deep sedative states and/or general anesthesia. Ketamine is not pharmacologically reversible.
Supplied	10 mg/mL, 50 mg/mL, 100 mg/mL

NALOXONE HYDROCHLORIDE (NARCAN)

Class	Opioid receptor antagonist
Clinical pharmacology	Naloxone hydrochloride is a pure opioid antagonist with no agonist activity. Through competitive inhibition at the opiate receptors, respiratory depression, hypotension, hypercapnia, sedation, and euphoria associated with the administration of narcotics are reversed. Naloxone has not been shown to produce tolerance or physical or psychological dependence. In the presence of physical dependence, naloxone will produce withdrawal symptoms. Requirement for repeat doses is dependent on the amount, type, and route of opioid administration.
Onset	IV = 2 minutes
Peak effect	5–15 minutes
Duration	30–45 minutes, dependent on dose and route of naloxone administration.
Indications	Complete or partial reversal of opioid depression (respiratory depression, sedation, and hypotension) induced by the administration of opioids. Additional indications include diagnosis of suspected acute opioid overdose. Unlabeled uses include reversal of alcoholic coma and improvement of circulation in refractory shock.
Contraindications	Known hypersensitivity to naloxone. Caution must be used when administering to patients with preexisting cardiac disease or patients with known or suspected physical dependence on opioids.
Half-life	30–60 minutes
Considerations	Titrate slowly to the desired effect. Excessive reversal with naloxone may result in total reversal of analgesia with additional side effects (e.g., hypertension, excitation). The short duration of action is presumed to be due to its rapid removal from the brain. Therefore, the duration of action of some opioids may exceed that of naloxone; therefore patients must be carefully monitored postsedation for signs of respiratory depression/arrest. Repeated doses of naloxone may be administered as required.
Respiratory effects	Reversal of respiratory depression. Rapid IV administration may induce pulmonary edema.
CV effects	Hypotension, hypertension, ventricular tachycardia, fibrillation.
CNS effects	Excitement, tremors, seizures.
Metabolism	Hepatic conjugation.
Excretion	Renal.
Overdose	Larger than necessary dosages of naloxone may result in significant reversal of analgesic effects (e.g., hypertension, tachycardia).
Dosage	1–4 µg/kg titrated in 0.1-mg increments promptly reverses opioid-induced analgesia and depression of ventilation.
Supplied	0.4 mg/mL, 1 mg/mL, 0.02 mg/mL

FLUMAZENIL (ROMAZICON)

Class	Benzodiazepine receptor antagonist
Clinical pharmacology	Flumazenil is used for complete or partial reversal of benzodiazepine sedation. It competitively inhibits the activity of the benzodiazepine receptor sites on the GABA-benzodiazepine receptor complex. Flumazenil has been shown to antagonize sedation and psychomotor impairment. The duration and degree of reversal of benzodiazepine effects are related to total dose administered and plasma benzodiazepine concentrations. Duration and degree of reversal are dose- and plasma content–related (both for amount of benzodiazepine and amount of flumazenil).
Onset	IV = 1–2 minutes. An 80% response will be achieved within 3 minutes of administration.
Peak	6–10 minutes
Duration	45–90 minutes. Duration of effect is dependent on the total benzodiazepine plasma concentration.
Indications	Complete or partial reversal of the sedative effects of benzodiazepines. Management of benzodiazepine overdose.
Contraindications	Known hypersensitivity to flumazenil or benzodiazepines. The use of flumazenil (Romazicon) has been associated with the occurrence of seizures. These are most frequent in patients who have been on benzodiazepines for long-term sedation or in overdose cases where patients are showing signs of serious cyclic antidepressant overdose. Practitioners should individualize the dosage of flumazenil and be prepared to manage seizures.
Half-life	41–79 minutes.
Considerations	Individualized dosage is required. Safety and effectiveness for reversal of sedation and analgesia induced with benzodiazepines have been established in patients 1 to 17 years of age. The major risk will be resedation because the duration of effect of a long-acting (or large dose of a short-acting) benzodiazepine may exceed that of flumazenil. Resedation may be treated by giving a repeat dose at no less than 20-minute intervals. For repeat treatment, no more than 1 mg (at 0.2 mg/min doses) should be given at any one time and no more than 3 mg should be given in any 1 hour.
Drug interactions	Flumazenil is not recommended in cases of tricyclic antidepressant overdosage.
Respiratory effects	Respiratory depression is related to the duration of effect of the benzodiazepine administered that has exceeded the therapeutic effects of flumazenil.
CV effects	Cutaneous vasodilation, sweating, and flushing. Arrhythmias (atrial, nodal, ventricular extrasystole, bradycardia, tachycardia), and hypertension.
CNS effects	Dizziness, headache, insomnia, abnormal or blurred vision, confusion, and benzodiazepine withdrawal–induced seizures.
Additional adverse reactions	Fatigue, pain at the injection site, thrombophlebitis, or rash.
Metabolism	Hepatic metabolism is dependent on hepatic blood flow.
Excretion	Inactive metabolites excreted via the urine.
Overdose	In the presence of benzodiazepine agonists, excessive doses of flumazenil result in anxiety, agitation, increase in muscle tone, and possibly benzodiazepine-induced seizure activity.
Dosage	Individualized dosage is required based on patient response: Adult reversal of sedation: 0.2 mg (2 mL) administered IV over 15 seconds. If the desired level of consciousness is not obtained after waiting an additional 45 seconds, a second dose of 0.2 mg (2 mL) can be injected and repeated at 60-second intervals, where necessary (up to a maximum of four additional times) to a maximum total dose of 1 mg (10 mL). The dosage should be individualized based on the patient's response, with most patients responding to doses of 0.6–1 mg. In the event of resedation, repeated doses may be administered at 20-minute intervals as needed. For repeat treatment, no more than 1 mg (given as 0.2 mg/min) should be administered at any one time, and no more than 3 mg should be given in any 1 hour. It is recommended that flumazenil be administered as the series of small injections described (not as a single bolus injection). Patients who have received flumazenil for the reversal of benzodiazepine effects (after conscious sedation or general anesthesia) should be monitored for resedation, respiratory depression, or other residual benzodiazepine effects for an appropriate period (up to 120 minutes) based on the dose and duration of effect of the benzodiazepine used.
Supplied	0.1 mg/mL in 5-mL vials, 0.1 mg/mL in 10-mL vials

ATROPINE SULFATE

Class	Anticholinergic, vagolytic, parasympatholytic, antimuscarinic, muscarinic antagonist, parasympathetic antagonist, parasympathetic blocker.
Clinical pharmacology	Atropine is a white crystalline alkaloid. Atropine antagonizes the action of acetylcholine at the muscarinic receptor, producing local, central, and peripheral effects. Atropine decreases salivary, respiratory, and gastrointestinal secretions. Bronchial and lower esophageal sphincter muscle tone is relaxed. As a parasympatholytic medication, atropine increases sinus node automaticity and atrioventricular conduction through a direct vagolytic mechanism of action.
	Relaxes bronchial smooth muscle, decreases gastrointestinal motility, decreases salivary gland secretion, dilates pupils.
Onset	IV = 45–60 seconds
	IM = 5–40 minutes
	Intratracheal = 10–20 seconds
	Oral = 30 minutes–2 hours
	Inhalation = 3–5 minutes
Peak	IV = 2 minutes
	Inhalation = 1–2 hours
Duration	IV, IM (vagal blockade) = 1–2 hours
Indications	To decrease salivary, bronchial, and gastric secretions. First-line treatment of symptomatic bradycardia and vagal episodes, and incorporated within the Advanced Cardiovascular Life Support (ACLS) algorithm.
Contraindications	Extreme care must be used in patients with tachydysrhythmias, congestive heart failure (CHF), acute myocardial infarction (MI), myocardial ischemia and MI. Second-degree atrioventricular (AV) block type II and third-degree AV blocks are unlikely to respond to atropine. IV infusion of a beta-adrenergic medication (dopamine, epinephrine, isoproterenol) is preferred in these situations.
Considerations	Large doses may produce mental disturbances, confusion, delirium, flushed hot skin, and blurred vision. Exercise caution in obstructive uropathy and obstructive diseases of the gastrointestinal (GI) tract. Transient decreases in heart rate (paradoxic) have been associated with the administration of low dosages or slow administration (<0.5 mg) due to weak peripheral muscarinic effects.
Respiratory effects	Respiratory depression in excessively large doses may be due to paralysis of the medullary center, smooth muscle relaxation, and suppression of secretions.
CV effects	Tachycardia is associated with high dosages; bradycardia is associated with low dosages, palpitations.
CNS effects	Confusion, hallucinations, drowsiness, excitement and agitation, blurred vision, dilation of pupils, psychosis.
Metabolism	Enzymatic hydrolysis.
Elimination	13%–50% of the drug is excreted unchanged in the urine.
Overdose	If marked excitement is present, a short-acting benzodiazepine may be used for sedation. Physostigmine salicylate (Antilirium) reverses most cardiovascular and CNS effects, but it may cause severe bradycardia, seizures, or asystole. Ice bags and alcohol sponges help reduce fever in the presence of hot flushed skin or febrile states, particularly in children.
Dosage	Bradycardia: 0.5 mg IV every 3 to 5 minutes as needed, not to exceed total dose of 0.04 mg/kg, total 3 mg. Use shorter dosing interval (3 minutes) and higher doses in severe clinical conditions.
Supplied	0.4–1 mg/1 mL, 0.4 mg/0.5 mL

EPHEDRINE

Class	Indirect acting, synthetic, noncatecholamine, sympathomimetic
Clinical pharmacology	Ephedrine causes endogenous catecholamine release via an indirect mechanism of action and stimulation of adrenergic receptors via a direct effect; a sympathomimetic drug, which is less potent than epinephrine. Through positive inotropic action, increased strength of myocardial contraction occurs. Through these combined effects (alpha and beta stimulation) blood pressure, heart rate, contractility, and cardiac output increase. Ephedrine is also a bronchodilator via beta stimulation. CNS stimulation occurs, and metabolic and respiratory rates are increased.
Onset	IV = 30–45 seconds (immediate)
	IM ≤ 5 minutes
Peak	IV = 2–5 minutes
	IM = < 10 minutes

EPHEDRINE—cont'd

Duration	10–60 minutes
Indications	Treatment of procedural hypotension, emergency treatment of hypotension of unknown origin. May be used to treat bronchospasm, bradycardia, and allergic disorders.
Contraindications	Cautious use in patients with hypertension, tachycardia, or unstable cardiovascular profile. Ephedrine is contraindicated in patients with narrow-angle glaucoma. Do not use to treat phenothiazine overdose; a further drop in blood pressure and irreversible shock may occur.
Considerations	Tachyphylaxis occurs with repeated doses, but temporary cessation of the drug restores its original effectiveness.
Drug interactions	Decreased responsiveness has been observed in patients treated with beta blockers. Unpredictable effects in patients with depleted catecholamine stores. Hypertensive crisis may occur in patients treated with MAO or tricyclic antidepressants.
Respiratory effects	Pulmonary edema, bronchodilation.
CV effects	Hypertension, tachycardia, dysrhythmias.
CNS effects	Agitation, anxiety, insomnia, tremors.
Metabolism	Hepatic.
Elimination	Renal.
Overdose	Signs and symptoms associated with an overdose (tachycardia, dysrhythmias, hypertension, agitation) generally dissipate within several minutes. Symptoms associated with an exaggerated pharmacologic response may be treated with alpha or beta blockade.
Dosage	Adults: IV = 2.5- to 10-mg increments titrated to effect. IM = 25–50 mg Supplemental doses may be increased to prevent the development of tachyphylaxis.
Supplied	50 mg/1-mL ampule

EPINEPHRINE HCL (ADRENALIN, EPINEPHRINE)

Class	Sympathomimetic, direct-acting, nonsynthetic catecholamine.
Clinical pharmacology	Epinephrine is a naturally occurring catecholamine secreted from the adrenal medulla. It possesses both alpha (peripheral vasoconstriction) and beta (increase in heart rate, bronchodilation) activity. However, its most prominent actions are on the beta receptors of the heart, vascular, and other smooth muscle. When given IV, it produces a rapid rise in blood pressure and direct stimulation of cardiac muscle (positive chronotropic and inotropic effects), which increase the strength of ventricular contraction and cardiac output.
Onset	IV = 30–60 seconds Subcutaneous = 6–15 minutes Inhalation = 3–5 minutes Intratracheal = 5–15 seconds
Peak:	2–3 minutes
Duration of action	IV = 5–10 minutes Intratracheal = 15–25 minutes Inhalational, subcutaneous = 1–3 hours
Indications	Cardiac arrest (ventricular fibrillation, pulseless ventricular tachycardia, asystole, pulseless electrical activity). Symptomatic bradycardia, severe hypotension, anaphylaxis, and severe allergic reactions. Conditions that require increased inotropy, bronchodilation, treatment of allergic reactions, and prolongation of local anesthetic activity.
Contraindications	Cardiac dilation, coronary insufficiency, cardiovascular disorders, thyroid toxicosis, diabetes mellitus, organic brain damage.
Considerations	Increases myocardial oxygen consumption and can cause ischemia secondary to hypertension and increased myocardial oxygen consumption. Caution in patients with hypertension, cardiovascular disease, diabetes, and hyperthyroidism. Contraindicated for IV regional anesthesia and local anesthesia supplement to end-organs (digits, ears, nose).
Drug interactions	The CV effects of epinephrine may be potentiated by tricyclic antidepressants and antihistamines (diphenhydramine). Use caution in patients taking MAO inhibitors. Vasodilators (alpha blocking agents) may counteract the pressor effects of epinephrine.
Respiratory effects	Pulmonary edema, bronchodilation, dyspnea.
CV effects	Hypertension, tachycardia, chest pain.

Continued

EPINEPHRINE HCL (ADRENALIN, EPINEPHRINE)—cont'd

CNS effects	Anxiety, headache, hemorrhage.
Metabolism	Enzymatic degradation (hepatic, renal, and GI tract).
Elimination	Kidneys.
Overdose	Excessive doses of epinephrine may result in precordial distress, vomiting, headache, dyspnea, and hypertension. Alpha or beta blockers may be required to counteract excessive dosage of epinephrine.
Dosage	Cardiac arrest: 1 mg (10 mL of 1:10,000 solution) administered every 3 to 5 minutes during resuscitation. Follow each dose with 20-mL flush; elevate arm for 10 to 20 seconds after dose.
	Higher doses (up to 0.2 mg/kg) may be used for specific indications (beta blocker or calcium channel blocker overdose)
	Continuous infusion: Initial rate, 0.1 to 0.5 µg/kg per minute (for 70-kg patient, 7 to 35 µg/kg per minute); titrate to response.
	Endotracheal: A diluted solution may be given through the endotracheal tube before an IV is established. American Heart Association recommends 2–2.5 mg diluted in 10 mL of normal saline.
	Hypersensitivity: 0.1–0.25 mg (1–2.5 mL of 1:10,000 concentration). Start with a small dose, giving only as much as required to alleviate undesirable symptoms, and repeat as necessary (usually every 20–30 minutes).
Supplied	0.01 mg/mL, 10 µg/mL; 0.1 mg/mL, 100 µg/mL; 0.5 mg/mL, 500 µg/mL; 1 mg/mL, 1000 µg/mL

BIBLIOGRAPHY

Aehlert B. *ACLS Study Guide.* (5th Ed) St. Louis, MO: Elsevier; 2017.

American Heart Association. Advanced Cardiovascular Life Support Provider Manual. Dallas. 2016.

Atkinson P, French J, Nice A. Procedural sedation and analgesia for adults in the emergency department. *BMJ.* 2014; 348.

Barash P, Cullen B, Stoelting R, et al. *Clinical Anesthesia.* 8th ed. Philadelphia: Wolters Kluwer Health/Lippincott Williams & Wilkins; 2017.

Biddle C, Aker J. Conscious sedation: between Scylla and Charybdis. Quality of Life—A Nursing. *Challenge.* 1995; 4(4):107.

Cummins R. *Textbook of Advanced Cardiac Life Support.* Dallas: American Heart Association; 1994.

Messinger J, Hoffman L, O'Donnell J, Dunworth B. Getting conscious sedation right. *American Journal of Nursing.* December 1999; 99(12):47.

Metzner J, Domino KB. Moderate sedation: a primer for perioperative nurses. *AORN Journal.* 2015; 102:526–535.

Miller RD. *Miller's anesthesia.* 8th ed. Philadelphia: Churchill Livingstone/Elsevier; 2015.

Nagelhout J, Elisha S. Nurse Anesthesia (6th ed.). St. Louis, MO: Elsevier; 2018.

Stoelting R, Flood P, Rathmell J, Shafer S. *Pharmacology & physiology in anesthetic practice.* Philadelphia: Lippincott Williams & Wilkins; 2016.

CHAPTER 5: REVIEW QUESTIONS

1. Which benzodiazepine has a half-life of approximately 30 to 50 hours?
   A. Diazepam
   B. Midazolam
   C. Ativan
   D. Temazepam

2. Which of the following benzodiazepines metabolizes into hydroxymidazolam?
   A. Diazepan
   B. Midazolam
   C. Ativan
   D. Temazepam

3. Which of the following benzodiazepines has an active metabolite, desmethyldiazepam?
   A. Diazepam
   B. Midazolam
   C. Ativan
   D. Temazepam

4. Which opioid analgesic is approximately 75 to 125 times more potent than morphine sulfate?
   A. Alfentanil
   B. Ketorolac
   C. Hydromorphone
   D. Fentanyl

5. Which pharmacologic antagonist reverses the clinical effects associated with benzodiazepine overdose?
   A. Ropivacaine
   B. Naropin
   C. Naloxone
   D. Flumazenil

6. Which opioid agonist possesses therapeutic actions with less spasm of smooth muscle, constipation, and suppression of the cough reflex than morphine?
   A. Hydromorphone
   B. Sufentanil
   C. Meperidine
   D. Naloxone

7. Which opioid agonist produces significant histamine release?
   A. Hydromorphone
   B. Meperidine
   C. Morphine
   D. Fentanyl

8. Which sedative-hypnotic agent produces augmentation of sedation and rapid hypnosis and possesses intrinsic antiemetic effects?
   A. Diazepam
   B. Midazolam
   C. Ketamine
   D. Propofol

9. Which sedative-hypnotic agent should only be used by health care providers skilled in advanced airway management and cardiac life support secondary to its ability to produce the development of deep sedative states and general anesthesia?
   A. Midazolam
   B. Diazepam
   C. Meperidine
   D. Propofol

10. A specific opiate receptor antagonist that reverses the respiratory depressant effects associated with narcotic use is identified as which of the following?
    A. Naropin
    B. Naloxone
    C. Flumazenil
    D. Ropivacaine

11. Select the appropriate initial dose of flumazenil required for pharmacologic reversal:
    A. 0.2 mg
    B. 0.4 mg
    C. 0.6 mg
    D. 1 mg

12. Which of the following medications exerts its pharmacologic effect on the N-methyl-D-aspartate (NMDA) receptor?
    A. Propofol
    B. Midazolam
    C. Ketamine
    D. Fentanyl

Answers can be found in Appendix A.

The Effects of Hypnotic Suggestions in Sedation and Anesthesia

Ron Eslinger

LEARNING OUTCOMES

At the completion of this chapter, the learner shall:
- Define hypnotic suggestions.
- Differentiate a positive hypnotic suggestion from a negative hypnotic suggestion.
- Classify sedative and anesthetic medications that are classified as hypnotic(s).
- Associate the effect of presurgical stress on the patient's intraoperative physiologic responses and postoperative outcomes.
- Relate the physiologic processes of the central nervous system that respond to hypnotic suggestion, in addition to moderate sedation and analgesic medications.

COMPETENCY STATEMENT

Health care practitioners caring for the moderate procedural sedation and analgesia patient will effectively incorporate a variety of hypnotic suggestion(s) into their sedation plan of care.

What is a hypnotic suggestion?

A hypnotic suggestion is the act of offering an idea for action or for consideration of an action.[1] Subjectively, hypnosis is a form of self-induced, focused attention. When focused on their anxiety and fear, patients meet the definition of focused attention or hypnosis.

It is easy to integrate the principles of therapeutic suggestion into daily conversations with patients and families. Unfortunately, it is just as easy to integrate toxic suggestions into the conversations with patients. As Mark Twain noted, "The difference between the almost right word and the right word is really a large matter. It is the difference between the lightning bug and the lightning."

By definition, hypnotic language is designed to produce a hypnotic trance; positive language is suggestive to patient safety, comfort, and wellness. Hypnosis or anything hypnotic has been considered by some to be dark and sinister, a magical power, and even mind control. In reality, it is a natural mental state of focused attention experienced when daydreaming, reading, watching television, or driving. Becoming highly focused in these types of activities can lead to zoning out and paying little or no attention to what is going on in the environment. The term *highway hypnosis* refers to a mental state in which a person can drive great distances, responding to external events in the expected, safe, and correct manner, but with no recollection of having consciously done so.[2]

In this state, the driver's conscious mind is apparently fully focused elsewhere, while seemingly still processing the information needed to drive safely. In this trancelike state, the automatic subconscious self is more open to suggestions.

When are patients most receptive to hypnotic suggestion?

During sedation and anesthesia, medications classified as hypnotics may be given to patients to decrease anxiety. Benzodiazepines (e.g., midazolam) and alkylphenols (e.g., propofol) are classified as hypnotics. Patients receiving hypnotic medications are more responsive to what they hear and see. Therefore, patients are more receptive to hypnotic suggestion during the procedural period when hypnotic medications are pharmacologically active. During this period, the brain responds to the suggestions, creating a biologic and physiologic reaction.

Has hypnosis been implemented successfully previously in the health care setting?

As noted, patients in an altered state of consciousness respond to words as hypnotic suggestions. A successful example includes a 34-year-old female patient referred for hypnosis with a 2-year history of painful chronic cystitis; this was related to a previous abdominal hysterectomy 2 years prior to initial hypnosis therapy. The patient regained consciousness in the postanesthesia care unit writhing in pain. This previous negative experience led to a personalized treatment plan, including 3 days of drug detoxification followed by hypnosis. Two initial treatment sessions per week were followed by once-weekly treatments as needed. However, after the first session, she asked, "Why didn't they send me to you 2 years ago? My pain is gone!"

During a later hypnosis session, the patient was asked if she was willing to uncover the cause of her pain. She agreed and, during her next session, it was discovered that while her surgeon was dissecting the uterus from the bladder, a surgical team member stated, "This will be one hurting bladder when she wakes up!" She had no conscious memory of the words, but her subconscious mind heard and did what it was told to do for over 2 years. Her hypnosis treatment included four total sessions. When she was contacted 3 years later, the pain had not returned.[3]

What are some positive and negative examples of hypnotic suggestion?

As noted in *Patient Sedation Without Medication*, Lang and Lasser noted the research of Rosabeth Moss Kanter related to self-confidence and how positive expectations can become self-fulfilling prophecies.[4] Nursing suggestions are also capable of creating positive or negative expectations. What is true for positive suggestions is also true for negative suggestions. Positive and negative suggestion direct comparators include the following:

- Positive
  - "You are looking comfortable. Can I get you anything?"
- Negative
  - "On a scale of 0 to 10, how much pain are you having?"

Many health care facilities are increasingly responsive to reframing potential negative suggestion into positive responses. Simple examples include changing the *pain scale* to *comfort scale*. Rather than asking, "On a scale of 0 to 10, with 0 being no pain and 10 being the most pain you've ever had, how much pain are you having now?" A more positive and effective inquiry could simply be stated as, "From 0 to 10, what is your comfort level currently?" The Joint Commission does not dictate how pain is measured, only that it is assessed and measured uniformly throughout an institution. Table 6.1 identifies additional examples of negative versus positive communication strategies.[5]

TABLE 6.1   Positive and Negative Communication Techniques

Negative Language	Positive Language
"Don't worry."	"What are your concerns?"
Hurt or pain	Comfort
"The doctor is cutting."	"This is an incision" or, "We're getting started."
"We're putting you to sleep."	"It's okay to take a nap."
"It won't be long."	"In a short time we'll be done."
"Are you having pain?"	"Are you comfortable?"
Labor pains or contractions	Baby hugs
"Are you feeling sick?"	"You should be hungry."

What factors increase preprocedure anxiety?

Factors that may increase preprocedure anxiety include fear of needles, pain, awareness during the procedure, infection risks, procedural length, and not waking up after the procedure.[4] Anxiolytics help decrease anxiety prior to the procedure, but it must be noted that both negative and positive suggestions respond to hypnotic class medications.

Anxiety is linked to greater pain, increased need for painkillers, and longer hospital stays after surgery. Anxiety increases the chances of postoperative pain, postoperative analgesic consumption, and hospital stay and recovery. As early as 2005, research demonstrated that hypnosis was an effective method for treating presurgery anxiety.[6] Additional evidence-based studies have shown that hypnosis, calming language, and therapeutic suggestions decrease postanesthesia care unit length of stay, nausea and vomiting, and required pain medications.

What is the relationship between anxiety and pain levels?

The connection between anxiety and pain has been well documented. Patients who demonstrate decreased anxiety experience less pain. The expectations that patients carry into surgery are critically important in how they respond to pain and the perioperative experience. As established through Montgomery's work in hypnosis, operating room staffers have reported that preprocedure hypnosis patients are calmer and require less effort to prepare for surgery, including induction.[7]

Additionally, a study by the Uniformed Services University of the Health Sciences implemented a guided imagery compact disk with biorhythmic music therapy prior to surgery. Their double-blind study demonstrated a significant reduction in preoperative anxiety, postoperative pain, and earlier discharge times after using guided imagery techniques.[8]

What is the history of therapeutic language in nursing?

As early as 1859, Florence Nightingale stated in her book, *Notes on Nursing*, "Volumes are now written and spoken regarding the effect of the mind upon the body." Her text provided a detailed discussion on the suggestibility of children and noted that nurses should encourage patients to vary their thoughts. Nightingale was more in tune with complementary and alternative medicine in 1859 than most contemporary nurses and physicians. She also discussed at length the advantages of using music, color, aroma, physical activity, fresh air, and exercise to help patients decrease their suffering. Stating that "words are great tools," her instincts told her that verbal dialogue is beneficial in healing and wellness.[9]

Self-selected music provided to sedated older patients during ophthalmic surgery has also been shown to decrease the patient stress response, cortisol levels, and amount of sedative agent required during the procedure. This research supports Florence Nightingale's original hypothesis that music has healing effects on patients. Moderate sedation and local anesthesia administration are quickly becoming the primary methods of anesthesia for a variety of outpatient surgical procedures. These surgical methods require the nurse to become aware of nonchemical adjuncts that can assist in providing a safe and comfortable atmosphere for patients. Furthermore, many patients now request nonchemical adjuncts for anxiolysis and sedation, as well as for analgesia, in the surgical suite.[10]

When were the benefits of positive suggestion initially described in the literature?

As early as 1906, Alice Magaw described the significance of suggestive language and its impact on decreasing drug dosages perioperatively. In her review of over 14,000 surgical anesthetics, Magaw noted the following[11]:

> Suggestion is a great aid in producing a comfortable narcosis…. The subconscious or secondary self is particularly susceptible to suggestive influence…. When patients are told what to expect and how to respond, the amount of stress is decreased to such an extent the anesthetic is decreased to about 10% of the normal dose, which in turn greatly increases patient safety…. The anesthetist should make those suggestions that will be most pleasing to this particular subject.

Her work reflected that hypnosis is simply a person's willingness to accept a suggestion given by another person. If that suggestion is realistic, believable, and achievable, and the person giving it is trusted, the acceptance of the suggestion is more likely.

What are the advantages of using hypnotic medication and hypnotic suggestion?

When hypnotic medications (e.g., benzodiazepines, propofol) are administered to patients for sedation and anesthesia, they also empower the health care practitioner to provide positive suggestions prior to the procedure.[12] Prehypnotic suggestion can have a profound effect on patients. Nursing can take advantage of this effect secondary to nursing being considered one of the most trusted professions.[13] Therefore, when the patient receives a suggestion from a nurse, that suggestion is more likely to be accepted and acted on. Combining the nurse's suggestions with a hypnotic drug, such as midazolam, greatly magnifies the response to the suggestion.

Unfortunately, some health care providers are not aware of the words that they use during patient conversations. Language creates perceptions, and those perceptions become truth to the patient. Lipton's biologic research has described how new studies in brain neuroplasticity explain how changing the way we think changes brain chemistry, which in turn can change behaviors and physiologic responses.[14] The brain responds equally to both negative (toxic) suggestions and positive reassuring (therapeutic) suggestions. Every suggestion creates a physiologic or biochemical response. Blushing, sweating, headaches, and digestive problems are only a few of the many possible responses.

What is the relationship between therapeutic suggestion and the limbic system?

Therapeutic talk is a simple communication tool used in developing rapport between two people—in this case,

between the health care provider and patient. Rapport is an early stage of hypnosis.[15] Therapeutic suggestions pass through the cortex and into the amygdala, which consists of a protective filtering system for suggestions entering into the limbic system. The limbic system is a part of the autonomic nervous system and responds to thoughts and suggestions that create emotions. The limbic system does not know the difference between reality and fiction. Whatever you are thinking, the limbic system responds to it as truth. That is why thinking of eating a lemon can create the same response as actually eating a lemon. To the limbic system, a memory is not a memory, but an actual happening. The limbic system consists of the following glands[16]:

- The amygdala filters information as a protective mechanism.
- The hippocampus is responsible for storing memories.
- The pituitary gland is the master gland and controls fight or flight.
- The hypothalamus is responsible for maintaining homeostasis.
- The thalamus filters information received from the spinothalamic tract. It is then distributed to other glands in the brain, depending on the person's emotional state.

Box 6.1 identifies symptoms associated with emotions. The limbic system responds to talking, thinking, and listening, creating an emotional response. When hypnotic medications are added that act in the limbic system, the effect becomes a hypnotic suggestion and can play a role in the patient's health, wellness, comfort, and healing. Benzodiazepines have sedative-hypnotic, anxiolytic, and anticonvulsive effects. It is their effect on the limbic system that produces a calm sedate state and amnesia.

What areas are affected by suggestive hypnotic language?

Every thought that a person has affects some organ or gland in the body. Imagine eating a lemon and experiencing the salivation and tart tanginess in your parotid gland. In the same way, negative thoughts (worry) can make an individual ill, whereas

---

BOX 6.1   Symptoms Associated with Emotions

Pain
Heart rate
Respiration
Contractions
Blood pressure
Bleeding
Inflammatory response
Itching
Bowel motility
Smooth muscle tension
Sweating
Allergic responses
Asthma
Immune response

positive thoughts can lead to wellness. Florence Nightingale directed nurses to use words to help patients change their thoughts. Words are a powerful tool. Lipton's and Pert's books[15,17] were based on the premise that changing thought patterns affects the protein neurotransmitters released by the limbic system, which can change emotions and behaviors. These behaviors can be negative or positive, depending on the thought. Thoughts create emotions; therefore, we can control our fears, anxieties, happiness, and even comfort by controlling our thoughts. Abraham Lincoln said, "Most folks are about as happy as they make their minds up to be." The limbic system does not choose the thought; rather, it just responds to the thought after it is filtered through the cortex and amygdala. This process allows the overwriting of self-sabotaging subconscious programming with hypnotherapy and positive affirmations.[15]

What is toxic language?

Toxic language is language or words that create affirmations, evoke emotional and/or physical responses, or alter perceptions in a negative manner. It is language that hurts. Examples of toxic language include the following:

- "This may burn."
- "You may feel an electric shock down your spine."
- "This is going to hurt."
- "It's noisy in the operating room."
- "This will feel like a bee sting."
- "That equipment is broken again!"
- "How much pain are you having, on a scale of 0 to 10?"
- "Do you feel sick?"
- "Are you having pain?"
- "We're going to put you to sleep."
- "Move over to the table."
- Nurse to a stroke victim: "If you do not take this pill, I am going to put a tube down your throat, crush this pill, and pour it down." The husband took the pill from the nurse and simply said, "Please take this; it will make you feel better."
- Physician to leukemia patient: "You have 5 years to live." In 5 years she died, even though she was in remission. She said to the family, "My doctor said, I had 5 years and it has been 5 years."

Words can paint mental pictures, change behaviors, and alter symptoms or sensations. The subconscious mind does not think or reason; it only responds to thoughts created by the words we speak and hear. Suggestions should be positive and affirming, clear and specific, firm, believable, rich in imagery, and beneficial. Suggestions should avoid anger or blame. In other words, don't say, "Boy, you really broke yourself up," or "How could you do something so stupid?" Also, avoid any negative words such as *pain* and *hurt*.

What are some examples for effective therapeutic communication?

In the presedation area, a health care provider may inquire, "Is there some place you would rather be than here?" If the

reply is "Yes," then ask, "Where would you rather be?" When the patient replies, simply state, "Use your imagination or remember a pleasant time when you were there." Another suggestion could be, "Close your eyes and describe it to me." These simple techniques create distraction and dissociation, decreasing the associated fight-or-flight response. Reassuring language that is easy to implement includes the following statements:

- "Just relax."
- "We are almost done."
- "You are doing fine."
- "Take a nice abdominal breath."
- "You look relaxed."
- "As I do this, you will probably feel this."
- "Some people feel this, and some do not."
- "Would you rather be someplace else?"

As stated earlier, propofol and midazolam are classified as hypnotic medications and may magnify comments made during sedation and anesthesia. Consider the following statements:

- "I will be with you during the entire procedure, doing everything needed to keep you safe and comfortable."
- "I will give you medications during your procedure to keep you comfortable and create good feelings in your stomach."
- "You should feel comfortable and pleasantly hungry when we are done."
- "Think of a happy place and imagine you are there."
- "You may feel some warmth in your IV as this medicine goes in. That feeling will help you relax."

Table 6.2 identifies therapeutic communication strategies that health care providers can implement to enhance patient outcomes simply by modifying the way they address and listen to patients.[17]

Are there specific questions or techniques I can use in the presedation area?

There are statements that the health care provider can make during admission to the presedation holding area. Rapport can be established with a proper introduction by listening carefully to the patient, responding appropriately to the patient's questions, and asking the patient if he or she has any concerns. Addressing the concerns of the patient and family will greatly decrease anxiety. Give the patient appropriate information and prepare the patient for noxious stimuli (e.g., IV start, noise, cold), and use positive suggestions in the process. Particular attention should be provided for those patients who wear glasses, hearing aids, or dentures. When patients do not see well or hear well, or are embarrassed because they do not have their dentures, anxiety increases. The higher the anxiety, the more medication required, and the more difficult the recovery.

Hypnotic language in the presedation holding area may be as simple as stating or doing the following:

- "Do you have a special vacation spot? Describe it to me."
- "Think water hoses." (This is a metaphor for enlarged veins, making IV starts easier.)

TABLE 6.2   Therapeutic Communication Strategies

Don't Say This	Say This!
"This isn't going to hurt."	"You might feel a slightly cool pressure as I…."
"Don't give up."	"Focus on what feeling good would feel like."
"Don't be afraid."	"What are your concerns?"
"This is like a little bee sting." (There is no such thing as a little bee sting.)	"You may or may not feel a little pinch."
"This is going to hurt."	"Some people feel this, and some people don't."
"Do you feel like vomiting?"	"You may have a warm hungry feeling in your stomach."
"We're going to put you to sleep."	"I am giving you some medication that will let you gently go to sleep."
"Don't worry, you will sleep during your sedation!"	"I will be with you the entire time to make sure you stay sedated during your surgery."
"Are you feeling better?"	"You look and sound like you are feeling better."
"See if this nitroglycerin tablet will help."	"Take this. It will make you feel more comfortable."
"Has the oxygen helped your breathing?"	"I see that the oxygen is making it easier for you to breathe."
"I'm not going to leave you."	"I will stay with you."
"It's not that bad."	"This will be more pleasant than you might think."
"Don't worry."	"What are your concerns?"
Hurt or pain	Comfort
"The doctor is cutting."	"This is an incision" or, "We're getting started."
"We're putting you to sleep."	"It's okay to take a nap."
"It won't be long."	"In a short time we'll be done."
"You're having labor pains or contractions."	"Are you having another baby hug?"
"Are you feeling sick?"	"You should be pleasantly hungry."

TABLE 6.3   Patient Benefits of Therapeutic Language

Positive Hypnotic and Therapeutic Language	Patient Benefits
Decrease in preoperative anxiety	Diminished blood loss
More positive attitude toward surgical experience	Better wound healing
More cooperative patient and family	Decreased pain
Greater rapport and trust	Decreased PONV
	Better overall experience and outcome

PONV, Postoperative nausea and vomiting.

What are the benefits of music in the sedation setting?

The benefits of music in health care have been widely reported in the literature. The use of headphones with biorhythmic music increases relaxation and decreases the noise and conversations in the procedure room. Adding subliminal suggestions for moderate sedation patients may also be beneficial. Examples should be in the first person and include the following:

- "I am relaxed and comfortable."
- "My surgery is going well."
- "I am healing more quickly than I thought I would."
- "I am feeling better than I thought I would."
- "My stomach is warm and comfortable."
- "All my body functions are normal."
- "I am pleasantly hungry."

SUMMARY

Incorporating many of the recommendations in this competency module provides the sedation practitioner with a variety of methods to improve patient care through the use of hypnotic suggestion. Each strategy suggested to a patient can affect their outcome positively or negatively. Patient benefits from incorporating positive hypnotic and therapeutic language outlined in this chapter are identified in Table 6.3.

REFERENCES

1. Miller BF, Keane CB, O'Toole MT. *Encyclopedia and Dictionary of Medicine, Nursing, and Allied Health.* 7th ed. Philadelphia, PA: Saunders; 2003.
2. Williams GW. Highway hypnosis: an hypothesis. *International Journal of Clinical and Experimental Hypnosis.* 1963; (103): 143–151.
3. Eslinger MR. Hypnosis and nursing: the perfect combination. *Beginnings.* 2009; 29:10–12.
4. Lang E, Lasser E. *Patient Sedation Without Medication: Rapid Rapport and Quick Hypnotic Techniques.* Victoria, Canada: Trafford; 2009.
5. Eslinger MR. *Hypnosis: Putting the Imagination to Work.* 2nd ed. Clinton, NJ: Healthy Visions; 2016.
6. Hitti M. Presurgery anxiety? Hypnosis may help. https://www.webmd.com/mental-health/news/20051025/presurgery-anxiety-hypnosis-may-help#2; 2005.

- "When I put this tourniquet on your arm, your arm may go to sleep. Can you remember what your arm or leg feels like when it's asleep?"
- "I'm going to wash this area with something cold that may make the area numb."
- When starting an IV, have the patient concentrate on the opposite hand and arm. This is a distraction away from the arm in which you're starting the IV and may help the vein in the IV arm dilate.
- Give a little pinch, or pull the hair near the IV site and say, "What I am going to do is going to feel much better than that." This gives a frame of reference away from the fear of needles and IV starts.

7. Montgomery, G.H. (2008). Hypnosis before surgery makes it faster, easier, less painful. https://bottomlineinc.com/health/surgery/hypnosis-before-surgery-makes-it-faster-easier-less-painful

8. Gonzales EA, Ledesma RJ, McAllister DJ, et al. Effects of guided imagery on postoperative outcomes in patients undergoing same-day surgical procedures: A randomized, single-blinded study. *AANA Journal.* 2010; 78:181–188.

9. Nightingale F. *Notes on Nursing: What It Is, and What It Is Not.* New York: Dover Publications; 1859.

10. Reilly M. Incorporating music into the surgical environment. *Plastic Surgical Nursing.* 1999; 19:35–38.

11. Magaw A. A review of over fourteen thousand surgical anaesthesias. *Surgery, Gynecology, and Obstetrics.* 1906; 3:795–799.

12. Kost M. *Moderate Sedation/Analgesia: Core Competencies for Practice.* St. Louis, MO: Elsevier; 2004.

13. Brenan, M. (2017, December 26). Nurses keep healthy lead as most honest, ethical profession. http://news.gallup.com/poll/224639/nurses-keep-healthy-lead-honest-ethical-profession.aspx

14. Lipton B. *The Biology of Belief: Unleashing the Power of Consciousness, Matter, and Miracles.* New York: Hay House; 2015.

15. Eslinger MR. *Hypnosis: Putting the Imagination to Work (2nd ed.).* Healthy Visions: Clinton, TN; 2016.

16. Pert CB. *Molecules of Emotion: The Science Behind Mind-Body Medicine.* New York: Touchtone; 1999.

17. Walsh BE. *Nurses Communication Skills Handbook: How Your Words and Actions Affect People in Your Care.* Victoria, BC: Walsh Seminars; 2013.

CHAPTER 6: REVIEW QUESTIONS

1. Who stated, "The difference between the right word and the almost right word is the difference between lightning and the lightning bug?"
   A. Mark Twain
   B. Florence Nightingale
   C. Bruce Lipton
   D. Rudyard Kipling

2. _____ is an example of a natural mental state of focused attention.
   A. Highway hypnosis
   B. Sleep patterns
   C. Toxic language
   D. Positive suggestive language

3. The act of offering an idea for action or for consideration of action is termed _____.
   A. Subjection
   B. Objection
   C. Hypnotic suggestion
   D. Therapeutic language

4. _____ is a biologic researcher who described how changing thinking changes the brain, which in turn changes a behavior or a physiologic response:
   A. Albert Einstein
   B. Candace Pert
   C. Bruce Lipton
   D. Rudyard Kipling

5. Which of the following statements is an example of toxic language?
   A. "This will feel like a little bee sting."
   B. "Take this. It will make you feel more comfortable."
   C. "You look and sound like you are feeling better."
   D. "You should be comfortable; if not, let us know."

6. Which area of the brain is responsible for storing memories?
   A. Brain stem
   B. Cerebral gray matter
   C. Cerebral white matter
   D. Hippocampus

7. During sedation and anesthesia, medications classified as hypnotics may be given to patients to decrease anxiety. Which of the following is used most frequently?
   A. Midazolam
   B. Ketamine
   C. Fentanyl
   D. Morphine

8. Which of the following health care professions has been identified as being the most trusted?
   A. Respiratory therapists
   B. Pharmacists
   C. Nurses
   D. Audiologists

9. _____ described the significance of suggestive language and its impact on decreasing drug dosages perioperatively.
   A. Florence Nightingale
   B. Alice Magaw
   C. Albert Einstein
   D. Bruce Lipton

10. Instead of saying, "Don't be afraid," a nurse should say:
    A. "Focus all your energy on healing."
    B. "What are your concerns?" Then address the concern(s).
    C. "Some people feel this; some people don't."
    D. "I will be with you the entire time during your procedure."

11. During the presedation assessment, the patient confides that the worst experience of the patient's last surgery was postprocedure nausea and vomiting. Which of the following positive suggestions would be most helpful?
    A. "I will give you medications during your procedure to keep you comfortable and create good feelings in your stomach."
    B. "I am sorry you got sick. Some people get sick and some don't. Maybe it won't happen this time."
    C. "You should feel comfortable and pleasantly hungry when we are done."
    D. A and C.

12. Instead of saying "This is going to hurt," a health care provider should say _____
    A. "We are well trained in how to take care of you."
    B. "Some people feel this and some people don't."
    C. "You may have a warm hungry feeling in your stomach."
    D. "This never hurts."

Answers can be found in Appendix A.

Airway Management Strategies
for the Sedation Provider

LEARNING OUTCOMES

At the completion of this chapter, the learner shall:
- Delineate the importance of the components of a presedation airway evaluation.
- Distinguish the clinical signs and symptoms associated with respiratory insufficiency and airway obstruction.
- Categorize the treatment modalities designed to relieve airway obstruction and restore airflow in the sedated patient.

- Demonstrate the proper technique for nasal and oral airway insertion.
- Identify the correct mask placement for a bag-valve-mask (BVM) device to deliver positive pressure ventilation effectively.
- Implement the components and treatment modalities associated with the sedation airway algorithm.
- Differentiate methods to effectively troubleshoot difficult BVM ventilation by applying the MOANS acronym.

COMPETENCY STATEMENT

Health care practitioners caring for the moderate procedural sedation and analgesia patient must demonstrate competency with airway management strategies and demonstrate proficiency in restoring ventilation using emergency resuscitative devices in the clinical setting.

The Joint Commission and the American Society of Anesthesiologists have promulgated standards related to the assessment and monitoring of the patient receiving moderate procedural sedation. Which factors identified during preprocedure patient assessment are associated with difficult airway management?

Respiratory depression or respiratory insufficiency may occur secondary to the administration of opioids, benzodiazepines, and sedative-hypnotic agents. Positive pressure ventilation, with or without tracheal intubation, may be necessary if respiratory compromise or airway obstruction develops during a procedure. Effectively managing the airway may be more difficult in patients with atypical anatomy. In addition, some airway abnormalities may increase the likelihood of airway obstruction during spontaneous ventilation. Factors associated with difficulty in airway management include the following:

- Presedation patient history
  - Previous problems with anesthesia or sedation
  - Stridor, snoring, or sleep apnea

  - Advanced rheumatoid arthritis
  - Chromosomal abnormality (e.g., trisomy 21)
- Physical examination
  - Habitus—significant obesity (especially involving the neck and facial structures)
  - Head and neck—short neck, limited neck extension, decreased thyromental distance (<3 cm in an adult), neck mass, cervical spine disease or trauma, tracheal deviation, dysmorphic facial features (e.g., Pierre-Robin syndrome)
  - Mouth—small opening (<3 cm in an adult), edentulous, protruding incisors, loose or capped teeth, dental appliances, high arched palate, macroglossia, tonsillar hypertrophy, nonvisible uvula
  - Jaw—micrognathia, retrognathia, trismus, significant malocclusion

What is respiratory insufficiency?

Respiratory insufficiency is a condition characterized by reduced gas exchange, which is inadequate to meet the body's metabolic demands. Use of sedative, hypnotic, and opioid medications, in conjunction with pathophysiologic disease processes, predisposes patients receiving sedation or analgesia to develop respiratory compromise. It should be noted that the synergistic respiratory depressant effects of opioids, sedatives, and hypnotics may produce respiratory insufficiency and airway obstruction in all patient populations, including the young healthy patient. Respiratory insufficiency may develop at any time during the procedure or in the postsedation period. It is imperative that health care providers participating in sedation patient care understand the principles of oxygen delivery and respiratory physiology. Providers must also demonstrate clinical competency in their ability to use oxygen delivery and mechanical airway devices. Attempts to decrease morbidity associated with the administration of sedation and analgesia are enhanced by the identification of patients at risk of respiratory complications with optimization of presedation medical therapy. Prior to the administration of sedation and analgesia, health care providers must be clinically competent with regard to airway management skills and treatment protocols used in case of airway obstruction or a respiratory event.

What specific features of the airway anatomy are pertinent to the health care provider administering moderate procedural sedation and analgesia?

To master airway management skills competently, it is important to understand the functional anatomy of the human airway. Air enters the pulmonary system through the nose, which has a bone and cartilage framework. The upper airway is defined as that portion above the vocal cords.

The oral cavity consists of the tongue and teeth. The pharynx is a 13-cm-long tube that begins at the internal nares and consists of the tonsils, uvula, and epiglottic structure. The pharynx is divided into three parts.

Nasopharynx. The nasopharynx begins just posterior to the internal nasal cavity. It extends to the soft palate. The nasopharynx contains the adenoids, located at the posterior pharyngeal wall.

Oropharynx. The oropharynx begins at the soft palate and extends to the level of the hyoid bone. It contains the paired palatine and lingual tonsils. The oropharynx serves as both a respiratory and food passageway.

Laryngopharynx. The laryngopharynx begins at the level of the hyoid bone and diverges posteriorly to connect with the esophagus and anteriorly into the larynx. Like the

oropharynx, the laryngopharynx also functions as a respiratory and gastrointestinal passageway.

Anatomy of the upper airway is depicted in Fig. 7.1. The glottic aperture (glottis) is the opening to the larynx, which is covered by the epiglottis. The epiglottis is a large, leaflike structure with its stem attached anteriorly to the thyroid cartilage, with no posterior attachment. The leaf portion of the epiglottis moves freely to prevent the aspiration of gastric contents from the oropharynx into the trachea. During swallowing, the epiglottis covers the glottic opening. To avoid gastric acid aspiration, it is advisable that the gag reflex be maintained during the administration of sedative and analgesic medications.

Is an understanding of the lower airway anatomy an important patient care aspect for the moderate procedural sedation provider?

The lower airway includes structures below the level of the vocal cords. The adult larynx (voice box) lies below the glottic opening anterior to the fourth through sixth cervical vertebrae. The larynx is composed of three single and three paired cartilages. The three single cartilages include the following:
- Thyroid
- Cricoid
- Epiglottis

The three paired cartilages include the following:
- Corniculate
- Cuneiform
- Arytenoid

Laryngeal cartilages are displayed in Fig. 7.2. The thyroid cartilage (Adam's apple) comprises the anterior portion of the larynx. The cricoid cartilage is the single complete cartilaginous ring, which comprises the lower border of the larynx. Of the three paired cartilages, the arytenoid cartilages control vocal cord function through pharyngeal muscle movement.

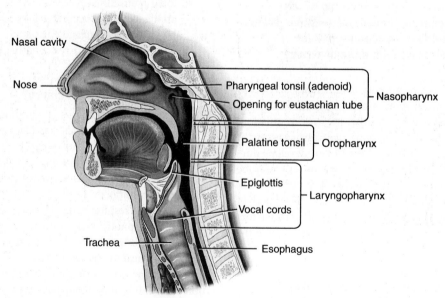

Fig. 7.1 Anatomy of the upper airway. (© Elsevier Collections.)

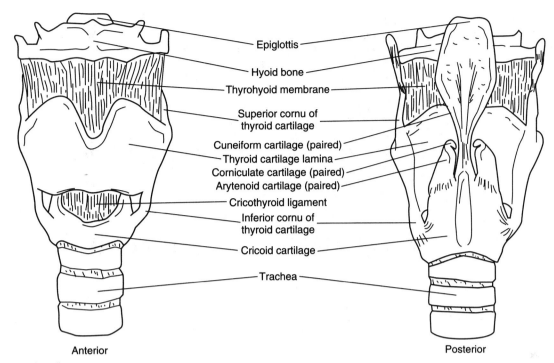

Fig. 7.2 Laryngeal cartilages.

The trachea (windpipe) is an air passageway, approximately 12 cm in length, which extends from the larynx to the fifth thoracic vertebra.[1,2] The trachea lies anterior to the esophagus and bifurcates into the right and left mainstem bronchi. The right and left bronchi progressively branch to form the terminal bronchioles eventually. The lungs consist of smooth muscle innervated by the autonomic nervous system. The lungs extend from just above the clavicles to the diaphragm and are housed within the rib cage. The function and purpose of the upper airway, larynx, trachea, lungs, and pulmonary circulation are to provide exchange of oxygen and carbon dioxide at the alveolar level. A primary concern of the health care provider participating in the administration of sedation and analgesia is to maintain and protect the integrity of respiratory processes. In the presence of comorbid states, synergistic pharmacologic effects, and individual patient variability, protection of the patient's airway may become tenuous during procedural sedation.

What are the essential components of the presedation airway evaluation?

Comprehensive presedation patient assessment is complemented by a focused physical examination, which includes the following:

- Oral cavity evaluation
- Temporomandibular joint evaluation
- Thyromental distance evaluation
- Atlantooccipital movement evaluation
- Physical characteristics related to airway management
- Assignment of a Mallampati airway classification

Equally important is the ability to identify patients with subtle physical anomalies, which may predispose them to the development of respiratory compromise. All patients presenting for sedation and analgesia should undergo a focused physical examination, which includes evaluation of the airway as a key component. A focused physical examination, including vital signs, auscultation of the heart and lungs, and evaluation of the airway, must be conducted on all patients prior to administering moderate procedural sedation and analgesia.

Is it important to inspect the oral cavity during the presedation airway assessment?

The oral cavity identified in Fig. 7.3 is assessed to identify loose, chipped, or capped teeth. Documentation of the presence of dental anomalies, crowns, bridges, and dentures should be completed before the start of the procedure. The oral cavity should also be examined for the presence of tumors or obstruction of airflow.

In the past, I have provided moderate procedural sedation and analgesia to patients with temporomandibular joint inflammation. What is the best way to assess the patient with a history of temporomandibular joint disease?

The assessment of the temporomandibular joint (TMJ; interincisor distance) identified in Fig. 7.4 is conducted with the patient's mouth opened as wide as possible. In the adult, the distance between the upper and lower central incisors is normally 4 to 6 cm (2.54 cm = 1 inch).[3,4] An adult should be able

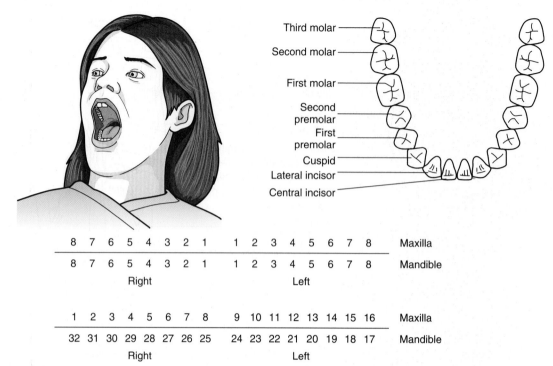

Third molar

Second molar

First molar

Second premolar

First premolar

Cuspid

Lateral incisor

Central incisor

8	7	6	5	4	3	2	1		1	2	3	4	5	6	7	8	Maxilla
8	7	6	5	4	3	2	1		1	2	3	4	5	6	7	8	Mandible

Right   Left

1	2	3	4	5	6	7	8		9	10	11	12	13	14	15	16	Maxilla
32	31	30	29	28	27	26	25		24	23	22	21	20	19	18	17	Mandible

Right   Left

Fig. 7.3 Oral cavity assessment. During this procedure, the patient is instructed to open the mouth wide for the health care practitioner. The oral cavity is then examined for the presence of anomalies that may obstruct airflow or impede instrumentation of the airway in case of an airway emergency.

to open the mouth at least 30–40 mm (two large finger-breadths) between the upper and lower incisors. An interincisor gap of less than two fingerbreadths may be associated with difficult endotracheal intubation. The presence of a clicking sound, pain associated with opening of the mouth, or a reduced

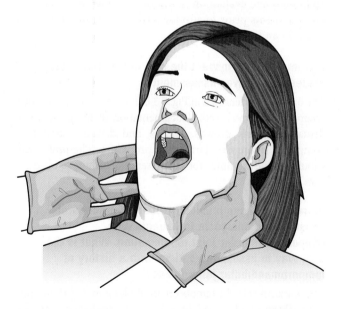

Fig. 7.4 Temporomandibular joint (TMJ) examination. While the patient's mouth is opened during this examination, the clinician may assess joint mobility by palpating the TMJ in an attempt to identify pain or limited range of motion.

ability to open the mouth indicates reduced TMJ mobility. Patients with preexisting TMJ disease may have limited airway mobility if mechanical conduits (e.g., oropharyngeal airways, endotracheal tubes, laryngeal mask airways) are required to treat respiratory distress during procedural sedation care.

Why is measuring the thyromental distance important during the presedation patient assessment?

Thyromental distance represents the straight distance, with the neck fully extended and the mouth closed. As demonstrated in Fig. 7.5, the distance between the prominence of the thyroid cartilage and the bony point of the lower mandibular border should be more than 7 cm (three fingerbreadths). As demonstrated in Fig. 7.6, a distance of less than 7 cm may indicate that the patient may be difficult to intubate, if needed during an airway emergency secondary to the inability to align the oral, pharyngeal, and laryngeal access, which is required for direct visualization and intubation of the larynx. Additionally, side to side movement, neck extension, and neck flexion must be assessed prior to the procedure. Alignment of the three axes required for successful endotracheal intubation—oral, pharyngeal, and laryngeal—requires a combination of flexion and extension with a goal of attaining the sniffing position. Limitations in the ability to achieve the sniffing position can impair laryngoscopy and endotracheal intubation during emergency airway maneuvers. Therefore, as demonstrated in Fig. 7.7, evaluation of the airway includes assessing atlantooccipital movement through full range of motion.

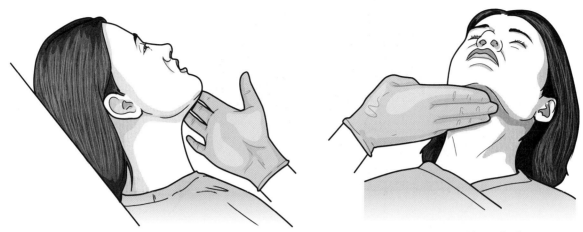

Fig. 7.5 Thyromental distance evaluation. Presedation patient assessment of the airway should reveal a thyromental distance of more than 7 cm (three fingerbreadths).

What physical characteristics are associated with difficult airway management?

The following physical characteristics may indicate the potential for difficult airway management:

- Hypognathous (recessed) jaw
- Prognathic (protruding) jaw
- Deviated trachea
- Large tongue
- Short, thick neck
- Protruding teeth
- High arched palate

Should a Mallampati airway classification be completed during the presedation patient assessment?

The modified Mallampati airway classification system, described in 1983, attempts to grade the degree of difficulty of endotracheal intubation from grades I to IV.[5] The examination is conducted with the patient in a sitting position. The patient's head is maintained in a neutral position, and the mouth is opened as wide as possible (50–60 mm).[6] Classification of the patient's airway is based on a description of the anatomic area visualized

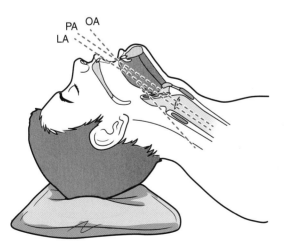

Fig. 7.6 Properly aligned axes. During a respiratory emergency, it is critically important for the health care provider responsible for intubating the patient to align properly three axes (oral axis [OA], pharyngeal axis [PA], laryngeal axis [LA]) for proper endotracheal placement.

(Fig. 7.8). During the examination, the patient is encouraged not to phonate because this maneuver may elevate the soft palate and interfere with accurate classification. The Mallampati classification system should not be used as the only method of airway evaluation and assessment. The system has been criticized secondary to false-positive and false-negative difficult airway identification associated with its use.

Which airway management skills are necessary for the sedation provider to identify and effectively manage a compromised airway during a procedure?

Skilled clinicians engaged in the administration of sedation and analgesia perform thousands of uneventful procedures annually. When complications do arise, the practitioner must immediately recognize the signs and symptoms of airway compromise and deal with them effectively. The pharmacologic effect associated with sedative, hypnotic, and analgesic medications in combination is synergistic. This synergism, or the pharmacologic effects of individual medications, alters airway muscle activity. Alterations in airway muscle activity may lead to airway obstruction. Signs and symptoms of airway obstruction include the following:

- Increased respiratory effort
- Sternal retraction
- Rocking chest motion (not in sync with respiratory effort)
- Inspiratory stridor (harsh, high-pitched inspiratory sounds)
- Hypoxemia
- Hypercarbia
- Absence of breath sounds

Although many clinicians believe that airway obstruction occurs from the base of the tongue occluding the airway, research studies have revealed that airway obstruction is a more complex phenomenon.[7] Airway patency is the result of an active mechanism associated with muscles that attach to the hyoid bone and thyroid cartilages. The tonic nature of muscle activity is responsible for maintaining airway patency by functioning as airway dilators, with a resultant increase in airflow and decrease in resistance of breathing. Airway obstruction is a very complex series of architectural changes that involve changes in pharyngeal and laryngeal

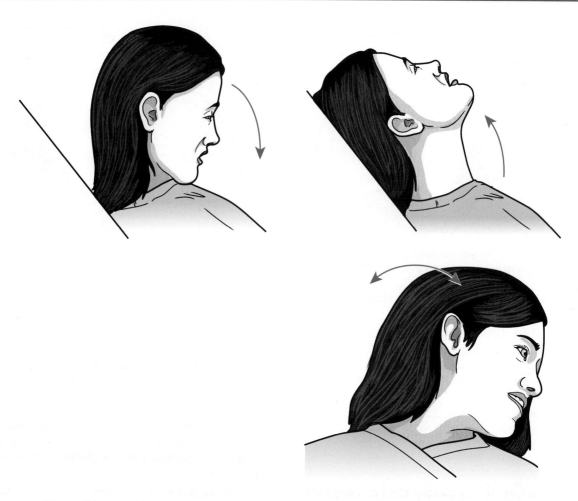

Fig. 7.7 Atlanto occipital movement assessment. This procedure evaluates range of motion through flexion, extension, and side to side movement.

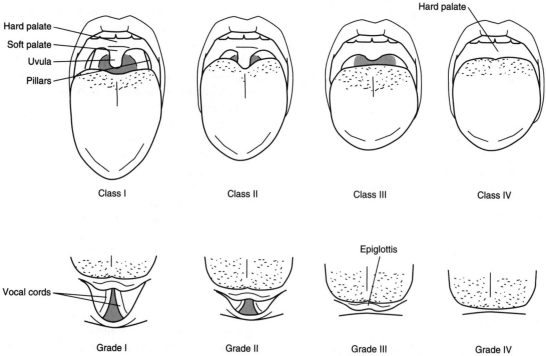

Fig. 7.8 Mallampati airway classification system. A difficult intubation (grade III or IV) may be predicted by the inability to visualize certain pharyngeal structures (class III or IV) during the presedation examination of a sedated patient.

muscle support.[8] The epiglottis or posterior movement of the soft palate is often the cause of airway obstruction. Relief of airway obstruction can be demonstrated through displacement of the hyoid bone anteriorly, with restoration of a patent airway. Therefore, clinical treatment of airway obstruction is not simply clearing the tongue from the posterior pharynx. Fig. 7.9 demonstrates forward displacement of the mandible, with resultant stretch of the front of the neck and elevation of the preepiglottic soft tissues anteriorly, which should restore effective ventilation.[7] Treatment modalities that may restore effective ventilation include the following:

- Auditory and tactile stimulation
- Head tilt
- Chin lift
- Jaw thrust
- Nasal and oral airway insertion
- Pharmacologic reversal of sedative or analgesic (e.g., flumazenil [Romazicon], naloxone [Narcan])

The goal of these interventions is to restore airflow. The sedation airway management algorithm featured in Fig. 7.10 should be used in the event of airway obstruction and respiratory compromise encountered during procedural sedation.

What are the most effective methods to restore airflow during a period of airway obstruction during a sedation procedure?

If verbal and tactile stimulation fail to relieve airway obstruction, the lateral head tilt depicted in Fig. 7.11 is a mechanical maneuver that moves the head from a neutral position to a lateral (side) position. This maneuver may result in tongue displacement from the posterior pharyngeal wall to the side of the oropharynx. Complete or partial relief of upper airway obstruction may occur after use of this maneuver. When the head tilt is unsuccessful, a chin lift may be used. The chin lift

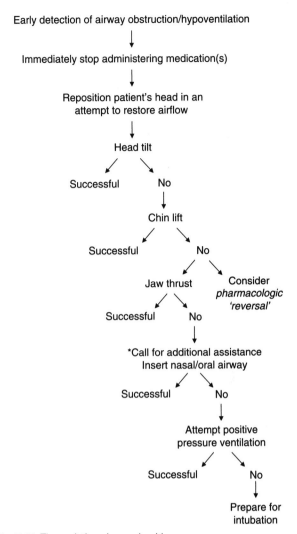

Fig. 7.10 The sedation airway algorithm.

depicted in Fig. 7.12 permits anterior movement of the mandible through superior displacement of the chin. This maneuver, combined with hyperextension of the head and neck and forward displacement of the mandible, will elevate the soft tissue anteriorly.

If verbal or tactile stimulation, head tilt, and chin lift do not produce relief of airway obstruction, the patient has entered a state of deep sedation or general anesthesia. Unless the obstruction is relieved and airflow restored, oxygen desaturation and hypoxemia will ensue. The jaw thrust maneuver depicted in Fig. 7.13 requires the use of both hands. A jaw thrust provides significant anterior displacement of the mandible, stretches the anterior aspects of the neck, and elevates the preepiglottic soft tissues anteriorly. In the event that these maneuvers do not relieve airway obstruction, pharmacologic reversal should be considered. Nonreversible medications may require the use of an oral or nasal airway to relieve obstruction. Airway obstruction not relieved by a head tilt, chin lift, and jaw thrust may require immediate consultation by a certified registered nurse anesthetist or anesthesiologist for additional airway support. See the Patient Safety box to review a situation when a patient obstructed during a routine procedure.

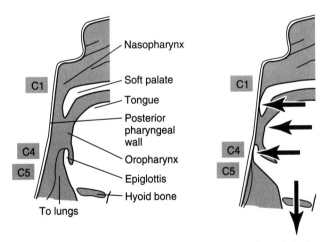

Fig. 7.9 Restoration of effective ventilation. The upper airway is in the sagittal plane. Left, the nasopharynx and oropharynx are patent due to proper tone and position of airway architectural structures. Right, significant posterior displacements of the soft palate and base of the tongue occur. Note also the downward displacement of the hyoid bone. Even with insertion of an oral airway, the soft palate and epiglottic obstructions would likely not resolve. Patient inspiratory effort in (right) could easily provoke even more soft tissue derangement, further exacerbating the airway distress.

Airway Management Strategies for the Sedation Provider

Situation

We recently had a patient that obstructed during a routine GI procedure. Midway through an uneventful procedure, the patient's oxygen saturation quickly decreased to 80%. Oxygen administered via nasal cannula was increased from 2 liters to 6 liters with no improvement in patient status.

Background

The moderate sedation provider observed the patient attempting to make an inspiratory effort; however there was no demonstrated air movement with each respiratory attempt. A jaw thrust eventually restored airflow. However, in the postsedation recovery area, it was noted that the patient had rales in both lung bases and only a slight improvement in oxygen saturation to 88%. Our nurse manager wanted us to discharge the patient to postsedation phase II in spite of the oxygen saturation because we had 27 GI procedures scheduled in our unit for the day.

Assessment

Postobstruction pulmonary edema (POPE) is a physiologic condition that occurs shortly after an airway obstruction. The extreme negative intrapleural pressure that is created by the airway obstruction increases pulmonary transvascular hydrostatic pressure moving fluid from the pulmonary vasculature to the interstitium. The pulmonary lymphatic system eventually cannot clear the fluid, leading to additional fluid movement into the alveoli. Timely diagnosis is dependent on recognition of the following possible symptoms:

- Hypoxia
- Exaggerated hemodynamic effects
  - Hypertension
  - Tachycardia
- Wheezing
- Rales
- Prolonged expiration
- Chest radiograph
  - Bilateral, perihilar, patchy infiltrates
  - Edema around major arteries
- Pink, frothy secretions

Inpatient management is dependent on the degree of POPE. Therapy may consist of endotracheal intubation, intravenous sedatives and muscle relaxants, vasoactive medications, diuretics, and invasive cardiovascular monitoring.

Recommendations

The sedation provider must be cognizant that an upper airway obstruction can quickly lead to the development of postobstruction pulmonary edema. Young, healthy athletic patients may demonstrate a higher incidence of developing POPE secondary to their ability to generate significant negative pressure against a closed glottis opening. Regardless of the etiology of airway obstruction, early recognition of the obstruction by the sedation provider is paramount to decrease the incidence of POPE.

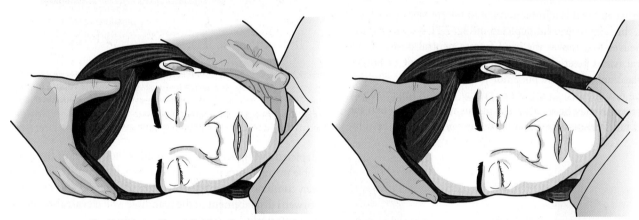

Fig. 7.11 Lateral head tilt. This allows the health care practitioner the ability to move the head from the neutral to the side position, which may result in relief of airway obstruction.

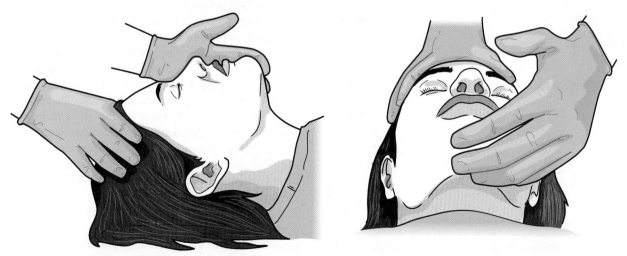

Fig. 7.12 Chin lift. This maneuver places traction on the mentum of the chin, providing forward displacement of the mandible in an attempt to restore air flow. It is important to apply pressure to the bony prominence of the mentum and not to the soft tissue.

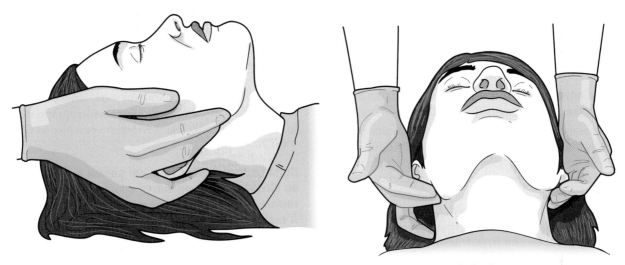

Fig. 7.13 Jaw thrust. This maneuver places significant anterior forward displacement on the jaw in an attempt to relieve obstruction and restore airflow.

If airway obstruction is not corrected with the maneuvers outlined, should a nasal airway be inserted to restore airflow?

If airway obstruction continues after the maneuvers outlined above, an airway conduit may be needed to displace the tongue physically from the posterior pharyngeal wall. In the sedated patient, nasal airways are generally better tolerated than oral airways. Oral airways frequently stimulate the gag reflex, with resultant vomiting or laryngospasm. However, nasal airways are not without risks. Inherent risks associated with nasopharyngeal airway use include epistaxis, hypertension, and difficult placement in patients with nasal deformity. Epistaxis in the presence of respiratory distress results in blood in the oropharynx, which may stimulate laryngospasm or bronchospasm. Nasopharyngeal airways are not recommended in the presence of anticoagulants, cerebrospinal fluid (CSF) rhinorrhea, septal deformity, or nasal polyps. They should not be forced in the presence of obstruction. Insertion of nasopharyngeal airways requires the assessment of nare size. Nasopharyngeal airways come in an assortment of adult sizes:

- 6.0 mm
- 6.5 mm
- 7.0 mm
- 7.5 mm
- 8.0 mm

These sizes for nasopharyngeal airways indicate the internal diameter in millimeters. The larger the internal diameter, the longer the airway.[9] As demonstrated in Fig. 7.14, the nasopharyngeal airway must be long enough to displace the base of the tongue physically from the posterior pharyngeal wall. Approximate length of the nasopharyngeal airway is measured from the tip of the nares to the angle of the jaw or to the earlobe (Fig. 7.15). Prior to insertion, the nasopharyngeal airway should be well lubricated. This can be accomplished with a water-soluble lubricant, such as 2% lidocaine (Xylocaine) jelly, or 5% lidocaine ointment. Lubrication also helps decrease the incidence of epistaxis. During insertion, gentle pressure may be used after initial insertion into the nare. However, one should never force a nasopharyngeal airway

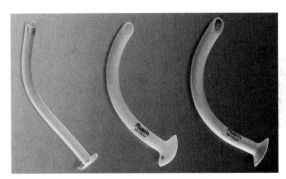

Fig. 7.14 Nasal airways. The nasopharyngeal airway (NPA) is a simple piece of equipment that is easy to use. It is effective and has several advantages when compared to the oropharyngeal airway. Traditional methods of sizing nasopharyngeal airways places emphasis on the width of the patient's nares or little finger, but these are inaccurate and must be abandoned; tube length is more important. Evidence clearly has demonstrated a relationship between nasal airway length and subject height, which is independent of gender. Average height females require a size 6 nasopharyngeal airway and males require a size 7. Optimal and rapid sizing of the NPA can be modified from these average sizes to take account of the subject's height. (From Harkreader H, Hogan MA, Thobaben M: *Fundamentals of Nursing: Caring and Clinical Judgment*. 3rd ed. St Louis: Saunders; 2007.)

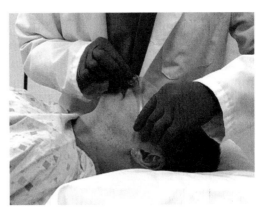

Fig. 7.15 A properly sized nasal airway extends from the tip of the patient's nose to the angle of the jaw or the earlobe. (From Roberts J: *Roberts and Hedges' Clinical Procedures in Emergency Medicine*. 6th ed. Philadelphia: Saunders; 2014.)

that is impeded in the posterior nasopharynx. The nasal airway must be inserted perpendicularly to the face. Fig. 7.16 demonstrates a properly positioned nasal airway, which provides a physical conduit for air passage.

Are there advantages associated with placing an oral airway in the sedation setting?

Just as a nasopharyngeal airway provides a mechanical passage for airflow, the oropharyngeal airway physically displaces the tongue off the posterior pharyngeal wall. The oropharyngeal airway may stimulate vomiting if the gag reflex remains intact. Additional complications associated with insertion of an oropharyngeal airway include the following:

*   Bradycardia secondary to vagal stimulation
*   Retching with resultant hypertension and tachycardia
*   Laryngospasm
*   Dental damage
*   Pharyngeal or lip lacerations

When indicated, insertion of an oropharyngeal airway must be performed carefully to avoid the complications noted previously. Proper placement of an oropharyngeal airway, depicted in Fig. 7.17, is outlined in Box 7.1. Patients who require and tolerate the insertion of nasal and/or oral airways have entered into a state of deep sedation or general anesthesia.

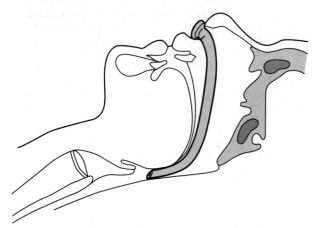

Fig. 7.16 The nasopharyngeal airway in place. The airway passes through the nose and extends to just above the epiglottis.

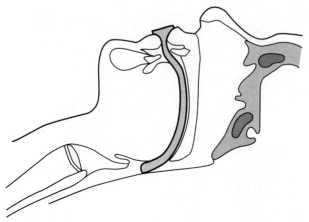

Fig. 7.17 The oropharyngeal airway in place. The airway follows the curvature of the tongue, pulling it in and the epiglottis away from the posterior pharyngeal wall and providing a channel for air passage.

When is it appropriate to reverse a patient pharmacologically?

Consideration should be given to the administration of pharmacologic antagonists to reverse the respiratory depressant effects associated with benzodiazepines and narcotic medications. A complete pharmacokinetic and pharmacodynamic profile of these medications and appropriate times to consider pharmacologic reversal are provided in Chapters 4 and 5.

During a recent procedure, our patient experienced an airway obstruction during which we could not restore effective airflow or reverse it pharmacologically. A rapid response team was called. When the anesthesia team arrived, they stated that the patient was experiencing a laryngospasm. What is a laryngospasm?

Laryngospasm is a spasm of the laryngeal musculature. It can be initiated by mucus, blood, or saliva irritating the vocal cords. Laryngospasm results in complete or partial closure of the cords, with inability of the patient to ventilate. Patients with total airway obstruction will often display "rocky" abdominal respirations with no air exchange. Untreated, laryngospasm predisposes the patient to the following:

*   Hypoxemia
*   Hypercarbia
*   Respiratory acidosis
*   Negative-pressure pulmonary edema
    *   Results from the patient attempting to breathe against a closed glottis opening, which generates a negative intrathoracic pressure (pulling fluid out of the intravascular fluid and into the alveoli)

Initial treatment for laryngospasm is positive pressure ventilation with 100% oxygen. A secure mask fit is required to generate positive pressure to break the spasm. If this maneuver is unsuccessful, an anesthesia provider or airway management expert should be summoned immediately. A nonparalyzing dose ($\approx 10\%$ of the full intubating dose) of succinylcholine is administered. Due to the need for advanced airway support associated with the use of muscle relaxants, this treatment modality should only be attempted by airway management experts. Coupled with ventilatory support, relaxation of the skeletal muscles of the larynx generally ensues. If necessary, endotracheal intubation is used as a last resort to break a laryngospasm.

Are there any additional treatment options for laryngospasm?

When head tilt, chin lift, jaw thrust, and pharmacologic reversal are not effective, there is a noninvasive maneuver that can also be implemented. In 1998, Dr. Philip Larson, in the journal *Anesthesiology*, described a physical maneuver that had been used for decades by Dr. N.P. Guadagni.[10] As outlined in Fig. 7.18, the laryngospasm notch is located behind the earlobe. The notch can be located by placing the middle (or index) finger toward the base of the skull and placing the tip of the finger on the mastoid process. Moving the finger anteriorly until the ascending ramus of the mandible is

1. Carefully open the patient's mouth, exercising caution to prevent finger injury to the clinician or dental damage to the patient.
2. Once the mouth is open, insert the tongue blade into the posterior pharynx.
3. Insert the tongue blade toward the base of the tongue. Apply pressure with the tongue blade to displace the base of the tongue anteriorly.
4. Insert the oropharyngeal airway into the oropharynx. The oropharyngeal airway is designed to follow the natural curvature of the oropharynx. The tongue blade should expose a clear view of the posterior oropharynx. Do not force or blindly position the oropharyngeal airway. Malpositioning the oropharyngeal airway can force the base of the tongue against the posterior pharyngeal wall, completely obstructing the airway.
5. After insertion, verify that the tongue and lips have not been inadvertently positioned between the teeth.
6. A patient who tolerates the insertion of an oropharyngeal airway is deeply sedated and, at this point, the practitioner is advised to consult an anesthesia practitioner to provide additional airway management assistance.

palpated may require moving the finger down and slightly caudad. The laryngospasm notch becomes apparent when cephalad pressure is applied in between the mastoid and the ascending ramus of the mandible. Treatment of a laryngospasm with the Larson maneuver requires the application of firm inward pressure at a point as superior as you can go in the notch.

Next, firmly push both sides inward toward the skull base. Finally, applying simultaneous anterior pressure, similar to a jaw thrust maneuver in the notch, should break the laryngospasm within one or two breaths.

It is unclear why the Larson maneuver works. Potential theories include the following:

- You are just performing a jaw thrust maneuver.
- You are providing deep and painful stimuli, which cause the vocal cords to relax.
- You are stimulating deep cranial nerves, which also happen to stimulate the vagus nerve.

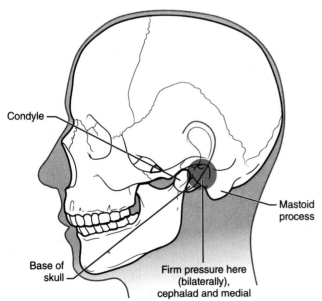

Fig. 7.18 The laryngospasm notch, first described by Dr. Philip Larson in 1998, becomes apparent when cephalad pressure is applied in between the mastoid and the ascending ramus of the mandible.

We have a physician who provides extremely deep sedation for procedures. The patients frequently become apneic. Many times during the procedure, I don't feel competent to manage the deeply sedated patient airway effectively. What is the most effective way to manage an obstructed patient's airway emergently?

Moderate sedation is typically the goal for most procedures. In most settings, if deep sedation or general anesthesia is required, a credentialed anesthesia provider must be consulted. However, it is common for moderate sedation to become deep sedation with only small incremental dosage increases. Therefore, all providers involved in moderate sedation must be familiar with deep sedation rescue approaches, including relief of upper airway obstruction and effective treatment modalities for respiratory insufficiency.

Upper airway obstruction and respiratory insufficiency should be recognized promptly and treated effectively. Mechanisms to relieve upper airway obstruction must be provided in a systematic manner, as outlined in the sedation airway algorithm (see Fig. 7.10). In the presence of respiratory depression, apnea, or airway obstruction, the health care provider must be prepared to ventilate the patient with a positive pressure breathing device. If all maneuvers previously outlined fail to relieve upper airway obstruction and do not restore effective ventilation, an airway management expert should be summoned emergently to correct the airway obstruction and administer positive pressure ventilation.

Commercially available bag-valve-mask devices are disposable systems for single-patient use. One disposable mask is generally packaged with this system for use with the bag-valve device. It is important to note that many of the masks packaged with these units are large adult sizes. However, the facial anatomy of each individual patient may be markedly different on the basis of factors such as patient weight, mandibular size, age, nutritional status, presence of facial hair, and dentition.

Therefore, it is important to select a properly sized mask based on these individualized patient factors. To account for patient variability, a variety of disposable masks sizes must be immediately available in each sedation area. It is critical to have an assortment of these masks on hand prior to the commencement of any sedation procedure. As identified in Fig. 7.19, a properly fitting mask should fit snugly between the bridge of the patient's nose, the mentum or the chin, and the medial aspects of the face. Masks that extend above the bridge of the nose, below the level of the mandible, or past the lateral aspects of the face are inappropriately sized. This results in ineffective positive pressure ventilation.

To secure an appropriate mask fit for positive pressure ventilation, the mask must form an effective seal between the skin of the face and the mask. Once the mask has been properly positioned (Fig. 7.20), the third and fourth or fourth and fifth fingers (depending on the clinician's hand size) are placed on the mandible. This maneuver elevates the jaw and the base of the tongue off the posterior pharyngeal wall. On delivery of the first positive pressure ventilation, there should be chest rise and fall, breath sounds, and no air escape around the mask. If the patient remains apneic, positive pressure ventilation should ensue at a rate of 16 to 20 breaths/min until additional assistance arrives. Preparation for a respiratory emergency is required whenever sedation or analgesia is administered. When summoned, anesthesia personnel or the attending physician will need specific equipment and supplies to secure the airway and establish effective ventilation. Therefore, it is important to maintain specific emergency airway equipment at each designated sedation location.

What is the most effective way to use a bag-valve-mask for a sedation patient who is hypoventilating?

It is important for the clinician participating in the administration of sedation to ventilate patients efficiently and effectively. As outlined earlier, the provider must be cognizant of airway obstruction and take definitive action when necessary. In the presence of apnea, hypoxemia, or respiratory

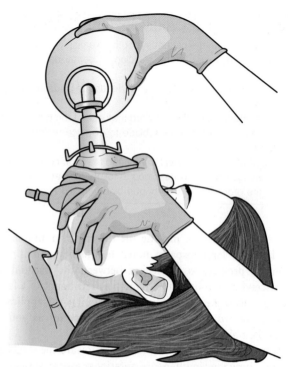

Fig. 7.20 Positive pressure ventilation. An effective seal is formed by placing the third, fourth, and fifth fingers below the mandible and exerting gentle pressure on the bridge of the nose. A proper mask does not allow oxygen to escape between the patient's face and mask seal. Note how the hands produce an effective mask seal and also extend the head to produce a patent airway.

distress, positive pressure ventilation must be used. In emergent situations, the bag-valve-mask is the ventilation system of choice to deliver oxygen-enriched positive pressure ventilation to the patient. Manual resuscitative devices are known by a variety of names, including the following:
- Bag-valve mask
- Bag-valve resuscitative device
- Respiratory bag
- Self-inflating resuscitator
- Ambu bag
  Advantages of bag-valve-masks include the following:
- Inexpensive
- Permit an enriched oxygen environment
- Portable
- Lightweight
The bag of the resuscitator is self-inflating and is coupled with a nonrebreathing valve to prevent rebreathing of exhaled gases. After oxygen is delivered into the self-inflating bag, inspired oxygen concentration increases. Some bags also have an additional reservoir, which allows an opportunity for oxygen to accumulate. Oxygen flows directly into the self-inflating bag when the refill valve opens. During a respiratory crisis, the oxygen flow rate should be 10 to 15 liters per minute in the adult patient. Positive pressure ventilation requires the clinician to grasp the self-inflating bag in the middle, with firm pressure,

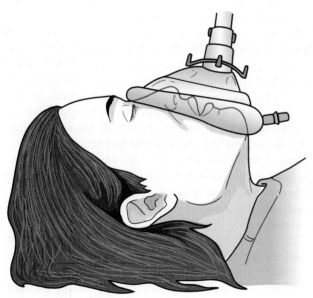

Fig. 7.19 Properly fitting mask.

and depress the bag to deliver effective ventilation. If the patient is not completely apneic, delivery of manual ventilation should be synchronized with the inspiratory phase of the patient. Complications associated with use of bag-valve-mask devices are generally related to valve failure, with resultant rebreathing of expired gases and decreased Fio_2. An additional complication is gastric insufflation secondary to attempted ventilation through a nonpatent airway. Since the advent of disposable single-use units, these complications occur with less frequency. A bag-valve-mask device that is self-inflating must be present with a backup source of oxygen available in each sedation practice setting. A backup oxygen source (E cylinder) should be present in the event that the regular tank system or hospital pipeline system fails.

What is the best method to troubleshoot difficulties encountered when managing a patient's obstructed airway with a bag-valve-mask device in the sedation setting?

Troubleshooting techniques to consider when using a bag-valve-mask (BVM) device are identified in Table 7.1. The table is organized using the MOANS acronym, which identifies difficulties that may be encountered when using a BVM, along with potential solutions.

In the event effective airflow is not restored with BVM ventilation, the SOAP-ME mnemonic is an effective preintubation checklist to ensure that all supplies are always immediately available in the event of a respiratory emergency in the sedation setting.[11] The SOAP-ME mnemonic is defined as follows:

- **S**uction: Yankauer suction catheter on the right side of the patient's head, within reach of the operator's right hand during laryngoscopy. When properly connected, the suction is audible and palpable when the tip of the Yankauer wand is touched against the hand.
- **O**xygen: BVM resuscitator with a positive end-expiratory pressure (PEEP) valve connected to an oxygen source turned all the way up (>15 L/min). The flow of oxygen should be audible and high enough to fill the reservoir bag or tubing. Squeeze the bag against the hand to verify positive pressure. A nasal cannula should be on the patient prior to intubation.
- **A**irways: Oral and nasal airways and rescue ventilation devices. The cuff of the tracheal tube should be checked and fully deflated. The tracheal tube should have a stylet inserted. The tip of the stylet should stop at or before the distal edge of the cuff, leaving the last 2 to 3 cm of the tube flexible.
- **P**ositioning and preoxygenation: Preoxygenation, 4 minutes, with nasal cannula and mask if possible. Position patient as upright as possible. A nasal cannula should be administered with the oxygen flow rate at 4 to 6 L/min in wide-awake patients, not hypoxic patients; 15 L/min should be administered in critically hypoxic, severely dyspneic patients.
- **M**onitoring equipment and medications: Sedation patients are monitored throughout the procedure. During emergent intubation, the laryngoscopist should clearly

TABLE 7.1 Troubleshooting Bag-Valve-Mask Problems[a]

Parameter	Difficulty	Solutions
Mask seal	Difficulty maintaining mask seal on patients with facial hair, large facial structures, or no teeth	Use water-soluble lubricant over facial hair to seal contact between mask and face. Use oral airway if having difficulty obtaining adequate seal with facial hair or no teeth. Consider two-hand, two-person ventilation.
Obese patient	Difficulty maintaining mask seal and providing adequate breaths due to increased redundant tissue (e.g., large tongue, thick neck, excess adipose tissue around face or neck) around upper airway, which can lead to obstruction	Use oral or nasal airway to displace redundant tissue and open airway. Place patient in reverse Trendelenburg position with a roll under patient's head when attempting to use BVM. This displaces excess abdominal and chest tissue weight, allowing improved chest expansion with ventilation. The goal is to achieve a horizontal line from the external auditory meatus to the sternal notch. In morbidly obese patients, the two-person technique works best.
Age > 55 years	Difficulty maintaining mask seal with older patients	Use an oral airway to open patient's airway. Leave dentures in place to improve mask seal.
No teeth	Difficulty maintaining mask seal on patients with poor dentition or no teeth	Use oral airway to improve mask seal. Leave dentures in place to improve mask seal.
Stiff	Difficulty providing adequate breaths to patients with asthma, COPD or ARDS or who are pregnant	Use albuterol or ipratropium to bronchodilate lungs; use PEEP valve, if available.

[a]This table, organized using the MOANS acronym, lists difficulties you might encounter when using a bag-valve-mask (BVM), along with potential solutions.
ARDS, Acute respiratory distress syndrome; *BVM*, bag-valve-mask *COPD*, chronic obstructive pulmonary disease; *PEEP*, positive end-expiratory pressure.
From Vo H, Park M, Wang S. Effective bag-valve-mask ventilation saves lives. Am Nurse Today. 12(2):8.

communicate with the team regarding the sequence and timing of intubation medications.

- *E*nd-tidal CO_2 device: End-tidal carbon dioxide monitoring is required for sedation procedures and to ensure that emergent intubation efforts were successful.

In addition to the SOAP-ME mnemonic, is there any additional information related to emergency airway equipment in the sedation setting that is helpful to the health care provider administering moderate procedural sedation and analgesia?

An assortment of endotracheal tubes must be kept on hand at all times for the variety of age groups receiving moderate procedural sedation and analgesia. Endotracheal tube sizes are designated in millimeters of internal diameter. Table 7.2 lists recommended endotracheal tube sizes according to patient age.

An endotracheal stylet (Fig. 7.21) is a polyvinylchloride or aluminum instrument that provides rigidity to the endotracheal tube. It enhances the clinician's ability to place the endotracheal tube in a variety of positions to aid in the intubation process. Stylets allow the endotracheal tube to be directed through the glottic opening and are frequently used for difficult intubations. Stylets are available in malleable aluminum or metal, with or without a rubberized cover. Adult and pediatric sizes are available, and the stylet should not extend past the tip of the endotracheal tube or into the Murphy eye. The Murphy eye is the eponymous name for a hole on the side of most endotracheal tubes (ETTs) that functions as a vent and prevents complete obstruction of the patient's airway should the primary distal opening of an endotracheal tube become occluded. To facilitate the insertion and easy removal of stylets from endotracheal tubes, a water-soluble lubricant should be applied along their axis before insertion.

The laryngoscope handle and blade are used to manipulate the oropharyngeal tissue and epiglottis. The blade

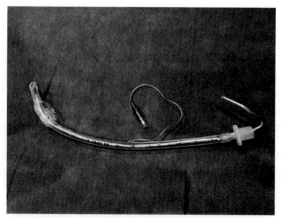

Fig. 7.21 Endotracheal tube stylet. Stylets should be well lubricated before insertion into the endotracheal tube. The stylet must be bent to prevent the proximal end from extending past the tip of the endotracheal tube.

provides the ability to visualize the glottic aperture and facilitates insertion of the endotracheal tube into the trachea. The laryngoscope handle serves a dual function. First, it acts as a power supply that is powered by NiCad or alkaline batteries. Its second function is to act as a receptacle for the blade. Various blades are available for use with the handle. Selection of a blade depends on patient age, anatomic variabilities of the patient, and clinician preference. Age-appropriate selection of blades listed in Fig. 7.22 should be followed in each practice setting. In most adults, intubation can be done successfully with a Macintosh no. 3 blade or a Miller no. 2 blade. Having both readily available significantly enhances the clinician's ability to secure endotracheal tube placement and a patent airway in emergent situations.

Magill forceps are ancillary airway tools used to direct an endotracheal tube during nasotracheal intubation. Endotracheal tubes inserted for nasotracheal intubation hug the posterior pharyngeal wall and may require use of the Magill forceps to direct the tube distally and anteriorly and through the glottic opening.

Various types of suction equipment are currently available. An ample supply of suction liners, filters, tubing, and suction tips must be readily available at each sedation location. In areas where sedation procedures are performed concurrently, one suction unit must be available for each patient. Yankauer suction tips aspirate large volumes of material from the oropharynx. They also offer the advantage of aspirating larger particulate matter. Disadvantages associated with the use of Yankauer suction tips include lip laceration, oropharyngeal damage, and dental trauma. No. 16-Fr suction catheters must be available to suction the oropharynx in case of a patient biting or clenching down. Advantages of 16-Fr suction catheters include insertion into small areas and the nasopharynx. Use of emergency airway equipment for respiratory resuscitation

TABLE 7.2 Recommended Endotracheal Tube Sizes Based on Patient Age	
Age	**Endotracheal Tube Size (internal diameter, mm)**
Newborn	3.0
6 months	3.5
18 months	4.0
36 months	4.5
5 years	5.0
6 years	5.5
8 years	6.0
12 years	6.5
16 years	6.5–7.0
Adult female	7.0
Adult male	8.0

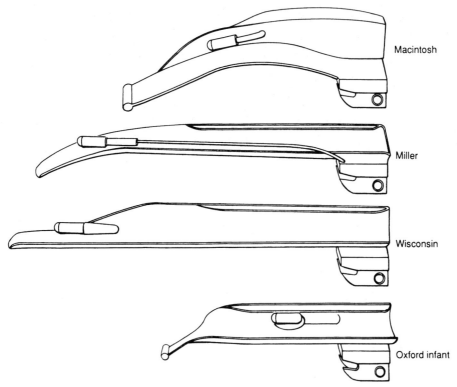

Macintosh

Miller

Wisconsin

Oxford infant

Fig. 7.22 Laryngoscope blades.

BOX 7.2 Minimum Recommended Emergency Airway Setup

- Nasopharyngeal airways (age-appropriate sizes)
- Oropharyngeal airways (age-appropriate sizes)
- Tongue blades
- Lidocaine (Xylocaine) ointment or jelly and water-soluble lubricant
- Two laryngoscope handles
- Two Macintosh blades (age-appropriate sizes)
- Two Miller blades (age-appropriate sizes)
- Spare blade light bulbs
- Endotracheal tubes (age-appropriate sizes)

- Two stylets (adult and pediatric)
- Magill forceps (adult and pediatric)
- Suction units
- Yankauer suction tips
- No. 16-Fr suction catheters
- Supplemental oxygen E cylinders
- Oxygen
- Bag-valve-mask device
- Face mask (age-appropriate size)

---

is dependent on clinician preference, degree of respiratory distress, and patient's anatomy. Box 7.2 outlines a minimum recommended emergency airway setup. An ample supply of respiratory equipment must be immediately available in all sedation locations.

Which methods of oxygen delivery are most effective in the sedation setting?

Supplemental oxygen may be administered by a variety of methods. The primary goal of oxygen therapy is the prevention of hypoxia, hypoventilation, and respiratory depression. Table 7.3 lists oxygen systems available to deliver an

enriched oxygen environment to the patient. Because of the respiratory depressant effects associated with all sedatives, hypnotics, and analgesics, serious consideration should be given to the administration of supplemental oxygen to all patients receiving sedation or analgesia unless specifically contraindicated.

Nasal cannulas are low-flow oxygen administration systems that increase the patient's inspired oxygen concentration. Comfortable and inexpensive, they increase the inspired oxygen concentration and allow the nasopharynx to serve as an oxygen reservoir. Inspired oxygen concentration increases 3% to 4% for each liter delivered through the nasal cannula.[12] Nasal cannulas are not recommended

TABLE 7.3   Methods of Oxygen Administration

Method	Fio_2	Flow (L/min)	Comments
Low-Flow Method			
Nasal cannula (prongs)	0.24–0.45	1–6	Comfortable to wear, patient can breathe orally or nasally and still raise Fio_2, humidification unnecessary
Simple face mask	0.4–0.6	10	Adjustable to fit face, may be hot for patients, poorly tolerated, potential for skin irritation from tight fit and oxygen contact
Face tent	0.3–0.55	4–10	Less confining, useful when extra humidity is needed
Partial rebreathing mask	0.35–0.6	6–10	Mask with attached reservoir bag, no valves on mask (exhalation ports open)
High-Flow Method			
Nonrebreathing mask	0.4–1.0	6–15	Mask with reservoir bag, one-way valves on mask, side ports of mask, one-way valve between mask and bag for inhalation
Venturi mask	0.24–0.55	2–14	Believed accurate delivery of desired Fio_2, may be less if patient is hyperpneic or unable to keep mask in position on face
T-piece or Brigg's	0.21–1	2–10	Used with endotracheal or tracheostomy tube, provides accurate delivery of desired Fio_2 and humidification, most often used in weaning patients from ventilator assistance before endotracheal tube removal
Mechanical ventilator	0.21–1	Direct from supply	Pressure, volume, flow, and oxygen percentage all adjustable

Fio_2, Fraction of inspired oxygen concentration.
From Odom-Forren J: *Drain's Perianesthesia Nursing: A Critical Care Approach*. 7th ed. St. Louis: Elsevier; 2018.

for flow rates exceeding 4 to 5 L/min. Flow rates greater than 4 L/min may lead to drying of mucous membranes, irritation, and bleeding.

Simple oxygen face masks permit delivery of inspired oxygen of 40% to 60%. This increase in Fio_2 occurs secondary to increased reservoir space and oxygen flow. An Fio_2 of 40% to 60% depends on oxygen flow rate, the patient's inspiratory flow, and mask fit. Nonrebreathing masks offer a distinct advantage of a reservoir bag to the oxygen face mask in that it allows delivery of up to 100% oxygen when a tight face seal is assured. Rebreathing is diminished through a combination of unidirectional valves and high inspiratory flow rates.

Clinicians engaged in caring for patients receiving any degree of sedation must be prepared to manage airway compromise. Airway obstruction, arterial desaturation, and respiratory insufficiency may develop secondary to the synergistic effects of the medication or untoward patient response. Health care providers who assume the responsibility of administering sedative and opioid medications must be clinically competent to respond to airway emergencies. A BVM device that is self-inflating must be available, along with a backup source of oxygen, in each sedation practice setting.

Our nurse manager recently informed our sedation team that we will be using a new oxygen delivery device to administer oxygen during interventional radiology procedures. Which new oxygen delivery devices have been released for patient use?

There are a variety of new oxygen delivery products available for use in the sedation setting. A current option for oxygen administration is the SuperNO$_2$VA™ (nasal oxygenation and ventilation apparatus). The device featured in Fig. 7.23 is a new solution to address the impact of sedation and general anesthesia on the patient's airway. It is designed to deliver positive pressure while providing access to the oral cavity.

The SuperNO$_2$VA™ is a nasal mask that was designed to create a tight seal, deliver gas, and provide positive pressure when placed over a patient's nose. The SuperNO$_2$VA™ only covers the patient's nose, making it ideal for all sedation cases, particularly intraoral procedures such as the following:

- Upper endoscopy
- Colonoscopy
- Bronchoscopy
- Fiberoptic intubation
- Laryngoscopy
- MRI procedures

Effective airway management

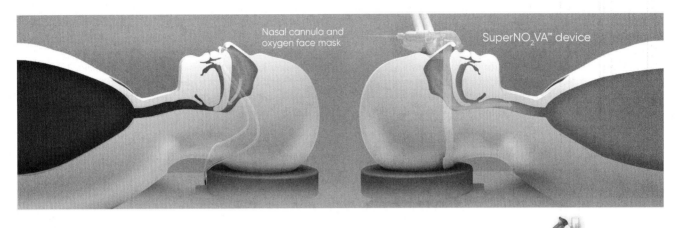

Competitive advantage

	Nasal cannula	High Flow nasal cannula	Anesthesia mask	Nasal CPAP	SuperNO₂VA™
Oral access	●	●	○	●	●
Passive oxygenation	●	●	●	●	●
High flow O₂	○	●	○	○	●
Rescue ventilation/RC	○	○	●	○	●
Additional capital equipment	Not required	●	Not required	●	Not required

Confident maintenance of perioperative airway patency

PRE-OP   INTRA-OP   POST-OP

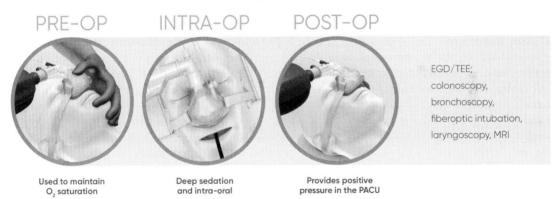

EGD/TEE;
colonoscopy,
bronchoscopy,
fiberoptic intubation,
laryngoscopy, MRI

Used to maintain O₂ saturation   **Deep sedation and intra-oral**   **Provides positive pressure in the PACU**

Fig. 7.23 The goal of the SuperNO₂VA device is to generate a positive nasal pressure that is capable of maintaining upper airway patency, deliver PEEP and ventilatory support, and provide rescue nasal ventilation during the procedural period. (© 2019 Vyaire Medical; Used with permission.)

SUMMARY

Clinicians engaged in caring for patients receiving any degree of sedation must be prepared to manage airway compromise. Airway obstruction, arterial desaturation, and respiratory insufficiency may develop secondary to the synergistic effects of the medication or an untoward patient response. Health care providers who assume the responsibility of administering sedative and opioid medications must be clinically competent to respond to airway emergencies. A self-inflating BVM device must be present, along with a backup source of oxygen in each sedation practice setting.

REFERENCES

1. Harjeet K, Sahni D, Batra YK, Rajeev S. Anatomical dimensions of trachea, main bronchi, subcarinal and bronchial angles in fetuses measured ex vivo. *Paediatric Anaesthesia*. 2008;18:1029–1034.
2. Skandalakis LJ, Skandalakis JE, Skandalakis PN. *Surgical Anatomy and Technique: A Pocket Manual*. 3rd ed. New York, NY: Springer; 2009.

3. Rose DK, Cohen MM. The airway: Problems and predictions in 18,500 patients. *Canadian Journal of Anaesthesia.* 1994;41:372–383.

4. Block C, Brechner VL. Unusual problems in airway management. II. The influence of the temporomandibular joint, the mandible, and associated structures on endotracheal intubation. *Anesthesia and Analgesia.* 1971;50:114–123.

5. Danielson DR. Management of the difficult airway. In: Lampert R, Ross A, Thorp D, eds. *Anesthesiology Review.* New York: Churchill-Livingstone; 2002:482–484.

6. Miller R, Cohen M, Fleisher L, et al. *Miller's Anesthesia.* 8th ed. Philadelphia: Elsevier; 2015.

7. Biddle C. Reflections on "maintaining an airway." *Current Review Perianesthesia Nursing.* 15:169–176.

8. Boidin MP. Airway patency in the unconscious patient. *British Journal of Anaesthesia.* 1985;57:306–310.

9. Butterworth JF, Wasnik JD, Mackey DC. *Clinical Anesthesiology.* 6th ed. New York: Lange Medical Books and McGraw-Hill; 2018.

10. Larson CP. Laryngospasm–the best treatment. *Anesthesiology.* 1998;89:1293–1294.

11. Levitan R. *Fundamentals of Airway Management.* 3rd ed. Irving, TX: Emergency Medicine Residents' Association; 2015.

12. McDonald CF. Low-flow oxygen: How much is your patient really getting? *Respirology.* 2014;19:469–470. https://doi.org/10.1111/resp.12290.

CHAPTER 7: REVIEW QUESTIONS

1. A pulmonary condition characterized by reduced gas exchange that is inadequate to meet the body's metabolic demand is identified as _____.
   A. Pulmonary embolus
   B. Pulmonary obstruction
   C. Respiratory arrest
   D. Respiratory insufficiency

2. Identification of loose, chipped, or capped teeth and observation of tumors or physical anomalies, which may interfere with procedural airway management, take place during which of the following presedation examinations?
   A. Temporomandibular joint examination
   B. Atlantooccipital movement examination
   C. Assignment of Mallampati airway classification
   D. Oral cavity inspection

3. During assessment of the temporomandibular joint (interincisor distance), the distance between the upper and lower central incisors is normally _____.
   A. 1–2 cm
   B. 3–4 cm
   C. 4–6 cm
   D. 15–18 cm

4. A normal thyromental distance during physical examination would reveal a distance of _____.
   A. <2 cm
   B. <4 cm
   C. >7 cm
   D. >28 cm

5. A mechanical maneuver used initially to restore airflow during airway obstruction, which moves the head from the neutral position to the side position, is identified as a _____.
   A. Chin lift
   B. Lateral head tilt
   C. Jaw thrust
   D. Finger sweep

6. Epistaxis (nasal bleeding) may be associated with which of the following airway maneuvers?
   A. Oral airway insertion
   B. Nasal airway insertion
   C. Chin lift
   D. Jaw thrust

7. Positive airway pressure may be delivered to the sedated patient in respiratory distress by which of the following devices?
   A. Nasal airway
   B. Oxygen cylinder
   C. Self-inflating bag valve mask
   D. Oral airway

8. One of the primary goals of oxygen therapy is the _____.
   A. Prevention of anoxia
   B. Treatment of airway obstruction
   C. Prevention of hypoxia, hypoventilation, and respiratory depression
   D. Elimination of carbon dioxide

9. Which of the following airway devices provides an increase in oxygen concentration of 3% to 4% for each liter delivered?
   A. Continuous positive airway pressure (CPAP) machine
   B. Oral airway
   C. Endotracheal tube
   D. Nasal cannula

10. Which of the following is not a sign of airway obstruction?
    A. Inspiratory stridor
    B. Hypercarbia
    C. Hypoxemia
    D. Hypocarbia

11. Which of the following respiratory complications results in rocky respirations and may be initiated by the presence of blood or mucus on the vocal cords requiring immediate intervention?
    A. Bronchospasm
    B. Laryngospasm
    C. Stridorous spasm
    D. Vagal episode

12. A presedation assessment Mallampati classification of IV indicates to the provider that the patient's airway anatomy should be easy to visualize in the event intubation is required.
    A. True
    B. False

Answers can be found in Appendix A.

Sedation Monitoring Modalities

LEARNING OUTCOMES

At the completion of this chapter, the learner shall:

- Delineate the rationale, advantages, and disadvantages associated with the following monitoring parameters used during sedation procedures:
  - Electrocardiogram (ECG)
  - Blood pressure
  - Pulse oximetry
  - Level of consciousness
  - End-tidal carbon dioxide
- Describe which ECG lead positions are best used in the detection of dysrhythmias versus ischemia.

- Interpret three types of dysrhythmias that may affect the patient's physiologic status during a sedation procedure.
- Analyze three factors that contribute to the development of hypotension.
- Apply recommended treatment protocols for hypotension and hypertension and their prescribed treatment protocols.
- Differentiate the advantages associated with the use of end-tidal carbon dioxide monitoring during sedation procedures.
- Describe components of the sedation and analgesia record.

COMPETENCY STATEMENT

The health care practitioner administering moderate procedural sedation and analgesia shall have no other responsibilities that compromise the continuous monitoring and assessment of the patient during diagnostic, therapeutic, or surgical procedures.

Occasionally, our interventional platform is short-staffed. Our manager frequently reassigns nurses from other units to administer moderate procedural sedation and analgesia within our interventional platform. Most of these nurses have not completed the moderate sedation education course offered by our hospital and have no working knowledge of the procedural medications administered to these patients. Is our manager exposing the hospital to additional risk by reassigning these nurses to our interventional platform?

To prevent patient harm, avoid catastrophic mishaps, and comply with promulgated practice standards, practice guidelines, position statements, and specific state statutes, all health care providers must demonstrate competency and critical thinking skills in the sedation setting. Completion of requisite sedation educational competencies is a mandatory requirement for all health care providers prior to accepting any patient assignment. The sedation skill set for purposes of this chapter includes familiarity with monitoring equipment and interpretation of the following monitoring processes:

- Observation and vigilance
- Interpretation of data
- Initiation of corrective action when required

How important is ECG monitoring during procedural patient care in the sedation setting?

The ECG is used during moderate sedation and analgesia procedures to assist in the detection of the following conditions:

- Dysrhythmias
- Myocardial ischemia
- Electrolyte disturbance
- Pacemaker function

How does the electrocardiogram detect cardiac rhythm disturbances and conduction disorders?

The ECG reflects the electrical activity of the heart in graphic form. Electrodes pick up electrical signals generated by the heart's conduction system. Electrodes may be placed on the four limbs and six areas on the chest. With time, it was recognized that the same recording could be made by placing the electrode on the shoulders and hips, which also resulted in less opportunity for noise to interfere with recordings. ECG monitoring is useful in the evaluation of the pathophysiologic condition of the entire heart, with detection of cardiac rhythm disturbances and conduction disorders. Most ECG monitors depict cardiac electrical activity through a single lead. Lead position is determined by the placement of positive and negative electrodes secured to the patient. The standard leads view the frontal plane of the heart, with differences in electrical potential recorded in the left arm, the right arm, and the left leg.[1] Standard bipolar limb leads include the following:

- Lead I. Difference in electrical potential between the left arm and the right arm
  - Heart surface viewed, lateral

- Lead II. Difference in electrical potential between the left leg and the right arm
  - Heart surface viewed, inferior
- Lead III. Difference in electrical potential between the left leg and the left arm
  - Heart surface viewed, inferior

Augmented limb leads reflect the electrical potential between the designated extremity lead and a neutral electrical point at the center of the heart.[1] The three augmented leads view the heart in the frontal plane by means of the same three limbs in different combinations. The augmented or unipolar limb leads include the following:

- aVR. Augmented voltage of the right arm. The right arm is positive compared with the reference electrode.
  - Heart surface viewed, none
- aVL. Augmented voltage of the left arm. The left arm is positive compared with the reference electrode.
  - Heart surface viewed, lateral
- aVF. Augmented voltage of the left foot. The left foot is positive compared with the reference electrode.
  - Heart surface viewed, inferior

Fig. 8.1 depicts the view of the standard limb leads and augmented leads. The unipolar precordial leads measure the heart's electrical activity in the horizontal planes.

- Lead V_1 is placed on the right side of sternum, fourth intercostal space.
  - Heart area viewed, interventricular septum
- Lead V_2 is placed on the left side of the sternum, fourth intercostal space.
  - Heart area viewed, interventricular septum
- Lead V_3 is placed midway between V_2 and V_4.
  - Heart area viewed, anterior surface
- Lead V_4 is placed on the left midclavicular line, fifth intercostal space.
  - Heart area viewed, anterior surface
- Lead V_5 is placed on the left anterior axillary line, same level as V_4.
  - Heart area viewed, lateral surface
- Lead V_6 is placed on the left midaxillary line, fifth intercostal space.

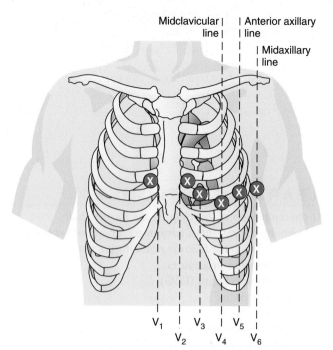

Fig. 8.2 Chest (precordial) leads V_1 through V_6. (From Banasik JL, Copstead-Kirkhorn LE. *Pathophysiology*. 6th ed. St. Louis: Elsevier; 2019.)

- Heart area viewed, lateral surface

Positioning of the precordial chest leads is depicted in Fig. 8.2.

When is cardiac monitoring indicated in the sedation setting?

Cardiac monitoring is indicated for patients in the early phases of acute coronary syndrome, unstable coronary syndrome patients, cardiac surgery patients, and those with implantable cardiac devices. Cardiac monitoring is required for all moderate procedural sedation and analgesia patients by professional practice organization guidelines, The Joint Commission, and specialty nursing organizations. ECG monitoring allows the health care provider to assess the effects of sedative and analgesic medications administered and the impact of the clinical procedure on the cardiac system.

Which lead should be used for patients in the moderate procedural sedation setting?

Lead I, II, or III of the standard bipolar limb leads is generally selected for procedural monitoring and recovery. Optimal ECG tracings depend on proper placement of two sensory electrodes and a ground or reference electrode. To obtain an accurate recording, gelled electrodes must be applied to clean dry skin. For sedation procedures, lead II is beneficial to detect the presence of dysrhythmias, primarily because of the increased visibility of the P wave in this lead. An important rationale for use of the ECG is to assess for the presence of myocardial ischemia. Indicators for myocardial ischemia are identified in Box 8.1.[2] In situations that afford only three lead monitoring systems, a modified chest lead (MCL) may be

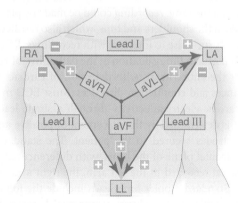

Fig. 8.1 View of the standard limb leads and augmented leads. *LA*, Left arm; *LL*, left leg; *RA*, right arm. (From Boron WF. *Medical Physiology*. 3rd ed. Philadelphia: Saunders; 2011.)

BOX 8.1   Indicators of Myocardial Ischemia[2]

1. Findings consistent with ST-elevation myocardial infarction: New ST elevation at the J point[a] in two anatomically contiguous leads using the following diagnostic thresholds: $\geq$0.1 mV (1 mm) in all leads other than V_2 and V_3, where the following diagnostic thresholds apply—$\geq$0.2 mV (2 mm) in men $\geq$ 40 years, $\geq$0.25 mV (2.5 mm) in men < 40 years, or $\geq$0.15 mV (1.5 mm) in women.

2. Findings consistent with non–ST-elevation myocardial infarction or unstable angina: New horizontal or downsloping ST depression $\geq$ 0.05 mV (0.5 mm) in two anatomically contiguous leads, or T inversion $\geq$ 0.1 mV (1 mm) in two anatomically contiguous leads with prominent R wave or R/S ratio > 1. Contiguous leads are defined as pairs or groups of leads that reflect the different walls of the heart. These are the inferior (II, III, aVF), lateral (I, aVL), and anterior leads (V_1 to V_6).

3. The findings on the ECG depend on several characteristics of the ischemia or infarction, including the following:
   - Duration—hyperacute, acute, evolving, or chronic
   - Size—amount of myocardium affected
   - Location—anterior versus inferior-posterior or right ventricle

[a]The J point is the junction between the termination of the QRS complex and the beginning of the ST segment.

used to monitor for the presence of myocardial ischemia. MCL electrode placement is depicted in Fig. 8.3. When indicated (e.g., for coronary artery disease, angina, left ventricular dysfunction), lead V_5 is used to detect ischemia. Because a large portion of the left ventricle is located beneath the V_5 position, it is a useful lead for the detection of myocardial ischemia.

Which cardiac dysrhythmias should the sedation practitioner be prepared to manage when providing moderate procedural sedation and analgesia?

The cardiac cycle is associated with five distinct waves or deflections, as defined in Box 8.2 and depicted in Fig. 8.4.

Fig. 8.5 demonstrates markings for measuring the amplitude and duration of waveforms using a standard ECG recording speed of 25 mm/s. Normal characteristics of the ECG are identified in Box 8.3. Alterations or variations of this cardiac cycle may represent dysrhythmias and lead to the associated symptoms presented in this chapter. The presentation of cardiac rhythms in Table 8.1 is intended to serve as a review of common and life-threatening dysrhythmias. It is strongly recommended that these materials be used as a reference tool and as a supplement to the American Heart Association Advanced Cardiac Life Support (ACLS) training and treatment protocols. Although many state statutes require ACLS course completion, and many specialty organizations

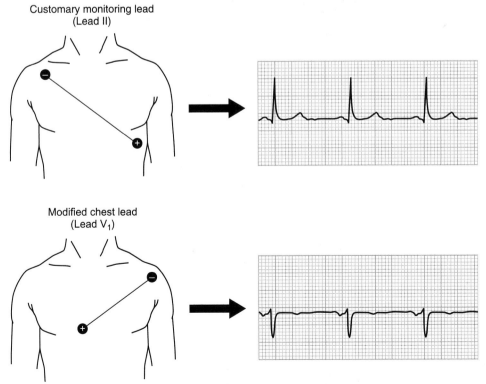

Customary monitoring lead
(Lead II)

Modified chest lead
(Lead V_1)

Fig. 8.3 Modified chest lead (MCL). Electrode positioning places the right arm lead under the left clavicle and the left arm in the V_5 position. The left leg lead is placed in the standard V_1 position (From Meltzer L. Intensive Coronary Care: A Manual for Nurses. 4th ed. East Norwalk, CT: Appleton & Lange; 1983:121.)

BOX 8.2 Elements of the Cardiac Cycle

P wave: The P wave is the first waveform in the cardiac cycle and represents atrial depolarization and impulse generation throughout the right and left atria (sinoatrial [SA] node through the atrioventricular [AV] node). It precedes the QRS complex and is positive (upright) in the standard limb leads.

PR interval: Represents the length of time required for the atria to depolarize and delay of the impulse through the AV junction; normally measures 0.12–0.20 s.

QRS complex: Represents ventricular depolarization and the spread of electrical impulse through the ventricles (ventricular depolarization).

Q wave = first negative deflection after P wave
R wave = first positive deflection after P wave
S wave = the negative deflection following the R wave
ST segment: Represents early repolarization of the right and left ventricles; begins at the end of the QRS complex and ends with onset of the T wave.

T wave: Represents ventricular repolarization. Peaked T waves are seen in patients with hyperkalemia.

QT interval: Represents total ventricular activity (depolarization and repolarization), measured from the beginning of the QRS complex to the end of the T wave; Normally measures 0.36–0.44 s (varies with heart rate, age, and gender).

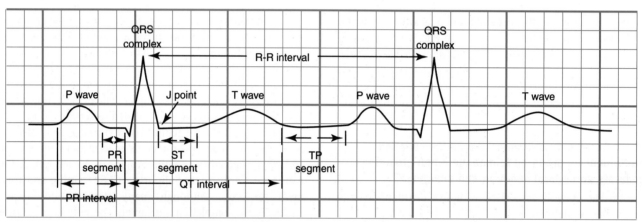

Fig. 8.4 Components of the electrocardiogram (ECG). (From Wesley K. *Huszar's ECG and 12 Lead Interpretation.* 5th ed. St. Louis: Elsevier; 2016.)

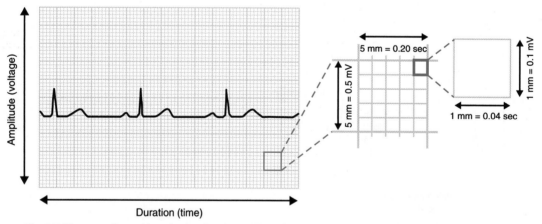

Fig. 8.5 Electrocardiographic strip showing the markings for measuring amplitude and duration of waveform, using a standard recording speed of 25 mm/s. (From Banasik JL, Copstead-Kirkhorn LE. *Pathophysiology.* 6th ed. St. Louis: Elsevier; 2019.)

recommend ACLS training, it is not a uniform requirement in all facilities. As eloquently stated in 1998 by Cummins, "ACLS is about preparing yourself to provide the best possible care for the most dramatic and emotional moment of a person's life."[3] It is strongly recommended that all team members participating in the administration of sedation and analgesia have ACLS course completion and a working knowledge of treatment algorithms.

What role does external cuff size play in the proper measurement of a patient's blood pressure?

The manual, externally applied blood pressure cuff provides an estimation of systolic and diastolic blood pressures. In 1905, Korotkoff, a Russian surgeon, first described turbulent blood flow sounds auscultated when deflating an external blood pressure cuff. Systolic blood pressure (SBP) is ascertained once the first Korotkoff sound is detected. Diastolic

BOX 8.3 Normal ECG Waveform and Segment Characteristics

P wave
- Rounded and smooth in appearance
- Height = 2.5 mm
- Duration = 0.12 s
- Positive complex in leads I, II, aVF, V_2, V_3, V_4, V_5, and V_6

Normal QRS complex
- Normal duration of 0.075–0.11 s for adult patients
- Amplitude of QRS complex varies in different leads

T Wave
- Negative in aVR
- Positive or negative in leads III, aVL, and V_1

- Upright in leads I, II, and V_3–V_6
- ≥0.5 mm in height in leads I and II
- ≤5 mm in height in the limb leads or ≤10 mm in the chest leads

PR segment
- Part of the PR interval, which is normally isoelectric

ST segment
- Normal ST segment begins at the isoelectric line, extends from the end of the S wave, and curves gradually upward to the beginning of the T wave.

---

blood pressure (DBP) is ascertained when the Korotkoff sounds change or disappear.

Technology has replaced the traditional sphygmomanometer device with oscillotonometers. Oscillotonometers are small microprocessor units that measure SBP, DBP, and mean arterial pressure (MAP).[4]

$$MAP = (SBP + 2[DBP])/3$$

Normal MAP ranges are between 70 and 110 mm Hg. A minimum of 60 mm Hg is needed to provide enough blood to nourish the coronary arteries, kidneys, and brain. When the MAP falls below 60 mm Hg for a considerable amount of time, organs may become deprived of the oxygen they need.

Automated blood pressure monitors electronically measure the pressures at which the oscillation amplitudes change. Cuff oscillations are obtained through the sensing unit at approximately 3-mm Hg increments. A microprocessor derives systolic, mean, and diastolic pressures using an algorithm (Fig. 8.6). To ensure accurate blood pressure measurement, it is important to select the proper size cuff. To avoid erroneous blood pressure measurement through what has been called *miscuffing*, appropriate cuff width sizes for patient use include the following:
- Small adult (22–26 cm arm circumference): 12 × 22 cm recommended cuff size
- Adult (27–34 cm arm circumference): 16 × 30 cm recommended cuff size
- Large adult (35–44 cm arm circumference): 16 × 36 cm recommended cuff size

The effect of blood pressure cuff width on accuracy is represented in Fig. 8.7. Additional factors that affect the accuracy of blood pressure measurement are outlined in Table 8.2.[5]

How should hypotension be treated in the sedation care setting?

There is no universal definition of hypotension. A systematic review by Bijker has found 140 definitions for hypotension in a review of 130 articles.[6] Acceptable blood pressure is dependent on a variety of factors, including patient age, comorbidities, and physiologic parameters required for the planned procedure. When procedural hypotension occurs, it may be caused by a variety of factors, including the following:

- Hypovolemia
- Myocardial ischemia
- Myocardial depressant effects of pharmacologic agents
- Acidosis
- Parasympathetic stimulation (pain, vagal response)
- Definitive treatment for hypotension includes the following:
- Administration of oxygen
- Administration of fluid challenge (300–500 mL of crystalloid)
- Correction of acidosis or hypoxemia
- Relief of myocardial ischemia
- Titration of sympathomimetic medications
  - Beta agonists (e.g., ephedrine)
  - Alpha agonists (e.g., phenylephrine)
  - Alpha and beta agonists (e.g., epinephrine, dopamine)
- Titration of inotropic agents
  - Calcium chloride

In the presence of hypotension, it is important for the health care provider monitoring the patient and the attending physician to arrive at a timely diagnosis. Close communication is required of all team members to identify and treat the underlying causative factor(s).

How should hypertension be managed in the sedation setting?

To prevent complications, hypertension must be treated in a timely fashion. Hypertension increases bleeding, predisposes the patient to hemorrhage, may lead to cardiac dysrhythmias, and increases myocardial oxygen consumption. Activation of the sympathetic nervous system (alpha and beta agonist stimulation) results in increased systemic vascular resistance and heart rate. Identification of the cause of hypertension is required to effectively return the blood pressure to baseline or normal values:
- Fluid overload requires diuresis.
- Noxious stimuli require analgesia or discontinuation of stimulation.
- Sympathetic nervous stimulation activation may require alpha and beta blockade.
- Myocardial ischemia may require nitrates and analgesia.

TABLE 8.1   Cardiac Rhythms

Parameter	Cause	Rate	Rhythm	P Waves
Normal sinus rhythm (NSR)	Normal sinus rhythm is the most common rhythm found in a healthy human heart. The electrical impulse originates in the sinoatrial (SA) node. The signal is then conducted through the atria to the atrioventricular (AV) node. Each complex is complete and consists of one P wave, QRS complex, and T wave. There are no wide, bizarre, ectopic, late, or premature complexes.	60–100 beats/min	Regular	Positive (upright) in lead II; one precedes each QRS complex; P waves look alike.

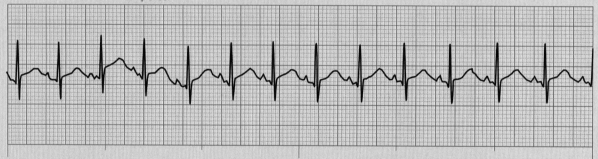

Normal sinus rhythm (NSR)

(From Wesley K. *Huszar's ECG and 12 Lead Interpretation*. 5th ed. St. Louis: Elsevier; 2016.)

Parameter	Cause	Rate	Rhythm	P Waves
Sinus tachycardia (ST)	The SA node in the atria discharges at a rate >100 beats/min. Very rapid rates decrease cardiac output secondary to reduced cardiac filling. Factors that increase heart rate include fever, pain, hypoxia, sepsis, anxiety, myocardial ischemia, exercise, and increased sympathetic nervous system activity. Each complex is complete, consisting of a P wave, a QRS complex, and a T wave. The P wave may be buried in the previous T wave. There are no bizarre, wide, ectopic, early, or late complexes.	Usually from 101–180 beats/min; alternatively, the upper ventricular rate limit may be calculated as 220 beats/min minus the patient's age in years.	Regular	Uniform and upright in appearance. One P wave precedes each QRS complex, 1:1 with QRS complex. The interval between P waves is constant.

(From Aehlert B: *ECG Study Cards*. St. Louis: Mosby; 2004.)

Parameter	Cause	Rate	Rhythm	P Waves
Sinus bradycardia (SB)	The SA node emits impulses at a rate <60 beats/min. Each complex is complete, consisting of a P wave, a QRS complex, and a T wave. All intervals are within normal limits, except heart rate. Parasympathetic dominance of the autonomic nervous system occurs. Sinus bradycardia is associated with pain, beta blockade, vagal stimulation, and myocardial infarction.	<60 beats/min	R-R and P-P intervals are regular.	Uniform and upright in appearance. One P wave precedes each QRS complex. 1:1 with each QRS complex, and the interval between the P waves is constant.

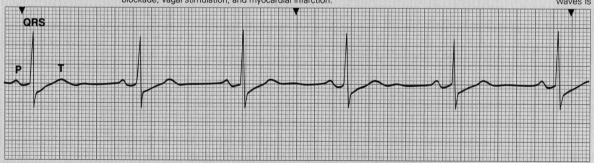

Sinus bradycardia

(From Wesley K. *Huszar's ECG and 12 Lead Interpretation*. 5th ed. St. Louis: Elsevier; 2016.)

PR Interval	QRS Duration	Signs and Symptoms	Treatment	Comments
0.12–0.20 s	≤0.11 s abnormally conducted.	—	None required	—
0.12–0.20 s and constant from beat to beat.	≤0.11 s abnormally conducted.	In most cases, sinus tachycardia is asymptomatic. An attempt must be made to ascertain the underlying cause. Once recognized, treatment is directed at the causative factor (e.g., fever, anxiety, hypovolemia).	Directed at correcting the underlying cause. Fever: ASA, acetaminophen, cooling. Pain: opioids, NSAIDs. Hypovolemia: volume infusion. Medications: reversal or washout. For additional treatment options for stable versus unstable tachycardia see ACLS treatment protocol	Normal response to factors such as increased demand for O_2 due to fever, pain, anxiety, hypoxia, congestive heart failure (CHF), fright, or stress.
0.12–0.20 s and constant from beat to beat.	≤0.11 s unless abnormally conducted.	May be asymptomatic. Fatigue, hypotension, and syncope are associated with decreased cardiac output.	Sinus bradycardia should be treated when signs and symptoms of decreased cardiac output occur (e.g., syncope, unconsciousness) or ventricular ectopy develops. If symptomatic, assess airway. Discontinue procedural or diagnostic stimulation (e.g., colonoscopy, endoscopy, hypoxia), which may correlate with the onset of bradycardia. The presence of severe pain may also enhance vagal tone. Stimulation may need to be decreased or discontinued, or additional analgesia may have to be administered. Atropine IV dose: • First dose = 0.5-mg bolus. Repeat every 3–5 min. • Maximum: 3 mg. Additional medications (dopamine, epinephrine) as per ACLS treatment protocol.	Normal in conditioned athletes. May be due to a variety of factors, which include enhanced vagal tone, parasympathetic dominance of the autonomic nervous system, vomiting, straining, SA nodal disease, increased intraocular pressure, or increased intracranial pressure. Often seen after acute inferior myocardial infarction (MI) or in patients taking beta blockers, quinidine or verapamil, and some calcium channel blockers.

Continued

TABLE 8.1   Cardiac Rhythms—cont'd

Parameter	Cause	Rate	Rhythm	P Waves
Sinus arrhythmia (SA)	The SA node discharges at an irregular rate. The rate of discharge is influenced by the respiratory pattern and the degree of parasympathetic nervous system (vagal) control over the SA node. Each complex is complete, consisting of a P wave, a QRS complex, and a T wave. All intervals are within normal limits except the R-R interval.	Usually 60–100 beats/min; however, the rate may be faster or slower. During inspiration, the heart rate increases, whereas expiration produces a decrease in heart rate.	Irregular	Uniform and upright in appearance. One P wave precedes each QRS complex. The interval between P waves is not constant.

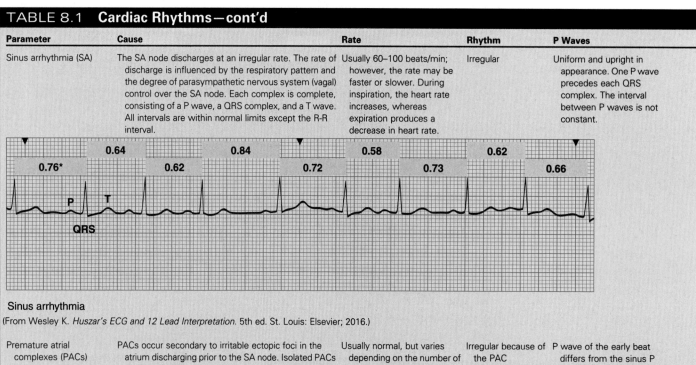

Sinus arrhythmia

(From Wesley K. *Huszar's ECG and 12 Lead Interpretation.* 5th ed. St. Louis: Elsevier; 2016.)

Parameter	Cause	Rate	Rhythm	P Waves
Premature atrial complexes (PACs)	PACs occur secondary to irritable ectopic foci in the atrium discharging prior to the SA node. Isolated PACs are frequently inconsequential. An increase in the rate of PACs may signify impending atrial fibrillation or flutter secondary to irritability of the atrial musculature.	Usually normal, but varies depending on the number of extra atrial beats that are created and the rate of the underlying rhythm.	Irregular because of the PAC	P wave of the early beat differs from the sinus P waves. The wave is premature and may be lost in the preceding T wave. 1:1 with the QRS complex.

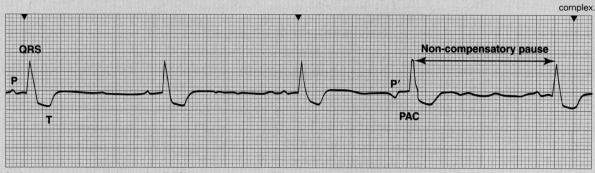

Isolated premature atrial complex (PAC)

(From Wesley K. *Huszar's ECG and 12 Lead Interpretation.* 5th ed. St. Louis: Elsevier; 2016.)

Parameter	Cause	Rate	Rhythm	P Waves
Supraventricular tachycardia (SVT)	Like PACs, SVT occurs secondary to atrial irritability. SVT occurs at an atrial discharge rate from 150–250 beats/min. Ectopic foci override the SA node with a corresponding ventricular response for each atrial impulse conducted. The rhythm can occur paradoxically (abruptly) at the site of reentry circuit in the AV junction.	150–250 beats/min	Regular	Atrial P waves differ from sinus P waves. P waves are generally identified at the lower end of the rate range but seldom are identified at rates >200.

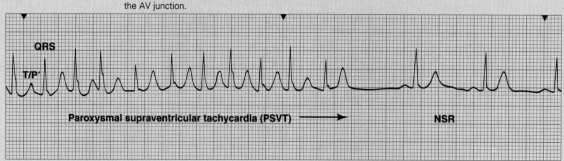

(From Wesley K. *Huszar's ECG and 12 Lead Interpretation.* 5th ed. St. Louis: Elsevier; 2016.)

PR Interval	QRS Duration	Signs and Symptoms	Treatment	Comments
0.12–0.20 s and constant from beat to beat.	≤0.11 s unless abnormally conducted.	The patient is generally unaware of the underlying rhythm. Although characterized by its irregularity, the rhythm possesses essentially normal waveform morphology.	Generally, no treatment is required. Continued procedural and postsedation monitoring as warranted by patient's condition.	Common in children and physically fit adults. Reflex vagal stimulation is related to the normal respiratory cycle. Sinus arrhythmia is a natural variation caused by normal breathing.
Varies from 0.12–0.20 s when the pacemaker site is near the SA node to 0.23 s when the pacemaker site is closer to the AV node.	Usually <0.12 s but may be prolonged if underlying bundle branch block or aberrant conduction.	The patient may be unaware of the underlying rhythm. Premature atrial complexes are frequently diagnosed when ECG monitoring commences immediately prior to the procedure. Ingestion of caffeine, tobacco, or alcohol, hypoxia, anxiety, or atrial enlargement may elicit PACs.	Identification of underlying cause. Rare PACs require no treatment. If PACs are increasing in frequency (>6/min), it may be beneficial to complete the procedure as soon as feasible. Medical consultation may be indicated to prevent the development of atrial tachycardia or atrial fibrillation or flutter and to ascertain the cause of the atrial irritability.	The most distinguishing feature of an ectopic beat arising in the atria (PAC) is that the configuration of the premature P wave differs from the other P waves. The P wave may also be obscured by the preceding T waves, particularly if the PAC occurs soon after the previous beat.
Usually not measurable because the P wave is difficult to distinguish from the preceding T wave. If measurable, the PR interval is 0.12–0.20 s.	<0.12 s but may be prolonged if bundle branch block or aberrant conduction.	Because of decreased ventricular filling time, signs and symptoms of decreased cardiac output (e.g., hypotension, syncope) may occur. Sudden feelings of palpitations, lightheadedness, and severe anxiety are common. Myocardial oxygen consumption increases in response to the tachycardic state.	Monitor patient for signs and symptoms of congestive heart failure or shock. Stable: Administer oxygen, establish IV line, vagal maneuvers, pharmacologic intervention. Unstable: Administer oxygen, IV medications. Additional treatment options, see ACLS treatment protocol.	Common causes are physical or psychological stress, hypoxia, epinephrine in the local anesthetic solution, and excessive caffeine intake. Also may occur in patients with rheumatic heart disease, coronary artery disease, digitalis toxicity, and respiratory failure.

Continued

TABLE 8.1   Cardiac Rhythms—cont'd

Parameter	Cause	Rate	Rhythm	P Waves
Atrial flutter (A-flutter)	Atrial flutter occurs secondary to rapid ectopic atrial discharge at a rate of 250–350 beats/min. Because of this rapid ectopic rate, the ventricle cannot respond to each impulse. However, the ventricle will selectively respond to impulses and contract. According to the number of atrial impulses discharged prior to ventricular contraction, atrial flutter is referred to as 2:1, 3:1, or 4:1 flutter.	Atrial rate is 250–350 beats/min. Ventricular rate is variable, depending on conduction through to the ventricle.	Atrial rhythm is regular. Ventricular rhythm is usually regular, with a constant conduction ratio, but may be irregular.	Sawtoothed, F or flutter waves.

II

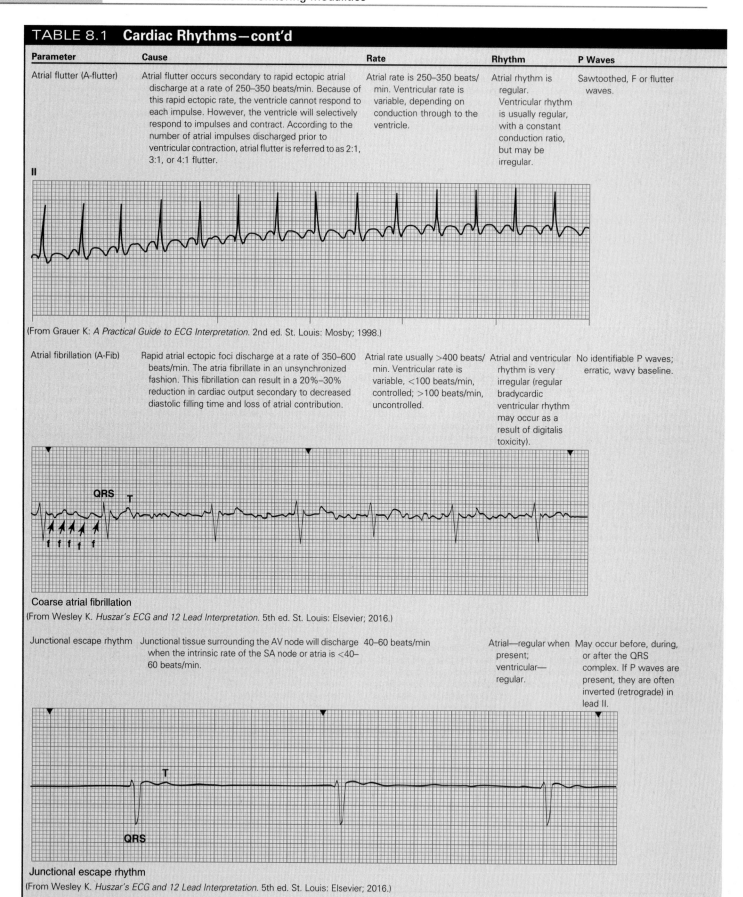

(From Grauer K: *A Practical Guide to ECG Interpretation.* 2nd ed. St. Louis: Mosby; 1998.)

Parameter	Cause	Rate	Rhythm	P Waves
Atrial fibrillation (A-Fib)	Rapid atrial ectopic foci discharge at a rate of 350–600 beats/min. The atria fibrillate in an unsynchronized fashion. This fibrillation can result in a 20%–30% reduction in cardiac output secondary to decreased diastolic filling time and loss of atrial contribution.	Atrial rate usually >400 beats/min. Ventricular rate is variable, <100 beats/min, controlled; >100 beats/min, uncontrolled.	Atrial and ventricular rhythm is very irregular (regular bradycardic ventricular rhythm may occur as a result of digitalis toxicity).	No identifiable P waves; erratic, wavy baseline.

Coarse atrial fibrillation

(From Wesley K. *Huszar's ECG and 12 Lead Interpretation.* 5th ed. St. Louis: Elsevier; 2016.)

Parameter	Cause	Rate	Rhythm	P Waves
Junctional escape rhythm	Junctional tissue surrounding the AV node will discharge when the intrinsic rate of the SA node or atria is <40–60 beats/min.	40–60 beats/min	Atrial—regular when present; ventricular—regular.	May occur before, during, or after the QRS complex. If P waves are present, they are often inverted (retrograde) in lead II.

Junctional escape rhythm

(From Wesley K. *Huszar's ECG and 12 Lead Interpretation.* 5th ed. St. Louis: Elsevier; 2016.)

PR Interval	QRS Duration	Signs and Symptoms	Treatment	Comments
None, not measurable.	Usually 0.04–0.12 s but may be widened. Flutter waves are buried in the QRS complex.	The patient may report a sense of palpitations. If ventricular filling and coronary artery blood flow are compromised, symptoms of decreased cardiac output may become clinically evident.	Hemodynamically stable patients generally require no initial treatment. Ventricular rates that are rapid may be terminated with cardioversion or beta blockade. Additional treatment options, see ACLS treatment protocol.	Clinical significance of this rhythm depends on the ventricular response rate. The more rapid the rate, the more serious the dysrhythmia. Seldom occurs in the absence of organic heart disease. Seen in association with mitral or tricuspid valve disorders, digitalis toxicity, pericarditis, and inferior wall MI.
None	Usually 0.04–0.12 s.	Asymptomatic, or the patient may sense palpitations. If underlying heart disease exists, then signs of decreased cardiac output may be present. In patients with a history of coronary artery disease, angina may manifest as the primary patient complaint.	Treatment is dependent on clinical presentation and ventricular rate. The goal of therapy is to convert to normal sinus rhythm, reduce the ventricular rate to less than 100, and restore atrial kick. Additional treatment options, see ACLS treatment protocol.	Erratic, wavy, chaotic baseline. Inefficient movement of blood in the atria predisposes the patient to stroke secondary to cardioembolism. May occur intermittently or as a chronic rhythm. Additional predisposing factors include MI, chronic obstructive pulmonary disease, coronary artery disease, CHF, cardiac valve disorders, and rheumatic heart disease.
Not measurable unless P wave precedes the QRS complex. When present, generally measures ≤0.12 s.	<0.12 s	A junctional rhythm seldom produces symptoms unless the rate is very slow (<40 beats/min).	Generally, no special drug therapy is indicated. Atropine may be successful in increasing the discharge rate of the SA node. If the slow heart rate compromises circulation, a transvenous pacemaker may be required to increase the ventricular rate and cardiac output. Additional treatment options, see ACLS treatment protocol.	The presence of a junctional rhythm (at a rate of ≈40 beats/min) indicates that the SA node is no longer discharging or is firing at a rate of <40 beats/min. A junctional rhythm is a safety mechanism that preserves the heart rate if higher pacemaker sites fail. The suppression of SA nodal discharge activity may permit lower pacemaker sites to develop. Junctional rhythm often results in response to excessive vagal activity. Additional factors include ischemic damage to the SA node and digitalis or quinidine toxicity.

Continued

TABLE 8.1   Cardiac Rhythms—cont'd

Parameter	Cause	Rate	Rhythm	P Waves
Premature ventricular contractions (PVCs)	Discharge from an irritable ventricular focus prior to discharge of the next impulse from the SA node. The resultant wide, distorted, and bizarre ventricular complex is a result of ventricular contraction outside the normal conduction pathway.	Atrial and ventricular rate dependent on underlying rhythm.	Irregular because of the premature ventricular complex.	There are no P waves associated with the PVC.

II

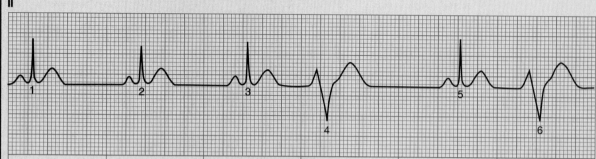

(From Grauer K: *A Practical Guide to ECG Interpretation*. 2nd ed. St. Louis: Mosby; 1998.)

Ventricular tachycardia (V-tach, monomorphic VT)	Ventricular tachycardia occurs when three or more PVCs occur at a rate >100 beats/min. These consecutive beats signify pronounced ventricular irritability. Persistent ventricular tachycardia leads to ventricular failure, cardiogenic shock, and decreased cardiac output and cerebral blood flow, with resultant cerebral ischemia.	Atrial not discernible; ventricular 100–250 beats/min.	Atrial not discernible, ventricular rhythm is essentially regular.	May be present or absent. If present, there is no set relationship to the QRS complexes. AV dissociation may be present during the ventricular tachycardia.

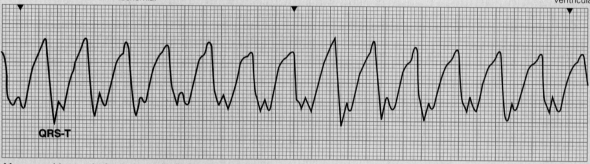

QRS-T

Monomorphic ventricular tachycardia (V-Tach)

(From Wesley K. *Huszar's ECG and 12 Lead Interpretation*. 5th ed. St. Louis: Elsevier; 2016.)

Ventricular fibrillation (V-fib)	Ventricular muscle fibers, which normally contract as a single unit, lose this inherent ability. Individual ventricular muscle fibers are stimulated so rapidly that there is no recovery phase between ventricular contractions. Fibrillation is ineffective in moving blood out of the ventricles, and circulation stops. If not corrected immediately, death ensues within minutes.	Cannot be determined because there are no discernible wave forms or complexes to measure.	Rapid and chaotic, with no pattern or regularity.	Not discernible.

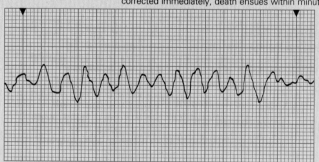

Coarse ventricular fibrillation

(From Wesley K. *Huszar's ECG and 12 Lead Interpretation*. 5th ed. St. Louis: Elsevier; 2016.)

PR Interval	QRS Duration	Signs and Symptoms	Treatment	Comments
None, because the ectopic beat originates in the ventricle.	<0.12 s. Wide and bizarre configuration is frequently in the opposite direction of the QRS complex.	Many patients are aware of PVCs and describe the sensation as "palpitations" or "skipping of the heart." When one is auscultating the heart or taking the pulse, a relatively long pause is noted immediately after the premature beat. This delay (complete compensatory pause) is characteristic and is particularly diagnostic of the arrhythmia.	Treatment of PVCs should be considered if the following occurs: (1) they occur at a rate of >6/min; (2) they are multifocal in appearance; (3) there are two or more in a row; or (4) an R on T phenomenon occurs (PVC falls on the T wave of the preceding beat). Supportive care aimed at the cause of the PVCs. Treatment protocol during sedation procedures requires airway assessment, procedural correlation, frequency of PVCs, and evaluation of the patient's pain threshold. For frequent PVCs (>6/min), common causative factors must be ruled out. Additional treatment options, see ACLS treatment protocol.	PVCs are among the most common of all arrhythmias associated with acute MI. PVCs signify ventricular irritability. PVCs are associated with hypoxia, electrolyte imbalance (hypokalemia), MI, stress, chronic heart disease, and medication overdosage. It is important to treat the underlying cause, not merely the symptom (PVC). Complications associated with PVCs rest in their ability to initiate ventricular tachycardia or fibrillation.
None	>0.12 s, with a bizarre configuration. Often difficult to differentiate between the QRS complex and the T wave. Three or more PVCs occurring sequentially are referred to as a run of ventricular tachycardia.	If conscious, the patient may complain of palpitations, chest pain, or shortness of breath. If ventricular tachycardia is prolonged or sustained, signs and symptoms of decreased cardiac output generally occur.	Additional treatment options, see ACLS treatment protocol.	May result in decreased cardiac output, with potential deterioration to ventricular fibrillation. VT is often precipitated by R on T phenomenon, PVC, myocardial irritability due to acute MI, coronary artery disease, congestive heart failure, or electrolyte imbalance. Development of ventricular tachycardia is also associated with toxicity from digitalis, quinidine, or procainamide.
Not discernible.	Not discernible.	Unconsciousness, absence of pulse.	Check vital signs; if none present, defibrillate immediately, begin CPR, establish IV line, institute ACLS protocol.	Life-threatening arrhythmia. If not converted, causes death within minutes.

Continued

TABLE 8.1   Cardiac Rhythms—cont'd

Parameter	Cause	Rate	Rhythm	P Waves
Asystole (flat line)	The absence of electrical impulse activity within the myocardium signifies massive myocardial ischemia. Development of asystole may be attributed to acute respiratory failure, myocardial rupture, or extensive ischemic damage.	None	None	None

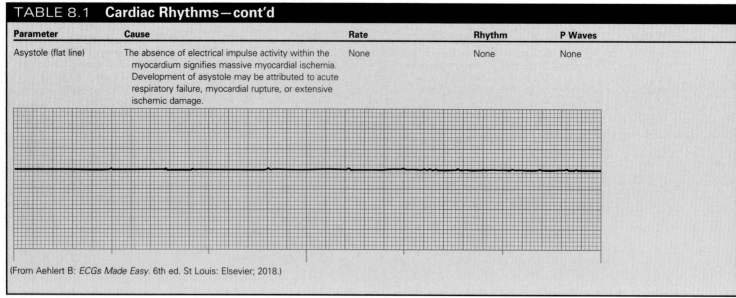

(From Aehlert B: *ECGs Made Easy.* 6th ed. St Louis: Elsevier; 2018.)

ACLS, Advanced Cardiac Life Support; *ASA,* acetylsalicylic acid; *NSAID,* nonsteroidal antiinflammatory drug.

PR Interval	QRS Duration	Signs and Symptoms	Treatment	Comments
None	None	Absence of pulse (check for carotid pulse), apnea, no signs of life.	CPR; again, verify rhythm in two leads; consider other causes, pacing, and pharmacologic therapy. Additional treatment options, see ACLS treatment protocol.	Always check "absence" of a rhythm in two leads and verification of lead placement.

⚡ PATIENT SAFETY SBAR FOCUS

Procedural Hypotension

Situation

A 23-year-old male patient presented to the emergency department for abscess drainage of the left forearm. Drainage of the abscess was uneventful. Following the procedure, significant hypotension occurred that required treatment.

Background

The patient presented to the emergency department with a superficial postoperative forearm abscess. Sedation was established with 3 milligrams of midazolam and 150 micrograms of fentanyl. Immediately prior to discharge, the patient's blood pressure dropped from 130/80 mm Hg to 70/40 mm Hg. Intravenous fluids were ordered to be "wide open," and nasal cannula oxygen was applied at a rate of 4 liters per minute. Blood pressure was unresponsive to these interventions and heart rate increased to 150 beats per minute. The patient required multiple doses of phenylephrine (50-microgram increments) until blood pressure stabilized and heart rate returned to a baseline rate of 94 beats per minute. The patient was admitted to the hospital. Further questioning revealed that the patient was allergic to multiple food groups including bananas, avocados, grapefruit juice, and chestnuts. A skin prick test was positive. A dermatology consult confirmed a diagnosis of latex allergy.

Assessment

Latex is a sappy milky substance that is used to manufacture natural latex products including surgical gloves, catheters, elastic bandages and surgical drains. Dermatology consultation revealed a genetic (atopic) predisposition. Cardiovascular collapse is the most common form of latex allergy presentation. However, skin rash and bronchospasm can precede cardiovascular collapse. Prevention of future reactions includes patient education and avoidance of all latex products. Immunotherapy protocol may be ordered by continued care by the dermatology service. Documented affirmative responses on a latex allergy prescreening questionnaire for specific food sensitivities may also cue the sedation provider to potential latex allergy prior to the procedure. The use of a latex allergy prescreening questionnaire with a focus on cross reactive foods may also be indicative of a preexisting patient latex allergy. Degree of food association or prevalence include:

High (4)

Banana, Avocado, Chestnut, Kiwi

Moderate (7)

Apple, Carrot, Celery, Papaya, Potato, Tomato, Melons

Low or undetermined (33)

Pear, Mango, Sweet Pepper, Peach, Rye, Cayenne Pepper, Plum, Wheat, Shellfish, Cherry, Hazelnut, Sunflower Seed, Pineapple, Walnut, Citrus Fruits, Strawberry, Soybean, Coconut, Fig, Peanut, Chick Pea, Grape, Buckwheat, Castor Bean, Apricot, Dill, Lychee, Passion Fruit, Oregano, Zucchini, Nectarine, Sage, Persimmon

Recommendation

Detailed latex allergy policies and procedures must be available in all sedation settings. Appendix D (AANA Latex Allergy Management Guidelines) features comprehensive preprocedural, procedural, and post-procedural care requirements associated with the latex allergy patient.

Data from American Latex Allergy Association (2014). *Cross Reactive Food.* Retrieved from http://latexallergyresources.org/cross-reactive-food; American Association of Nurse Anesthetists (2014). AANA Latex Allergy Protocol. Retrieved from https://www.aana.com/docs/default-source/practice-aana-com-web-documents-(all)/latex-allergy-management.pdf?sfvrsn=9c0049b1_2

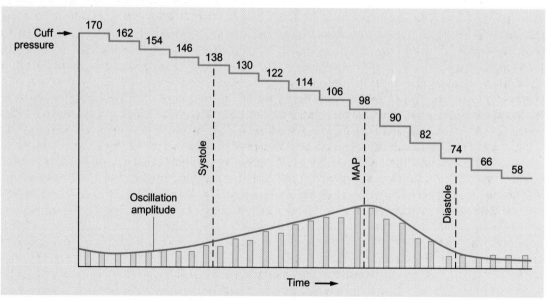

Fig. 8.6 Oscillometric determination of blood pressure (in mm Hg). (From Butterworth JF. *Morgan and Mikhail's Clinical Anesthesiology.* 5th ed. New York: McGraw-Hill; 2013.)

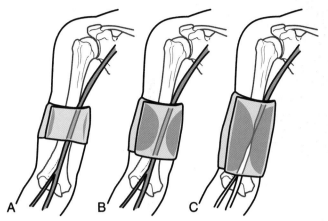

Fig. 8.7 Blood pressure cuff width influences the pressure readings. Three cuffs, all inflated to the same pressure, are shown. The narrowest cuff (A) will require more pressure, and the widest cuff (C) less pressure, to occlude the brachial artery for the determination of systolic pressure. Too narrow a cuff may produce a large overestimation of systolic pressure. Whereas the wider cuff may underestimate the systolic pressure, the error with a cuff 20% too wide is not as significant as the error with a cuff 20% too narrow.

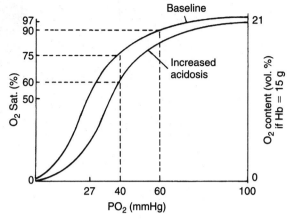

Fig. 8.8 Oxyhemoglobin dissociation curve. (From Custalow CB, Roberts JR, Todd W, Thomsen TW, Jerris R, Hedges JR. *Roberts and Hedges' Clinical Procedures in Emergency Medicine.* 6th ed. Philadelphia: Elsevier; 2014.)

TABLE 8.2 Factors Affecting Accuracy of Blood Pressure Measurement	
Factor	Magnitude of Systolic/Diastolic Blood Pressure Discrepancy (mm Hg)
Talking or active listening	10/10
Distended bladder	15/10
Cuff over clothing	5–50/
Cuff too small	10/2–8
Smoking within 30 min of measurement	6–20/
Paralyzed arm	2–5/
Back unsupported	6–10/
Arm unsupported, sitting	1–7/5–11
Arm unsupported, standing	6–8/

From Handler J, The importance of accurate blood pressure measurement, Perm J. 2009;13(3):51–54.

What impact has pulse oximetry had in the sedation setting?

The advent of pulse oximetry in the 1980s has provided the clinician with a simple, safe, and inexpensive method to assess patient oxygenation. Pulse oximetry is a standard of care in all sedation settings. It is a clinical assessment tool used to decrease the incidence of unrecognized hypoxic events. Through its noninvasive technology and continuous monitoring capabilities, oxygen and respiratory system function are assessed in patients.[7,8] Oxygen saturation is recorded as an SpO_2 parameter; and 98% of oxygen is transported throughout the body in combination with hemoglobin, whereas 2% is dissolved in plasma. The oxyhemoglobin dissociation curve depicted in Fig. 8.8 assists the clinician in determining the correlation between oxygen saturation and PO_2. Hemoglobin saturation is determined by a light absorbance technique across a pulsating vascular bed. Examination of the oxyhemoglobin dissociation curve reveals the development of hypoxemia at an SaO_2 of 90%, which equals a PO_2 of 60 mm Hg.

Severe hypoxemia develops when the SaO_2 decreases to 75%, with a resultant PO_2 of 40 mm Hg. The height and slope of the curve depend on a variety of factors that influence a left or right shift in the oxyhemoglobin dissociation curve (Box 8.4).[9-14] Factors that shift the curve to the left result in a decreased release of oxygen at the tissue level. Factors that shift the curve to the right result in an increase in the amount of oxygen released at the tissue level. When providing sedation, it is important to understand the principles of pulse oximetry to recognize the development of hypoxic episodes and take corrective action as needed. Pulse oximetry provides a noninvasive continuous monitoring parameter to assess the percentage of oxygen combined with hemoglobin. This convenient monitoring modality should be used for all patients receiving moderate procedural sedation and analgesia.

How does pulse oximetry technology actually work?

Pulse oximetry combines the principles of optical plethysmography and spectrophotometry to ascertain hemoglobin oxygen saturation. As depicted in Fig. 8.9, pulse oximeters use two light-emitting diodes (LEDs), which are placed opposite each other across an arterial vascular bed. These LEDs measure the intensity of transmitted light across the vascular bed. The critical feature of pulse oximetry is that it measures the difference in the intensity of light absorption at each wavelength caused by oxygenated and deoxygenated hemoglobin (Fig. 8.10). The signal is then transmitted to the pulse

BOX 8.4   Physiologic Factors Affecting Hemoglobin-Oxygen Affinity[9-14]

Left Shift: Increased Oxygen Affinity

This allows less oxygen to be available to the tissues.

- Alkalosis
- Anemia
- Carboxyhemoglobin
- Decreased 2,3-diphosphoglycerate (2,3-DPG)
- Decreased pco_2
- Fetal hemoglobin
- Hypothermia
- Hypothyroidism
- Methemoglobin

Right Shift: Decreased Oxygen Affinity

This allows more oxygen to be available to the tissues.

- Acidosis

- Increased pco_2
- Increased 2,3-DPG
- Hyperthermia
- Sulfhemoglobin
- Fever
- Corticosteroid administration
- Hyperthyroidism
- Hyperaldosteronism
- Polycythemia

A right shift indicates decreased oxygen affinity of hemoglobin, allowing more oxygen to be available to the tissues. A left shift indicates increased oxygen affinity of hemoglobin, allowing less oxygen to be available to the tissues.

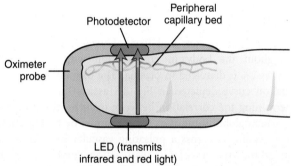

Fig. 8.9 Pulse oximetry technology. Two light-emitting diodes (LEDs) measure the intensity of transmitted light across the vascular bed. (From Bonewit-West K. *Clinical Procedures for Medical Assistants.* 10th ed. St. Louis: Elsevier; 2018.)

oximetry unit for determination of arterial hemoglobin oxygen saturation. Pulse oximeter sensors come in a variety of types. A variety of pulse oximeter sensors are available, which include the following:

- Single-patient use
- Two-piece
- Reusable
- Specialty

Sensors are chosen according to the patient's body weight, exposed site of application, patient activity level, and expected duration of patient monitoring.

Pulse oximeters in our sedation setting seem to have a high incidence of interference or inaccurate readings. What causes interference or contributes to inaccuracy in pulse oximetry measurement?

The importance of an accurate pulse oximetry reading in the sedation setting cannot be overstated. Without accuracy, the ability to detect hypoxemia associated with the deterioration of respiratory function is compromised.[8] Patient movement and low perfusion states affect accurate Spo_2 measurement.[7] Because pulse oximetry units were introduced into clinical practice in the 1980s, manufacturers continue to focus their development of motion tolerant pulse oximetry using

software algorithms to account and correct for motion artifact.[15] Additional conditions that result in pulse oximetry readings that are unreliable, incorrect, or less informative are identified in Box 8.5.[16]

Is carbon dioxide monitoring required for moderate procedural sedation patients?

The Joint Commission, Centers for Medicare & Medicaid Services, state licensing and medical boards, and specialty-specific governing bodies have established guidelines to address provider education and qualification requirements and other patient care standards related to sedation.[17-19] In 2011, the American Society of Anesthesiologists (ASA) approved modifications to its Standards for Basic Anesthetic Monitoring. A significant change to these standards included the recommendation for capnography to monitor the adequacy of ventilation during moderate and deep sedation procedures. It last affirmed these standards on October 28, 2015. Additionally, "Practice Guidelines for Moderate Procedural Sedation and Analgesia 2018" were published in March 2018.[18] These practice guidelines included new recommendations, which included continual monitoring of ventilatory function with capnography to supplement standard monitoring by observation and pulse oximetry.

The ASA guidelines represent expert consensus, based on research findings and best evidence available. However, some medical societies have stated little value for the universal adoption of capnography for moderate sedation.[20,21] The sedation provider monitoring the patient and the attending physician are required to adhere to monitoring guidelines as outlined by the institutional policy and procedure, regulatory bodies, and licensing agencies.

Office-based surgery settings and outpatient facilities must also abide by regulatory guidelines related to end-tidal carbon dioxide ($Etco_2$) monitoring as well. New York State recently issued a new $Etco_2$ monitoring regulation that requires compliance, effective January 31, 2018. "Office-based surgery practices located in New York State will be required to provide continual (repeated regularly and frequently in steady rapid succession) end-tidal carbon dioxide monitoring using

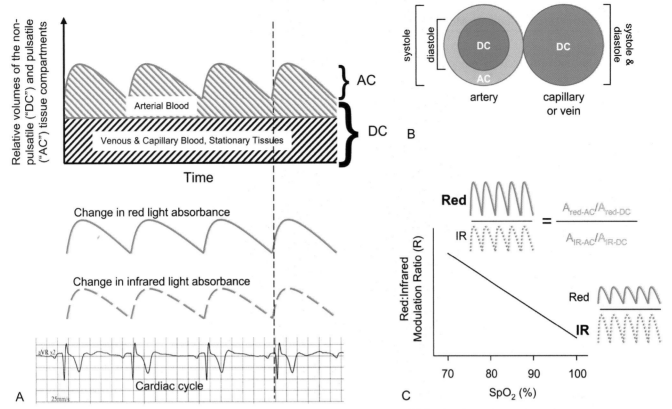

Fig. 8.10 Pulse oximetry technology. Shown is a schematic diagram of light absorbance by a pulse oximeter. (A) In a person with good cardiac function, the onset of the cardiac systole, as denoted by the onset of the QRS complex, coincides with the onset of the increase of the arterial blood volume. The amount of red and infrared (IR) light absorbed in the arterial compartment also rises and falls with systole and diastole, respectively, due to the increase and decrease in blood volume. The volume that increases with systole is also known as the *pulsatile* or *alternating current* (AC) compartment, and the compartment in which the blood volume does not change with the cardiac cycle is known as the *nonpulsatile* or *direct current* (DC) compartment. (B) A cross-sectional diagram of an artery and a vein displaying the pulsatile (AC) and nonpulsatile (DC) compartments of the blood vessels. Note that only the artery has a pulsatile (AC) component. (C) Diagram of a calibration (standard) curve of the red IR modulation ratio in relation to the Spo2. Increased red light absorbance (increased R) is associated with increased deoxyhemoglobin (i.e., lower Spo2). (From Chan ED, Chan MM, Chan MM. Pulse oximetry: Understanding its basic principles facilitates appreciation of its limitations. Resp Med. 2013;107(6):789–799.)

BOX 8.5 Recommendations for Improving Pulse Oximetry Readings

Anemia

Anemia causes decreased arterial oxygen content by reducing the level of hemoglobin that is available to bind with oxygen. Although Spo2 readings may be considered in the normal range, an anemic patient may be hypoxic due to reduced hemoglobin levels. The pulse oximeter may fail to provide an Spo2 reading if hemoglobin levels fall below 5 g/dL. Correcting the cause of the anemia may improve arterial oxygen content.

Dyshemoglobins

Dysfunctional hemoglobins such as carboxyhemoglobin, methemoglobin, or sulfhemoglobin are unable to carry oxygen. However, Spo2 values only report functional saturation—oxygenated hemoglobin as a percentage of functional hemoglobin. Therefore, although the Spo2 values reported by a pulse oximeter may appear normal when dysfunctional hemoglobin levels are elevated, oxygenation may be compromised due to decreased arterial oxygen content. A more complete assessment of oxygenation beyond pulse oximetry is recommended whenever dysfunctional hemoglobins are suspected.

Edema

Position the sensor on nonedematous application sites. Otherwise, the fluid in the edematous tissue may cause the light from the light-emitting diodes (LEDs) to scatter and affect the Spo2 readings.

Intravascular Dyes

Use care when interpreting Spo2 values after injection of IV dyes, which may affect the reading.

Light Interference

In the presence of bright lights, cover the sensor with an opaque material. Avoid direct sunlight, surgical lamps, infrared warming devices, and phototherapy lamps.

Low Perfusion States

Consider the use of an adhesive digit sensor, protection of sensor site from heat loss, and rewarming the sensor site.

Motion

Motion artifact in a clinical setting such as the obstetric unit (laboring women or women with neuraxial anesthesia undergoing cesarean delivery), intensive care unit, and postanesthesia care unit, where patients experience voluntary and involuntary movement, including tapping, rubbing, shivering, and seizures in adult and pediatric patients and kicking and crying in neonates.[16] When motion artifact impacts accurate readings, consider moving the sensor to a less active site or replace adhesive.

Nail Polish

Remove all nail polish, particularly brown, blue, and green shades. The sensor may also be applied to a digit that has no polish.

capnography for patients receiving moderate sedation, deep sedation, and general anesthesia."[22]

How does pulse oximetry compare to end-tidal carbon dioxide monitoring?

There is a significant difference between pulse oximetry and $Etco_2$ monitoring. The most significant difference includes the immediate recognition of apnea or hypoventilation when using capnography compared to pulse oximetry. In 2011, a meta-analysis by Waugh et al. demonstrated that respiratory depression is more than 17 times more likely to be detected when capnography is used.[23] Pulse oximetry measures the quantity of arterial blood oxygen saturation and pulse rate, whereas capnography is a direct measure of ventilation that measures the concentration of carbon dioxide exhaled by the patient. An easy way for the sedation provider to remember differences in technology includes the following:

- Pulse oximetry measures oxygen deficiency or the development of a hypoxic state.
- Capnography measures ventilation or the concentration of carbon dioxide in exhaled air.

Capnography is acknowledged as a superior method for the evaluation of ventilation in patients. It is theoretically more sensitive to alveolar hypoventilation than SpO_2 and has been clinically demonstrated to be an earlier indicator of respiratory distress than SpO_2. In lieu of waiting additional time for the pulse oximeter to identify a hypoxic state, the sedation provider using capnography can immediately initiate protocols to correct airway obstruction, apnea, or hypoventilation syndrome.

Our unit manager informed us that we "don't need capnography in our practice setting." Many of our practitioners believe that this is related more to the difficulty in implementing capnography monitoring in our facility and not a fair evaluation of the patient benefits. What is the best way to convince management to consider implementing capnography for the sedation patient?

As noted, monitoring $Etco_2$ is far superior to using pulse oximetry for the immediate detection of an obstructed airway, apnea, and other airway problems that manifest much later when pulse oximetry is used alone. Carbon dioxide monitoring provides a useful, objective clinical assessment parameter. Functioning as a physiologic indicator, it demonstrates the following:

- Ventilation is sufficient to carry oxygen into the lungs.
- Oxygen is being transported to the mitochondria (cardiovascular function).
- Aerobic metabolism is consuming this oxygen and producing carbon dioxide.
- Carbon dioxide is being transported to the lungs (cardiovascular function).
- Carbon dioxide in the expired air gives an indication of adequate ventilation.

It should be reiterated to administrators that oximeters only measure the oxygen saturation of peripheral blood hemoglobin, and capnography continuously and nearly instantaneously measures pulmonary ventilation. Capnography allows for the detection of small changes in cardiorespiratory function before oximeter readings change. Escalating departmental concerns to the hospital administration level does not make anyone popular, but it is important to address all elements of patient safety when providing moderate procedural sedation and analgesia.

How does capnography actually measure end-tidal CO₂?

Capnography measures carbon dioxide in expiratory gases. Most capnographs use infrared absorption techniques. Infrared absorption analysis provides quantitative respiratory monitoring data in the sedation setting. When the patient exhales, a beam of infrared light is passed over the gas sample on a sensor. The presence or lack of carbon dioxide is inversely indicated by the amount of light that passes through the sensor:

- High CO_2 levels are indicated by low infrared amounts of light.
- Low CO_2 levels are indicated by high infrared amounts of light.

What are considered normal end-tidal CO₂ levels?

$Etco_2$ is the partial pressure or maximal concentration of carbon dioxide (CO_2) at the end of an exhaled breath, which is expressed as a percentage of CO_2 or mm Hg. The normal values are 5% to 6% CO_2, which is equivalent to 35 to 45 mm Hg (normal arterial blood gas reading).[24] CO_2 reflects cardiac output (CO) and pulmonary blood flow as the gas is transported by the venous system to the right side of the heart and then pumped to the lungs by the right ventricles.[25]

What are the differences in available capnographs on the market for use in the sedation setting?

When CO_2 diffuses out of the lungs into the exhaled air, a device called a *capnometer* measures the partial pressure or maximal concentration of CO_2 at the end of exhalation. There are a variety of capnography sampling devices available, including sidestream, mainstream, and microstream.

First-generation sidestream capnography samples a fixed amount of gas from the side of the main respiratory gas flow. The rate of gas sampling is generally from 50 to 500 mL (typical amounts = 150 mL, which precludes their use in neonatology and pediatrics). The gas sample is processed through sample tubes and adapters to an infrared light source and detector. Complications associated with sidestream capnography include contamination and clogging by respiratory secretions unless sample tubes are frequently replaced.

Second-generation mainstream capnography mounts the infrared head in close proximity to the endotracheal tube. Although mainstream capnography has resolved some of the technical problems associated with capnography use, its major limiting factor is that it can only be used on intubated patients. Additional limiting technical factors associated with mainstream capnography include optical pathway clouding and disruption by moisture and respiratory tract secretions, costly damage secondary to optical sensor mounting, and bulkiness associated with sensor assemblies that predisposes to kinking of ventilator lines. Therefore, mainstream

BOX 8.6 Advantages of Microstream Capnography

Liquid and Secretion Handling
Position-independent adapters, vapor-permeable tubing, and submicron multisurface filters minimize the frequency of filter line replacement and instrument contamination. There are no water traps to service.

Transportability and Ruggedness
It may be used with intubated or nonintubated patients. Rugged compact units are highly mobile and are not position-dependent. The low-power $Etco_2$ sensor is protected in the instrument.

Cross Sensitivity to Non-CO_2 Gases
A microbeam infrared sensor is inherently specific for CO_2 and does not require user corrections, recalibration, or software compensation for nitrous oxide, oxygen, or other common anesthetic gases.

Support for Neonatal Applications
Measuring the cell volume is similar to that of other technologies, making microstream capnography inherently suitable for low flow and for many neonatal applications, as well as for adult use.

Sample Line Compatibility
Microstream adapters and filter lines can be used with inpatients and outpatients, whether intubated or not, allowing for standardization of patient connections.

Additional Advantages
This ensures effective oral and nasal sampling at low tidal volumes, with no dilution of the waveform during oxygen delivery. It enables effective oxygen therapy and reduces any oxygen drying effect on sensitive mucous membranes. It prevents moisture from entering the monitor while maintaining easily displayed waveforms and laminar flow. It meets all clinical needs, including long-term monitoring and in high-humidity environments.

---

capnography has no clinical use in the nonintubated sedation patient.

Microstream capnography technology is based on *molecular correlation spectroscopy* (MCS), which uses a unique, laser-based technology as the infrared emission source. Operating at room temperature, an emitter is electronically activated and self-modulating, which eliminates the need for moving parts. This respiratory monitoring system is suitable for all patients, including neonates and pediatric and adult patients. The advantages associated with microstream capnographs are identified in Box 8.6.

What affects end-tidal carbon dioxide values in the sedation setting?

A capnogram is the graphic waveform depicting the carbon dioxide concentration throughout respiration. $Etco_2$ refers to the measurement of carbon dioxide concentration at the end of exhalation. A normal range for $Etco_2$ is 35 to 45 mm Hg (4.5%–6%) Elevated levels of carbon dioxide (>45 mm Hg) can result from hypoventilation, respiratory acidosis, fever, bronchospasm, ventilation of a previously unventilated lung, or an adrenergic response. Decreased levels of carbon dioxide (<35 mm Hg) can result from hyperventilation, respiratory alkalosis, partial airway obstruction, pulmonary embolus, cardiac arrest, hypotension, hypovolemia, or hypothermia. During each breath, the alveoli exchange carbon dioxide and oxygen. At the inhalation, the alveoli receive oxygen, which diffuses into the pulmonary capillaries. Then, at exhalation, carbon dioxide diffuses into the alveoli and is eliminated via ventilation. Capnography waveforms reflecting a normal waveform, partial airway obstruction, hypoventilation, and apnea are identified in Fig. 8.11.

What are the components of a comprehensive moderate sedation patient record?

The purpose of a comprehensive, moderate procedural record, as depicted in Fig. 8.12, is to provide a legible and complete record of patient care during the administration of moderate procedural sedation and analgesia that also functions as a historical procedural record for quality and risk management review. The record should be neat, accurate, clear, and concise.

The moderate sedation record must provide proof of continuous care that is reflective of appropriate standards of care and regulatory guidelines. The components of any moderate sedation record should include all aspects—presedation, procedural, and postsedation—of patient care.

What presedation information should be recorded on the patient record?

Basic presedation patient care information is initially recorded on the sedation flowsheet and includes the patient's name, address, and hospital administrative identification number, as well as other pertinent information. Physical characteristics (height, weight) may be recorded directly on the moderate sedation record. If premedication has been administered, it should be documented on the patient record prior to the procedure. The effect of the sedative should be noted and is characteristically recorded, for example, as cooperative, calm, and sleeping. The time of administration of the premedication should also be noted. Patient medications are recorded on the sedation flowsheet with the last dose administered noted prior to the procedure. Allergy status should also be recorded on the flowsheet. The patient's allergies should be documented, and an attempt should be made to elicit the type of reaction (e.g., hives, gastrointestinal upset), and the data recorded on the flowsheet.

Presedation vital signs or the first set of vital signs obtained immediately before the procedure should be recorded on the sedation flowsheet. A presedation Aldrete score should also be recorded prior to commencement of the procedure. Although initial vital signs may be falsely elevated because of anxiety, they provide a baseline prior to the therapeutic, diagnostic, or minor surgical procedure. Monitors used and site of application are recorded before the procedure. The site of IV catheter insertion and the size of the catheter should be

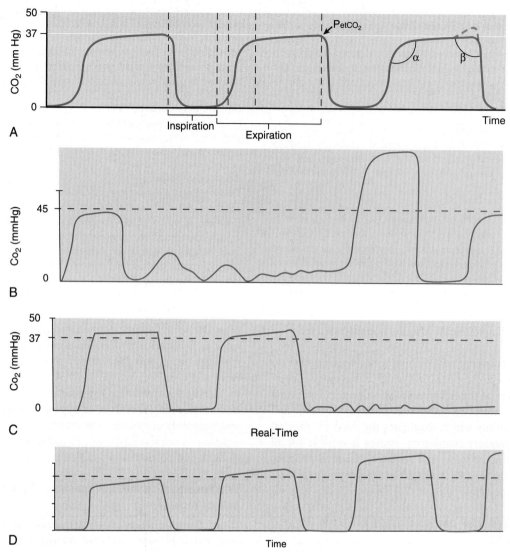

Fig. 8.11 End-tidal carbon dioxide waveforms. (A) The capnogram corresponds to the patient's respiratory cycle. An almost square waveform indicates a nonobstructed airway. (B) Partial airway obstruction. A nonsquare waveform indicates impaired ventilation secondary to partial airway obstruction or oversedation. (C) Sudden loss of a waveform indicates that no carbon dioxide is present secondary to total airway obstruction or respiratory arrest. (D) Hypoventilation is seen when end-tidal CO_2 levels start to rise; however, the waveform still possesses a somewhat normal resemblance. Decreased respiratory drive, CNS depression, and excessive sedation result in a patient who is not breathing fast or deeply enough to adequately remove CO_2 from the lungs. (From Miller RD, ed. *Miller's Anesthesia.* 8th ed. Philadelphia: Saunders; 2015.)

recorded. The type and amount of IV solution administered must be recorded and should be totaled at the conclusion of the procedure. A column for blood loss (if applicable) allows an accurate mechanism for postsedation assessment.

What procedural patient care information should be recorded on the patient record?

Recording of procedural patient care includes documentation of monitoring modalities and medications administered during the procedure. Depending on the pharmacologic technique used, medications are recorded in incremental doses or as a continuous infusion. The total dose administered should then be recorded in a total dose column. If reversal agents are required to counteract the pharmacologic effects

of sedative medications, their dosage and time of administration must be recorded. Information on the time of administration and total dose of reversal agent used assists the clinician with postprocedure monitoring and discharge planning. The patient's sedation level must also be documented.

What assessment scales are available for use to assess the postsedation level of consciousness?

The Ramsay Scale was originally used to quantitate the level of drug-induced sedation and measure patient responsiveness and drowsiness in the intensive care unit. It is, however, difficult to quantify a degree of agitation and oversedation with this scale.[26] The Ramsay Scale is represented in Table 8.3. The Observer's Assessment of Alertness/Sedation (OAA/S) Scale

DOWNTIME
☐ Entered into electronic record after downtime

date   time

initials

MODERATE (CONSCIOUS) SEDATION RECORD 1 of 4

Patient Name

Date of Birth   Admission/Visit Date   Site

Medical Record Number   Financial Number

Patient ID Area

NURSING TO FILL OUT

DATE_____ UNIT_____ Plan of care: ☐ Inpatient ☐ Outpatient Transfer from:_____
Accompanied by a responsible adult: ☐ No ☐ Yes Contact name:_____ Phone/Family pager:_____

NURSING PATIENT ASSESSMENT & FOCUSED HISTORY

PROCEDURE: AGE: WEIGHT: kg   HEIGHT: cm   ☐ NPO @

ALLERGIES ☐ NKA ☐ Latex ☐ Contrast ☐ Meds / Food / Product_____
    ☐ **ALLERGY BAND ON**

☐ Procedure Prep: ☐ Isolation, type: **Patient pregnant** ☐ No ☐ Yes, LMP_____

☐ History of Adverse Reaction to Sedation / Anesthesia, describe:_____
☐ Previous Anesthesia / Operations:_____

☐ Medical History in chart, if not-complete focused history   ☐ History of anticoagulation, Medication & Last Dose:_____

☐ Angina/MI ☐ CHF ☐ Cardiac Dysrhythmia ☐ Cardia surgery ☐ Pacemaker/AICD ☐ Murmur ☐ HTN ☐ Infectious disease:_____
☐ Chronic Lung Disease ☐ Obstructive sleep apnea ☐ CPAP/home settings_____ ☐ Asthma ☐ Smoker, packs/day_____
☐ GERD ☐ Dysphagia/motility issue/nausea/vomiting ☐ Liver disease/hepatitis/jaundice ☐ ETOH ☐ Renal Disease ☐ CRI/CRF/Dialysis ☐ Diabetes
☐ CVA/TIA ☐ Epilepsy ☐ Developmental Delay ☐ Chronic pain ☐ Depression ☐ Cancer ☐ Substance abuse, type_____
☐ Transplant:_____ ☐ Thyroid disease ☐ Glaucoma ☐ Bleeding disorder ☐ Implants:_____ ☐ Jehovah's Witness
☐ Other:_____

PRE OP VS: BP   HR   RR   T   O$_2$ SAT

RN Signature: Date: Time:

PROVIDER TO FILL OUT

HISTORY AND PHYSICAL EXAM BY PHYSICIAN OR LICENSED INDEPENDENT PRACTITIONER

HPI (History of Present Illness) / Indication for Procedure:

☐ See H&P if **Updated within 24 hours of procedure (must complete sedation assessment below if not on H&P)**

Medication Reconciliation: ☐ See Inpatient or Observation OR ☐ See Outpatient Medication Reconciliation form(s)

Area	WNL	Abn	FOCUSED Abnormal Findings
General appearance	☐	☐	☐ Obese ☐ Malnourished ☐ Infection ☐ Pressure ulcer (stage ____) ☐ Tracheostomy ☐ Cooperative
HEENT	☐	☐	
Cardiovascular	☐	☐	☐ Cyanotic ☐ Murmur
Lungs	☐	☐	
Abdomen	☐	☐	
Neurologic	☐	☐	
Other	☐	☐	

SEDATION ASSESSMENT ☐ **Provided on H&P or**
    ASA Classification: ☐ I ☐ II ☐ III ☐ IV ☐ V ☐ E **Mallampati Airway Assessment:** ☐ I ☐ II ☐ III ☐ IV
    Mental / Emotional ☐ Alert, oriented to name, place and time ☐ Calm ☐ Anxious ☐ Agitated ☐ Restraint

APPROPRIATENESS FOR SEDATION - Based on H&P, airway assessment, and planned procedure, this patient is an appropriate candidate for procedural sedation.
☐ Risks/Benefits/Complications explained & understood   ☐ Moderate Sedation   ☐ Deep Sedation
☐ Emergency Procedure - see chart for risk/benefit statement

Provider Signature_____   Date_____ Time_____

Attending Signature_____   Date_____ Time_____

OP-PROC EPISODE

Fig. 8.12 Moderate (conscious) sedation record.

Continued

Patient Name _____

Date of Birth _____ Admission/Visit Date _____ Site _____

Medical Record Number _____ Financial Number _____

Patient ID Area

MODERATE (CONSCIOUS) SEDATION RECORD 2 of 4

*Intra-procedure documentation completed by RN/RT for moderate sedation & credentialed LIP for deep sedation, all medications given IV unless specifically indicated.

TIME (I / P)*	TEMP °C	BP	HR ☐EKG monitored during case	RR	O₂ SAT	O₂ L/min	End tidal CO₂ ☐N/A	PAIN SCORE**	SEDATION SCORE	Midazolam mg	Fentanyl mcg	Meperidine mg				Initials
										PRE-PROCEDURE						

(Left margin, vertical text: NURSING TO FILL OUT)

Type of Fluid	Intravenous Amount	Fluids/Boluses		
		Date	Time	Initials

*I = intra-procedure; P = post-procedure   **Reminder: Circle TOTAL amount MEDICATION given INTRA-PROCEDURE**

**Document pain scale used to score patient pain: ☐ Wong-Baker® FACES Pain Scale 0-10 ☐ Numerical rating score (0-10) ☐ Peds FLACC Behavioral Pain Scale ☐ Other_____

Pasero Sedation Scale

Sedation Classification	Sedation Score	Description	Signature / Credentials	Initials	Date
Minimal	S	Sleep, easy to arouse			
Minimal	1	Awake and alert			
Moderate	2	Slightly drowsy, easily aroused			
Moderate	3	Frequently drowsy, arousable, drifts off to sleep during conversation			
Deep	4	Somnolent, minimal or no response to physical stimulation			

OP-PROC EPISODE

Fig. 8.12, cont'd

Continued

DOWNTIME

☐ Entered into electronic record after downtime

_____ _____
date   time

_____
initials

MODERATE (CONSCIOUS) SEDATION RECORD 3 of 4

Patient Name _____

Date of Birth _____ Admission/Visit Date _____ Site _____

Medical Record Number _____ Financial Number _____

Patient ID Area

COMMENTS: ☐ See Pentax ☐ See Sensis

_____
_____
_____
_____
_____
_____

PATIENT DISCHARGE FROM SEDATION

Temp: _____ Mental status ☐ Calm ☐ Oriented ☐ Anxious ☐ Disoriented Amount IV fluids infused: _____ mL Output: _____ mL

IV discontinued at_____ by_____ Condition of IV site ☐ No apparent problem ☐ Other_____

☐ Discharge instruction given to ☐ Patient ☐ Family ☐ Friend

☐ Patient meets criteria for recovery from sedation (see Sedation Scale on page 2)

☐ Patient has NOT recovered from effect of sedation, plan ☐ Transfer to ICU ☐ Other:_____

BP_____ HR_____ RR_____ T_____ SaO$_2$ _____

PATIENT'S POSSESSIONS ☐ NA ☐ Glasses ☐ Contacts ☐ Hearing aid(s) ☐ Ring(s) ☐ Watch ☐ Earring(s) ☐ Other:_____
☐ Xray / CD ☐ _____ Patient belongings returned to/or sent with: ☐ patient ☐ family member

☐ **Reversal agent administered, patient recovered for 90 minutes**

☐ **Patient transfer time:** _____ **Report given to RN:** _____ **Unit:** _____
  Discharging RN: _____ **Date:** _____ **Time:** _____

PATIENT LEAVING HOSPITAL / CLINIC - RESPONSIBLE ADULT
Discharge RN_____ Time_____ ☐ Home Other:_____
☐ Ambulatory ☐ Wheelchair ☐ Ambulance Accompanied by ☐ Self ☐ Family ☐ Friend ☐ EMS ☐ Other

SEDATION RECOVERY

☐ Complication_____
Follow up care_____
BP_____ HR_____ RR_____ T_____ SaO$_2$ _____
Hydration ☐ Acceptable ☐ Hydrating
Nausea/Vomiting ☐ None ☐ Nausea ☐ Nausea and Vomiting
Pain Score_____
Mental Status ☐ Return to baseline ☐ Other_____
Appropriate for DC ☐ Yes ☐ No
Provider Signature: _____ Date: _____ Time: _____

PATIENT DISCHARGED FROM DEEP SEDATION; COMPLETE DEEP SEDATION PROVIDER ASSESSMENT

☐ Complication_____
Follow up care_____
BP_____ HR_____ RR_____ T_____ SaO$_2$ _____
Hydration ☐ Acceptable ☐ Hydrating
Nausea/Vomiting ☐ None ☐ Nausea ☐ Nausea and Vomiting
Pain Score_____
Mental Status ☐ Return to baseline ☐ Other_____
Appropriate for DC ☐ Yes ☐ No
Provider Signature: _____ Date: _____ Time: _____

OP-PROC EPISODE

Fig. 8.12, cont'd

Continued

Patient Name _____
Date of Birth _____ Admission/Visit Date _____ Site _____
Medical Record Number _____ Financial Number _____
Patient ID Area

MODERATE (CONSCIOUS) SEDATION RECORD 4 of 4

CLINICIAN RESOURCES

Normal	Abnormal	American Society of Anesthesiologists Classifications
Mouth opening > 3 cm	Micrognathia	I Normal healthy patient
Chin to thyroid cartilage distances = 3 finger breadths	Retrognathia	II Mild systemic disease, no limitation of activity
	Trismus	III Severe systemic disease, limitation of activity
	Mallampati Class III*	IV Severe systemic disease that is constant threat to life
Normal neck flexion and extension	High arched palate	V Moribund, patient is not expected to survive 24 hours with or without procedure
Mallampati Class I*	Limitation in mouth opening or neck motion	E Emergency

Airway Assessment

Mallampati Classification: Have the patient perform the following in the upright sitting position: a. Open mouth as wide as possible; b. Protrude tongue as far as possible (no phonation). Identify the following structures: a. Uvula; b. Tonsillar pillars; c. Soft palate

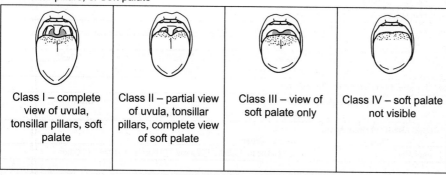

Class I – complete view of uvula, tonsillar pillars, soft palate	Class II – partial view of uvula, tonsillar pillars, complete view of soft palate	Class III – view of soft palate only	Class IV – soft palate not visible

Nothing by Mouth (NPO) Guidelines for Sedation / Analgesia – 2011

Clear Liquids	Breast Milk	Non-human Milk/Formula	Light Meal (toast/clear liquids)	Solids	Upper Gastric Tube Feeding
Stop 2 hrs prior to procedure for otherwise health children and adult	Otherwise healthy neonates and infants < 44 gestational weeks stop 4 hrs before procedure	Otherwise healthy stop 6 hours before procedure	Stop 6 hours before procedure	Stop 8 hours before procedure	Stop transpyloric feed 2 hours before procedure

NOTES:	1. Medication may be taken with one sip of water.	4. Clear, carbonated soft drink is permitted. Alcohol is not a clear liquid.
	2. Oral contrast, if required for the procedure, may be given according to the Department of Radiology protocol.	5. **All patients with documented delayed gastric emptying should be NPO at least 8 hours. This includes patients with diabetes, obesity, pregnancy, gastric bypass patient, trauma or chronic renal failure.**
	3. If patient is emergent, see risk / benefit statement.	

OP-PROC EPISODE

Fig. 8.12, cont'd

TABLE 8.3   Ramsay Sedation Scale

Clinical Score	Patient Characteristics
1	Awake, agitated or restless or both
2	Awake, cooperative, oriented, and tranquil
3	Awake but responds to commands only
4	Asleep, brisk response to light glabellar tap or loud auditory stimulus
5	Asleep, sluggish response to light glabellar tap or loud auditory stimulus
6	Asleep, no response to glabellar tap or loud auditory stimulus

Adapted from Ramsay MA, Savege TM, Simpson BR, Goodwin R. Controlled sedation with alphaxalone-alphadolone. Br Med J. 1974;2:656–659.

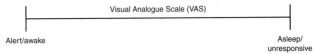

Fig. 8.13 Sedation visual analogue scale. (From McCaffery M, Pasero C. *Pain: Clinical Manual*. St. Louis, Mosby; 1999.)

was developed to quantify the CNS effects of benzodiazepines.[27] The OAA/S assesses patient responsiveness, speech, facial expression, and ocular appearance. The OAA/S provides a higher level of discrimination for various levels of sedation. However, a major disadvantage of this level of consciousness (LOC) assessment technique is that the patient needs to be stimulated to perform the testing procedure. The OAA/S is represented in Table 8.4. The Sedation Visual Analogue Scale has been used to quantify the level of sedation during monitored anesthesia care cases.[28-30] The Sedation Visual Analogue Scale uses a 100-mm visual analogue scale, which is displayed at one end as "awake and alert" and at the opposite end by "asleep." A distinct disadvantage associated with this scale is that it requires the patient to be alert and stimulated throughout the procedure. A sample of the Sedation Visual Analogue Scale is represented in Fig. 8.13.

Use of a level of consciousness scoring tool or monitor (Ramsay Scale, OAA/S, or Sedation Visual Analogue Scale) provides the clinician with the ability to monitor the level of CNS depression more objectively while attempting to

adhere to the goals and objectives of moderate procedural sedation and analgesia. Additional information recorded on the sedation flowsheet includes the name or signature of the attending physician, health care provider monitoring the patient, diagnosis, procedure, and start and stop time.

What postsedation aspects of care should be recorded on the patient record?

The postsedation phase of care includes vital signs, pain assessment scores, treatment protocols implemented (e.g., nausea, vomiting), discharge recovery scoring (Aldrete score), and the administration of any pain medications. The condition of the patient at the time of discharge, responsible adult accompanying the patient home, and documentation that discharge education and instructions have been provided.

SUMMARY

Patients receiving sedation are monitored on a continuous basis throughout the procedure. Although generally a safe practice, there is a degree of morbidity and mortality associated with sedation practice. Sedation monitoring standards continue to evolve. Although vital sign parameters are recorded at regular intervals, subjective and objective monitoring modalities are conducted throughout the procedure. A wide variety of differential diagnoses associated with sedation and postsedation complications are outlined in Box 8.7. Monitoring parameters outlined in this chapter are effective tools when used in conjunction with vigilant health care provider assessment strategies.

TABLE 8.4   Observer's Assessment of Alertness/Sedation Scale (OAA/S)

Responsiveness	Speech	Facial Expression	Eyes	Composite Score (Level)[a]
Responds readily to name spoken in normal tone	Normal	Normal	Clear, no ptosis	1 (alert)
Lethargic response to name spoken in normal tone	Mild slowing or thickening	Mild relaxation	Glazed or mild ptosis (<50% of the eye)	2
Responds only after name is called loudly and/or repeatedly	Slurring or prominent slowing	Marked relaxation (slacked jaw)	Glazed and mild ptosis (≥50% of the eye)	3
Responds only after mild prodding or shaking	Few recognizable words			4
Does not respond to mild prodding or shaking				5 (deep sleep)

[a]Assign the composite score corresponding to the highest level at which any statement is checked. Responsiveness should be evaluated first.

BOX 8.7   Differential Diagnosis of Moderate Procedural Sedation and Analgesia Postsedation Complications

Restlessness
- Hypoxemia ($\downarrow$ SpO$_2$)
- Pain
- Hypotension
- Bladder distention, urinary retention
- Emotional response
- Shivering, feeling of being cold
- Hypercarbia ($\uparrow$ CO$_2$)
- Emergence delirium
- Gastrointestinal distress, distention
- Psychotropic effects of sedative medications
- $\uparrow$ Intracranial pressure, intracranial event

Hypotension
- Decreased preload
- Hypovolemia from prolonged or inadequate fasting or inadequate fluid replacement
- Excessive urinary losses, bleeding
- Peripheral vasodilation ($\downarrow$ resistance)
- Effects of sedative and narcotic drugs
- Decreased myocardial contractility
- Orthostatic effects of progressive ambulation

Hypertension
- Pain, surgical stimulation
- Hypoxemia ($\downarrow$ SpO$_2$)
- Bladder distention, urinary retention
- Shivering, vasoconstriction due to hypothermia
- Preexisting disease (e.g., hyperthyroidism, essential hypertension, renal disease)
- Emergence delirium, emotional response
- Hypercarbia ($\uparrow$ CO$_2$)
- Retching or vomiting
- Fluid overload
- Effects of medications (e.g., vasopressors, naloxone, ketamine, anticholinergics, cocaine, ephedrine, epinephrine)

Dysrhythmias
- Pain
- Hypoxemia ($\downarrow$ SpO$_2$)
- Procedural myocardial infarction
- Catecholamine release
- Metabolic changes (e.g., acidosis, alkalosis)
- Preexisting disease
- Hypercarbia ($\uparrow$ CO$_2$)
- Failure of artificial pacemaker
- Side effects of sedative-analgesia medications
- Electrolyte imbalance (e.g., potassium, calcium)

Tachycardia
- Pain
- Hypovolemia
- Emergence delirium
- Fever (e.g., malignant hyperthermia, sepsis)
- Hyperthyroidism
- Effects of medications (e.g., atropine, glycopyrrolate)

Bradycardia
- Oculocardiac reflex
- Stimulation of baroreceptors
- Hypoventilation, especially in children
- Cardiac effects of heavy athletic activity
- Sedative, analgesic drugs

Respiratory Depression
- Obstructed airway
- Splinting, secondary to pain
- Pulmonary congestion
- Positioning, especially in the obese
- Mechanical failure of equipment (bag, valve, mask)
- Preexisting disease, chronic obstructive pulmonary disease, reactive airway

Modified from Burden N. *Ambulatory Surgical Nursing.* 2nd ed. Philadelphia: WB Saunders; 2000:413.

REFERENCES

1. Mirvis DM, Goldberger AL. Electrocardiography. In: Mann DL, Zipes DP, Libby P, Bonow RO, Braunwald E, eds. *Braunwald's heart disease: A textbook of cardiovascular medicine (10th ed.).* Philadelphia: Saunders; 2015:114–154.
2. Thygesen K, Alpert JS, Jaffe AS, et al. Third universal definition of myocardial infarction. *Circulation.* 2012;126(16):2020.
3. Cummins R. *Advanced Cardiac Life Support.* Dallas: American Heart Association; 1998.
4. Butterworth JF. *Morgan and Mikhail's Clinical Anesthesiology.* 5th ed. New York: McGraw-Hill Education/Medical; 2013.
5. Handler J. The importance of accurate blood pressure measurement. *Permanente Journal.* 2009;13(3):51–54.
6. Bijker JB, van Klei WA, Kappen TH, et al. Incidence of intraoperative hypotension as a function of the chosen definition: Literature definitions applied to a retrospective cohort using automated data collection. *Anesthesiology.* 2007;107:213–220.
7. Jubran A. Pulse oximetry. *Crit Care.* 2015;19:272.
8. Nitzan M, Romem A, Koppel R. Pulse oximetry: Fundamentals and technology update. *Med Devices (Auckl).* 2014;7:231–239.
9. Lake C. *Clinical Monitoring.* Philadelphia: WB Saunders; 1991:589.
10. Bohr C, Hasselbalch K, Krogh A. Concerning a biologically important relationship—the influence of the carbon dioxide content of blood on its oxygen binding. *Scand Arch Physiol.* 1904;16:402.
11. Severinghaus JW. Simple, accurate equations for human blood O2 dissociation computations. *Journal of Applied Physiology.* 1979;46(3):599–602.
12. Mills Frederick C, Ackers Gary K. Quaternary enhancement in binding of oxygen by human hemoglobin. *Proceedings of the National Academy of Sciences.* 1979;76(1):273–277.
13. Eaton William A, Henry ER, Hofrichter J, et al. Evolution of allosteric models for hemoglobin. *IUBMB life.* 2007;59(8-9):586–599.
14. Dash RK, Bassingthwaighte JB. Erratum to: Blood HbO2 and HbCO2 dissociation curves at varied O2, CO2, pH, 2,3-DPG and temperature levels. *Annals of Biomedical Engineering.* 2010;38(4):1683–1701.
15. Giuliano KK, Higgins TL. New-generation pulse oximetry in the care of critically ill patients. *Am J Crit Care.* 2005;14:26–37.
16. Tobin RM, Pologe JA, Batchelder PB. A characterization of motion affecting pulse oximetry in 350 patients. *Anesthesia and Analgesia.* 2002;94(1 Suppl):S54–61.

17. The Joint Commission. *The Joint Commission Standards and Elements of Performance Standards for Sedation and Anesthesia Care. Provision of Care, Treatment, and Services.* Oakbrook Terrace, IL: The Joint Commission; 2018.

18. Practice guidelines for moderate procedural sedation and analgesia 2018: a report by the American Society of Anesthesiologists Task Force on Moderate Procedural Sedation and Analgesia, the American Association of Oral and Maxillofacial Surgeons, American College of Radiology, American Dental Association, American Society of Dentist Anesthesiologists, and Society of Interventional Radiology. *Anesthesiology.* 2018;128:437–479.

19. AORN. Guideline for care of the patient receiving moderate sedation/analgesia. In *Guidelines for Perioperative Practice.* Denver, CO: Association of periOperative Registered Nurses; 2016:617–648.

20. Vargo JJ, DeLegge MH, Feld AD, et al. Multisociety sedation curriculum for gastrointestinal endoscopy. *Gastrointestinal Endoscopy.* 2012;76(1):e1–e25.

21. Jarzyna D, Jungquist CR, Pasero C, et al. American Society for Pain Management Nursing. Guidelines on monitoring for opioid-induced sedation and respiratory depression. *Pain Management Nursing,* 12 (3), 118-145.

22. The Joint Commission Perspectives. Capnography monitoring required in NY office-based surgery practices. https://www. jointcommission.org/capnography_monitoring_required_in_ny_office-based_surgery_practices/...

23. Hiroshi A, Mitsuru K, Kazuki S, et al. Does pulse oximetry accurately monitor a patient's ventilation during sedated endoscopy under oxygen supplementation. *Singapore Med J.* 2013;54(4):212–215. https://doi.org/10.11622/smedj.2013075.

24. Trillo G, von Planta M, Kette F. ETCO2 monitoring during low flow states: Clinical aims and limits. *Resuscitation.* 1994;25 (6):412.

25. Sanders A. Capnography in emergency medicine. *Ann Emerg Med.* 1989;18:1287–1290.

26. Ramsay MA, Savage TM, Simpson BR, et al. Controlled sedation with alphaxalone-alphadolone. *BMJ.* 1974;2:656.

27. Chernik DA, Gillings D, Laine H, et al. Validity and reliability of the observer's assessment of alertness/sedation scale: Study with intravenous midazolam. *J Clin Psychopharmacol.* 1990;10:244.

28. White PF, Negus JB. Sedative infusions during local and regional anesthesia. *J Clin Anesth.* 1991;3:32.

29. Ramirez-Ruiz M, Smith I, White PF. Use of analgesics during propofol sedation: A comparison of ketorolac, dezocine, and fentanyl. *J Clin Anesth.* 1995;7:481.

30. Borgeat A, Wilder-Smith OH, Saiah M, et al. Subhypnotic doses of propofol possess direct antiemetic properties. *Anesth Analg.* 1992;74:539.

CHAPTER 8: REVIEW QUESTIONS

1. Which ECG monitoring lead is useful in the detection of dysrhythmias secondary to the increased visibility of the P wave in this lead?
   A. Lead I
   B. Lead II
   C. Lead III
   D. Lead IV

2. Which of the following ECG monitoring leads is useful in the detection of dysrhythmias because a large portion of the left ventricle is located beneath its position and is a useful lead in the detection of myocardial ischemia?
   A. Lead I
   B. Lead II
   C. Lead III
   D. Lead V_5

3. Which of the following is the monitoring lead of choice for a patient with a significant past medical history of severe coronary artery disease and myocardial ischemia?
   A. Lead I
   B. Lead II
   C. Lead III
   D. Lead V_5

4. Which of the following is a cardiac dysrhythmia characterized by fluctuations in heart rate influenced by the respiratory pattern and the degree of parasympathetic nervous system control over the sinoatrial node, and features a heart rate increase during inspiration?
   A. Sinus tachycardia
   B. Sinus bradycardia
   C. Sinus arrhythmia
   D. Premature atrial contraction

5. Which of the following cardiac dysrhythmias is characterized by a rapid ectopic atrial discharge at a rate of 250 to 350 beats/min, with inability of the ventricle to respond to each impulse?
   A. Premature atrial contractions
   B. Atrial flutter
   C. Ventricular fibrillation
   D. Ventricular tachycardia

6. A life-threatening dysrhythmia that results in the inability of the ventricle to contract, with no recovery phase between ventricular contractions, is identified as which of the following?
   A. Ventricular tachycardia
   B. Ventricular fibrillation
   C. Atrial fibrillation
   D. Atrial tachycardia

7. Which of the following statements most accurately reflects the effect of blood pressure cuff size on measurement?
   A. Blood pressure cuff size has no impact on the accuracy of blood pressure readings.
   B. A blood pressure cuff that is too large for the patient results in an excessively elevated measurement.
   C. A blood pressure cuff that is too large for a patient results in an excessively low measurement.

D. A blood pressure cuff that is too small for a patient results in an excessively low measurement.

8. All of the following are treatment protocols for managing procedural hypotension except _____.
   A. Administration of hydralazine (alpha blocker)
   B. Correction of acidosis or hypoxemia
   C. Administration of oxygen
   D. Administration of ephedrine

9. Patient movement and a low perfusion state affect the accuracy of which of the following monitors in the sedation setting?
   A. Pulse oximeter
   B. Capnography
   C. Continuous positive airway pressure (CPAP) mask
   D. Nonrebreather mask

10. An SaO_2 of 90% correlates with an approximate PO_2 of ___ mm Hg on the oxyhemoglobin dissociation curve.
    A. 30
    B. 40
    C. 50
    D. 60

11. Which of the following monitors almost instantaneously detects total airway obstruction or a state of respiratory arrest?
    A. Pulse oximeter
    B. Capnography
    C. CPAP mask
    D. Nonrebreather mask

12. When the patient is maintained in a state of moderate procedural sedation, which of the following procedural monitoring tools requires a patient's response to commands?
    A. Assessment of vital signs
    B. Level of consciousness monitoring
    C. Pulse oximetry measurement
    D. ECG monitoring

Answers can be found in Appendix A.

Intravenous Insertion Techniques and Procedural Fluid Selection

At the completion of this chapter, the learner shall:
- Delineate the principles of intravenous therapy.
- Describe the proper technique for intravenous cannula insertion required for moderate sedation patients.
- Analyze common complications of peripheral intravenous therapy and treatment options for these complications.
- Identify common intravenous solutions used during the administration of moderate procedural sedation and analgesia.
- Demonstrate the appropriate patient care requirements associated with intravenous fluid therapy requirements for presedation and procedural and postprocedural patient care.

COMPETENCY STATEMENT

The sedation health care practitioner initiates intravenous catheterization and selects appropriate intravenous fluid(s) for the patient scheduled for therapeutic, diagnostic, or surgical procedures requiring moderate procedural sedation and analgesia.

What is the purpose of intravenous (IV) cannulation?

There are a variety of reasons for IV cannulation, including the following:
- To replace fluids and electrolytes and maintain fluid and electrolyte balance
- To administer medications, anesthetics, diagnostic dyes and testing agents, and antibiotics
- To deliver nutrients and nutrition

In the moderate procedural sedation setting, the purpose of IV cannulation is to provide direct vascular access for the administration of medications and supplemental fluid during therapeutic and diagnostic procedures requiring sedative and analgesic agents. IV access provides immediate uptake and distribution for sedative medications and serves as a lifeline in the event of patient decompensation or crisis. Placement of the IV cannula is critical to the success of the planned procedure. Whenever there is doubt regarding successful cannulation or possible infiltration, the clinician should err on the side of caution and replace the catheter.

What are the basic components of preparing for IV insertion?

Supplies and equipment must be assembled before the application of a tourniquet and selection of a vein. Supplies and equipment required for IV insertion are listed in Box 9.1. Often, sedation providers personally select the IV solution and rate of administration in the presedation holding area. However, the health care provider performing the procedure is required to order the following IV therapy parameters:
- Type of solution
- Rate of infusion
- Duration
- Date
- Time

Once equipment is gathered, and the IV solution is ordered by a health care provider, a variety of administration sets are available for use. Administration sets are selected on the basis of the following criteria:
- Length
- Location of access ports used to infuse sedative, hypnotic, and analgesic medications
- Size of drop chamber—microdrip versus macrodrip (Fig. 9.1)
- Type of flow regulator to regulate the speed of administration and stop an IV gravity infusion (Fig. 9.2)
- Back-check valve to prevent backflow of IV solution

Which peripheral vein is ideal for IV catheter insertion for moderate procedural sedation and analgesia procedures?

Once in the presedation holding area or procedure room, the patient is assessed for identification of a vascular access site. Veins that are generally selected for peripheral cannulation are depicted in Fig. 9.3. Selection of a vein for vascular access depends on a number of variables, including the following:
- Planned therapeutic or diagnostic procedure
- Patient positioning
- Patient status
  - Inpatient versus outpatient
- Anticipated postsedation activity level
- Length of time that IV access is required

BOX 9.1 Intravenous Insertion Supplies

- Disposable gloves
- Alcohol swabs, antiseptic solution
- Tourniquet
- Selection of IV catheter
  - 18 gauge
  - 20 gauge
  - 22 gauge
- 1% lidocaine (optional)
- EMLA cream—eutectic mixture of local anesthetics (EMLA) cream (lidocaine 2.5%, prilocaine 2.5%); emulsion in which the oil phase is a eutectic mixture of lidocaine and prilocaine in a ratio of 1:1 by weight
- Extension tubing and sterile cap(s)
- Normal saline flush
- Adhesive, paper tape
- Tuberculin syringe with 29- or 30-gauge needle
- For local anesthetic injection (optional)
- Assortment of syringes
  - 3 mL
  - 5 mL
  - 10 mL
- IV solution of choice
  - Ringer's lactate
  - Normosol
  - Normal saline
- Flush solution (0.9% sodium chloride, preservative-free)
- Sharps container
- Arm board
- 1-inch nonallergic tape
- Sterile, transparent, semipermeable dressing (e.g., Tegaderm)

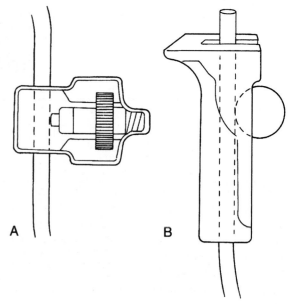

Fig. 9.2 Administration set—fluid-regulating clamps. (A) Screw clamp. (B) Roller clamp. (From Booker MF, Ignatavicius DD: *Infusion Therapy: Techniques and Medications*. Philadelphia: WB Saunders; 1996.)

Previous mastectomy, lymph node dissection, or the presence of renal access grafts is a contraindication for vascular access in the affected extremity. Anatomically, areas for venipuncture include the following:

- Dorsum of the hand
- Veins of the wrist
- Forearm veins
- Major veins of the antecubital fossa

Advantages and disadvantages of peripheral vein selection are listed in Box 9.2. Inpatients receiving prolonged IV fluid therapy benefit from IV insertion at the most distal portion of the upper extremity.

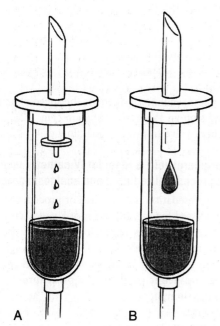

Fig. 9.1 Administration of Venoset drip chambers. (A) Microdrip. (B) Macrodrip. (From Booker MF, Ignatavicius DD: *Infusion Therapy: Techniques and Medications*. Philadelphia: WB Saunders; 1996.)

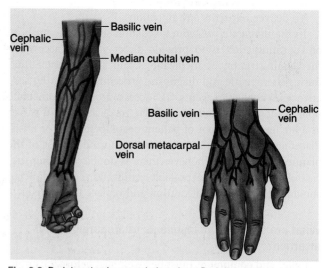

Fig. 9.3 Peripheral vein cannulation sites. Peripheral veins are appropriate for vascular access in older children and adults. (From Potter PA, Perry AG, Stockert P, Hall A. *Essentials for Nursing Practice*. 9th ed. St. Louis: Elsevier; 2019.)

BOX 9.2 Advantages and Disadvantages of Peripheral Vein Selection

Dorsum of the Hand
Dorsal Digital Veins
Dorsum of the hand veins are formed from the adjacent sides of the fingers and converge to form three dorsal metacarpal veins, which end in a dorsal venous network opposite to the middle of the metacarpus.

Advantages
Preferred site for venipuncture by many health care providers
Reside very superficial to the surface of the skin
Very visible
Easy to palpate
Splinted by metacarpal bones
Allow use of more proximal veins in the same limb for future catheter insertions
Cannula easily accessible

Disadvantages
Veins smaller than veins found more proximally
Superficial veins more mobile, may roll

Veins of the Wrist
Dorsal Venous Network
Veins of the wrist that continue proximally, draining subcutaneously along the margins of the hand and wrist; the lateral (radial) aspect of the wrist, where the intern or resident vein is located.

Advantage
Highly visible vein(s)

Disadvantages
Immobilization difficult
Veins not as large as those on the dorsum of the wrist
Presence of arteries, nerves, and tendons—makes the area more sensitive, increases risk of catheter placement

Forearm Veins
Cephalic Vein
This is a forearm vein formed from the convergence of veins at the base of the thumb and that passes upward along the radial (lateral) aspect of the forearm to enter the lateral part of the antecubital fossa.

Advantages
Easily accessible for insertion and routine care
Easy palpation and visualization above and below antecubital fossa
Splinted by the forearm bones
Cannula easily secured

Disadvantages
Smaller than basilica
Pathway in upper arm and thorax variable and unknown
Can be more difficult to cannulate than the metacarpal veins
May be confused with an aberrant radial artery

Basilic Vein
This is a forearm vein formed from the convergence of veins on the posteromedial aspect of the wrist; it passes upward slightly posterior to the medial border of the forearm but winds around over the ulnar to enter the medial aspect of the antecubital fossa.

Advantages
Largest vein
Straight pathway in upper arm and thorax

Disadvantages
Awkward placement—may be located too far to the posterior side for sterile procedure and routine care
May only be able to palpate a short segment
Prone to the development of phlebitis
Cannula port can get caught in bed linens

Major Veins of the Antecubital Fossa
Cephalic Vein
This is the continuation of the vein from the anterolateral aspect of the forearm onto the anterolateral aspect of the arm over the bicep muscle to the deltoid to join the brachial vein, ending in the axillary vein.

Basilic Vein
This is continuation of the vein from the anteromedial aspect of the forearm; it joins the deep veins to branch into the brachial vein or traverses the antecubital fossa.

Median Vein
This is a superficial vein that connects the basilica and cephalic vein; it lies close to the surface of the arm and becomes extremely prominent when direct pressure is applied.

Advantages
Joins with larger basilica
Easily accessible for insertion and routine care
Tends to stay patent longer than peripheral veins
Generally first choice in emergency situations

Disadvantages
Valve may be located at junction with basilica, causing obstruction to cannula advancement
Can be uncomfortable due to flexion and extension of the elbow

What size IV catheter is appropriate for the sedation patient?

The peripheral catheter selected for IV cannulation for short-term care is generally 3/4 to 1 inch (2–2.5 cm) in length, with a 20- or 22-gauge diameter. However, larger gauge catheters may be required to facilitate hydration or for specific diagnostic or therapeutic procedures. As identified in Table 9.1, the larger the peripheral IV catheter, the greater the flow rate.[1] Physical principles related to IV solution flow rate include the following:

- The larger the IV catheter size, the greater the increase in velocity of flow.

TABLE 9.1   Intravenous Catheter Size and Fluid Flow Rate

Gauge	Length	Water Flow Rate (mL/min)
14	50	236.1
16	50	154.7
18	45	98.1
20	33	64.4
22	25	35.7

- Shorter IV catheters offer less resistance to flow.
- Consider plugging a drip directly into the catheter hub instead of into flow-restricting connectors, such as needle-free adapters and saline locks.
- Increase IV solution bag height to optimize pressure differences between the bag and sleeve.

Is there a quick reference guide that can be used to assist the health care provider in selecting a properly sized catheter for the procedure?

Properly sized catheters and their use are indicated in Table 9.2.

What is an effective method to initiate insertion of a peripheral IV catheter for procedural sedation?

Application of a tourniquet approximately 6 inches above the insertion site (Fig. 9.4) distends the peripheral blood vessels. Periodic clenching of the patient's hand distends the vessel more fully. Warm cloths and rubbing of the extremity provide vasodilation and venous filling in patients who are peripherally vasoconstricted. Prior to insertion, the area should be cleansed in a circular fashion (Fig. 9.5) within a 2- to 2.5-inch radius from the intended insertion site. The cleansing agent (e.g., iodine, alcohol) is allowed to air-dry to provide antibacterial action.

When a local anesthetic is used to anesthetize the skin, it should be injected superficially. A small intradermal skin wheal (0.1 mL of plain lidocaine, 30-gauge needle) anesthetizes the local tissue. Care must be taken not to insert the local needle deeply into the skin, or venous perforation and hematoma formation may occur. Once the area has been localized, traction on the vein is applied by the nondominant hand to

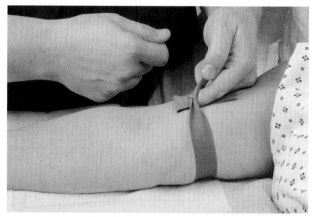

Fig. 9.4 Application of venous tourniquet provides venous engorgement before IV cannulation. (From Potter PA, Perry AG, Stockert P, Hall A. *Essentials for Nursing Practice*. 9th ed. St. Louis: Elsevier; 2019.)

secure or anchor the vein. This prevents the vein from rolling and excessive movement when one is preparing to insert the IV catheter.

When the appropriately sized IV catheter is selected, it should be inserted through the small skin wheal of local anesthesia. The needle is then advanced at a 30- to 40-degree angle in the direction of the vein to be cannulated. Once a so-called flash of blood is noted in the catheter chamber (Fig. 9.6), the needle should be advanced slightly (several millimeters). This maneuver ensures that the plastic catheter is situated in the vein and is not positioned superficially over the vein. At this point, extreme care must be taken not to advance the needle through the back wall of the vein. Malpositioning of the catheter may result in local tissue trauma, hematoma formation, and a nonfunctional IV site. If the attempt to secure an IV line is unsuccessful, it is beneficial to leave the plastic catheter in place while an attempt is made at another IV access to avoid hematoma formation. After venous access is established, the unsuccessful IV catheter may then be removed. Pressure is then applied until hemostasis is achieved.

TABLE 9.2   Properly Sized Catheters and Their Use

Size (gauge)	Color	Recommended Use
14	Orange	Massive trauma, shock-like state
16	Gray	Trauma, surgery requiring large volume infusion
18	Green	Blood transfusion, large volume infusion
20	Pink	Sedation procedures, multiple routine uses for medications and fluids
22	Blue	Chemotherapy infusions, geriatric, small-vein candidates
24	Yellow	Patients with very fragile veins (e.g., older adults, pediatric patients)

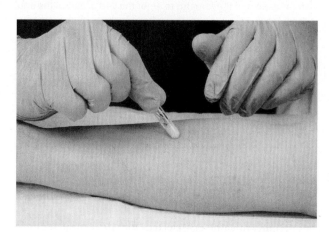

Fig. 9.5 Preparation of IV cannulation site. Prior to vascular access, alcohol or an antiseptic agent is applied in a circular fashion within a 2- to 2.5-inch radius and permitted to dry. (From Potter PA, Perry AG, Stockert P, Hall A. *Essentials for Nursing Practice*. 9th ed. St. Louis: Elsevier; 2019.)

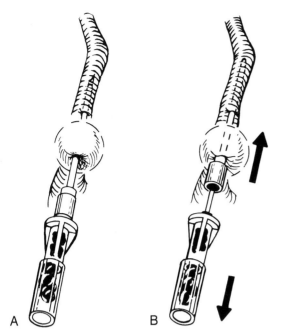

Fig. 9.6 Presence of venous flash with advancement of catheter. (A) Venous access is ascertained with the presence of a flash followed by advancement of the catheter into the peripheral blood vessel (B). (From Butterworth J. *Atlas of Procedures in Anesthesia and Critical Care.* Philadelphia: WB Saunders; 1991.)

Once the IV line is established, the health care provider advances the catheter over the stylet with the index finger of the dominant hand or opposite hand. Either technique is acceptable for positioning the IV catheter into the vein. Contemporary systems for IV access incorporate needleless technology, which includes self-retracting trocars on systems that cover the sharp tip of the needle. The Venoset is then connected with pressure applied between the male Venoset connector and the female catheter connector. Firm pressure should be applied at this junction to avoid unintentional disconnection. It is important to secure the catheter and tubing with a sterile dressing, tape, or transparent dressing. Transparent dressings afford direct visualization of the IV site. Redness, swelling, edema, or leakage around the site may be evaluated directly through the presence of the clear Tegaderm dressing (transparent medical dressing).

Are there any devices available to help identify veins prior to attempting catheter insertion?

Vein identification devices (e.g., Veinlite LED Transilluminator, Venoscope II Transilluminator, Illumivein) are available for patients whose veins are not readily identifiable. Vein identification devices are beneficial in a variety of patient populations, which include the following:
- Older patients
  - Thin, friable veins
- Pediatric patients
  - Small veins
- Presence of fatty tissue
- Patients with dark complexions
- Obese patients

Blood contains oxygen and nutrient-carrying hemoglobin molecules, which readily absorb infrared light. When an active infrared vein finder is applied to the skin, the vessels become visible because the absorbed light in the hemoglobin makes the veins appear darker secondary to the high contrast when compared to the surrounding tissue. The vein finder emits light waves that penetrate into the skin, and superficial veins become easily identifiable.

What complications are associated with peripheral IV cannulation?

Local complications associated with IV catheter insertion include infiltration, extravasation, phlebitis, hematoma formation, catheter embolism, local infection, and venous irritation. Local and systemic complications associated with IV therapy are listed in Table 9.3.

What IV fluid should be administered in the sedation setting?

IV fluid replacement is typically accomplished with crystalloid solutions during the administration of conscious sedation. IV solutions maintain fluid and electrolyte balance. Body fluids are divided into intracellular and extracellular fluids. Intracellular fluids are contained within the cells of the body; extracellular fluid is divided into three compartments:
- Interstitial
- Intravascular
- Transcellular

Interstitial fluid is located between cells, whereas intravascular fluid lies within blood vessels or plasma. Transcellular fluid is secreted by epithelial cells and constitutes cerebrospinal fluid, intraocular fluid, and digestive fluids. Factors that have an impact on intravascular fluid replacement include the presence of concomitant disease states (e.g., hypertension, dehydration), procedural fluid losses, and the patient's cardiovascular status. In emergency situations, restoration of intravascular volume restores plasma volume and optimizes cardiac output to ensure adequate tissue oxygen delivery.

Crystalloid solutions can be differentiated according to their osmolality. *Osmolality* is a term used to identify the number of particles in 1 L of solution. Measured in milliosmoles per liter (mOsm/L), the osmolality of the extracellular fluid is determined by measuring the solute concentration of the blood (normal serum osmolality = 280–300 mOsm). Electrolyte solutions (crystalloid) are capable of conducting an electrical charge. Cations (e.g., potassium, sodium) maintain a positive charge, and anions (e.g., chloride) produce a negative charge. Anions and cations of intracellular, interstitial, and intravascular fluids are identified in Fig. 9.7.

The tonicity of crystalloids is also a major factor in the selection of IV fluids. Crystalloid solutions are therefore divided into the following classifications:
- Hypotonic—lower osmotic pressure than plasma
- Isotonic—same osmotic pressure as plasma
- Hypertonic—greater osmotic pressure than plasma

TABLE 9.3   Intravenous Therapy
Local and Systemic Complications

Complication	Cause	Signs and Symptoms	Treatment	Prevention
Local Complications				
Infiltration	Infusion of seepage of IV fluid into extravascular tissue caused by partial or complete venous access dislodgement	Decreased infusion rate Localized edema Complaints of burning, pain, and tenderness at IV site	Remove catheter. Apply warm, moist heat to enhance fluid absorption.	Stabilize catheter insertion site. Avoid catheter insertion at points of flexion. Frequently assess catheter site.
Extravasation	Accidental administration of medication or solution, which results in tissue destruction (e.g., dopamine, diazepam)	Patient complaint of: • Stinging or localized burning at the catheter insertion site • Swelling • Localized tissue destruction (blister formation)	Stop infusion. Related to amount of concentration of medication or solution Physician notification Catheter remains in place	Monitor insertion site frequently. Stabilize catheter insertion site. Administer IV push medications via free-flowing IV insertion site.
Phlebitis	Inflammation along the course of the vein. Contributing factors in the development of phlebitis include: • Insertion technique • Type of medication • Catheter size and length	Pain at the catheter site Red, inflamed "knotty" cordlike vein Temperature	Catheter removal Warm compresses	Change catheter site every 48–72 hours Use large veins when irritating solutions (highly osmolar) are used. Use strict aseptic handling of catheter during insertion.
Hematoma formation	Leakage of blood into the surrounding tissue	Bruising around the IV insertion site Pain at the site	Removal of catheter Application of direct pressure at insertion site Warm soaks applied if hematoma site is stable	Select small-gauge catheter. Carefully advance catheter parallel to patient's skin.
Local infection	Contamination at the IV insertion site secondary to a break in aseptic technique	Red, swollen, warm area or presence of purulent exudate at the insertion site	Catheter removal Catheter tip may be sent for culture. Site cleansed with antibacterial solution, covered with a sterile dressing	Use strict aseptic technique. Change infusion containers after minimum of 24 hours Change Venoset every 48–72 hours
Catheter embolization	A piece of the IV catheter breaks off and floats freely in the blood vessel. Embolization can occur when the needle is reinserted into the catheter and advanced once a flash has been obtained.	Cardiovascular compromise: • Hypotension • Tachycardia • Cyanosis Pain along the vein	Catheter removal Tourniquet placement proximal to the insertion site Radiograph to locate catheter tip Surgical excision of catheter tip	Never reinsert the needle into the catheter during Jelco catheter insertion. During medication administration, use the shortest needle to puncture the injection port (1 inch).
Systemic Complications				
Systemic infection, sepsis	Pathogenic organism entrance into the systemic circulation Results from poor aseptic technique, contaminated solution, or catheter insertion	Early • Fever • Chills • Headache • Malaise	Change entire infusion system. Notify physician. Obtain cultures as ordered.	Strictly adhere to aseptic technique. Change infusion containers at a minimum of every 24 hours

TABLE 9.3   Intravenous Therapy—cont'd

Local and Systemic Complications

Complication	Cause	Signs and Symptoms	Treatment	Prevention
		Late • Cardiovascular collapse • Death		Change Venoset every 48–72 hours
Air embolism	Air entrains into the systemic circulation. Entrainment may occur secondary to empty solution container, air in Venoset tubing, and loose IV connections.	Chest, shoulder pain Back pain Dyspnea Hypotension Cyanosis	Position patient on left side in the Trendelenburg position to contain air in right atrium. Notify physician. Administer oxygen, cardiovascular support as ordered.	Use of Luer-Lok connectors Carefully monitor IV volume infused. Use electronic control device to detect presence of air.
Circulatory overload	Excess fluid in the circulatory system at a rate greater than the patient's cardiovascular system can accommodate	Shortness of breath Rales on auscultation Engorged neck veins Dependent edema	Reduce IV flow rate. Administer oxygen, monitor vital signs as ordered. Administer diuretics as ordered.	Monitor intake and output.
Allergic reaction	A localized or systemic reaction to an allergen	Skin wheals Redness, edema Hypotension, tachycardia Bronchospasm Wheezing Cardiovascular collapse	Remove allergen. Redress with hypoallergenic tape. If medication is suspected allergen, discontinue medication. Systemic treatment is dependent on presenting symptoms, including administration of: • Oxygen • Antihistamines • Epinephrine • Steroids	Carry out careful preprocedure assessment to elicit allergy status. Assess for medication cross-reaction.

With the administration of hypotonic solution (0.45% [half-normal] saline), cells begin to swell. As hypotonic solution is added to the extracellular fluid, the osmolality decreases, forcing water to enter the cells in an area of higher osmolality. Hypertonic solution (3% saline) increases the osmolality of the surrounding extracellular fluid and forces water to leave the cell and enter the extracellular fluid, with resultant cellular shrinkage. In comparison, isotonic solutions (0.9% normal saline, lactated Ringer's) produce no change in the osmolality of body fluids. The infusion of isotonic solutions results in equal distribution throughout the extracellular compartment because the tonicity is similar to that of plasma (300 mOsm). Characteristics of commonly administered IV solutions are provided in Table 9.4. Table 9.5 shows the amount of volume expansion of each compartment that can be expected from commonly administered IV fluids.[2] Isotonic solutions are generally the crystalloid of choice for IV maintenance during the administration of sedation and analgesia.

At times, our interventional platform patients are admitted after moderate procedural sedation. Are there specific protocols or algorithms that can be used by the health care provider who is ordering continuous IV fluid therapy for their patients?

There are a variety of guidelines that health care providers use when ordering continuous IV fluid administration. Some providers write orders based on scientific guidelines, whereas some providers write orders based on where they were trained or current facility practices. Although inappropriate fluid therapy is rarely reported as being responsible for patient harm, a 1999 report from the National Confidential Enquiry into Perioperative Deaths (NCEPOD) suggested that as many as one in five patients receiving IV fluids in the hospital suffered complications or morbidity due to their inappropriate administration.[3] A NCEPOD 2011 report highlighted that patients were at an increased risk of death within 30 days of having

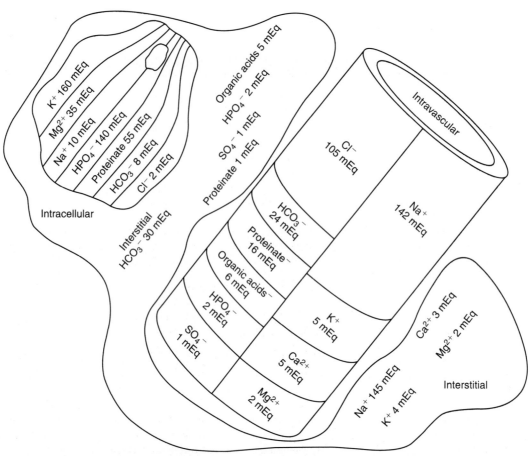

Fig. 9.7 Anions and cations of intracellular, interstitial, and intravascular fluids. (From Alexander M, Corrigan A, Gorski L, et al, eds: *Infusion Nursing: An Evidence-Based Approach.* 3rd ed. St. Louis: Saunders Elsevier; 2010.)

TABLE 9.4	Commonly Administered Intravenous Solutions[a]							
Solution	**Osmolality**	**Tonicity**	**Na⁺**	**Cl⁻**	**K⁺**	**Mg²⁺**	**Ca²⁺**	**Buffer[b]**
Plasma	288	Reference	140	103	4.5	1.25	2.5	24
0.9% NaCl	308	Isotonic	154	154	0	0	0	0
Lactated Ringer's	279	Hypotonic	130	111	4.0	0	2.7	29
Plasma-Lyte	N/A	Isotonic	140	98	5.0	1.5	0	50
Sterofundin	309	Isotonic	140	127	4.0	1.0	2.5	29
5% Glucose	278	Hypotonic	0	0	0	0	0	0
1.4% NaHCO₃	333	Hypertonic	167	0	0	0	0	167

[a]All in mmol/L, except for osmolality in mOsm/kg. [b]Buffers consist of bicarbonate (plasma, NaHCO₃), lactate (lactated Ringer's), acetate (27 mmol/L in Plasma-Lyte, 24 mmol/L in Sterofundin), gluconate (23 mmol/L in Plasma-Lyte), and maleate (5 mmol/L in Sterofundin). From Hoorn EJ, Intravenous fluids: balancing solutions. J Nephrol 2017;30(4):485–492.

TABLE 9.5	Compartmental Volume Expansion from Common IV Fluids				
Fluid	**Expansion of IVF (mL)**	**Expansion of ISF (mL)**	**Expansion of ICF (mL)**	**Na Content (mmol/L)**	**Osmolarity (mOsm/L)**
NaCl 0.9%	250	750	0	154	308
NaCl 0.45%	167	500	333	77	154
Glucose 5%	83	250	667	0	252
Glucose 5% with NaCl 0.45%	167	500	333	77	432
Albumin 5%	1000+	0	0	154	310
Hetastarch 6% in NaCl 0.9%[a]	1000+	0	0	154	310

ICF, Intracellular fluid; *ISF,* interstitial fluid; *IVF,* intravascular fluid; *NaCl,* sodium chloride; *Na,* sodium.
[a]The values for hetastarch in NaCl and albumin solutions indicate their ability to expand the volume in IVF by more than the amount of fluid administered.
Staples A, Dade J, Acomb C. Intravenous fluid therapy-what pharmacists need to monitor. *Hospital Pharmacy.* 2008; 15:277–282.

an operation if they had received inadequate or excessive IV fluids in the preoperative period.[4] In 2013 (updated, 2016), the National Institute for Health and Care Excellence (NICE) guidelines were published, featured in Fig. 9.8. These guidelines were published because no standardized guidance existed on the management of IV fluid therapy in hospitalized patients.[5]

The guidelines reviewed the available scientific evidence and relied on the fundamental principles of physiology and pathophysiology of fluid balance. Guidelines and algorithms based on scientific evidence provide the health care provider with standardized fluid replacement therapy options to optimize patient outcomes. See the Patient Safety box.

PATIENT SAFETY SBAR FOCUS

Unsafe Injection Practices: A NEVER Event

Situation

Our endoscopy center recently had an outbreak of hepatitis C. The State Department of Health is investigating our GI center to identify a source of the outbreak. I recently spoke to the center director who stated that it "couldn't possibly be anything that we are doing here."

Background

The State Department of Health visited our endoscopy center last week. Four patients treated at our center in the last six months have contracted hepatitis C. Our staff believes that this is merely a coincidence. However, the State Department of Health has identified this as a trend at our facility. Approximately six months ago, a new physician was appointed as Chief Operating Officer at the center. A number of cost savings measures have been implemented during that time period. Our new policy on midazolam administration includes using 10-milliliter vials of 5 milligrams per milliliter solution. Previously we used 2 milliliter, 1 milligram per milliliter vials. Departmental staff now draw up 1 milliliter (5 milligrams) of solution from the multi-dose vial. In the event that more than 5 milligrams of midazolam are required, additional medication is drawn up from the multi-dose vial.

Multiple staff stated that they feel "uncomfortable" using a multi-dose midazolam vial and were more comfortable using the single use 1 milligram, 2-milliliter vial. The Department of Health confiscated six multi-dose midazolam vials from our facility.

Assessment

Bloodborne diseases such as hepatitis B, hepatitis C, and HIV/AIDS can be transmitted through unsafe injections due to poor injection practices. Unsafe injections place patients at risk of morbidity that may culminate in mortality secondary to outbreaks related to poor injection technique. A *safe injection* does not harm the recipient, does not expose the health care worker to any avoidable risk, and does not result in waste that is dangerous for the community. Medications administered in the sedation setting must be administered safely. These safe injection practices include the use of *sterile single-use needles and syringes*.

Recommendations

The diagram featured below demonstrates the need to follow current safe injection practices for needle and syringe use at all times to prevent infection.

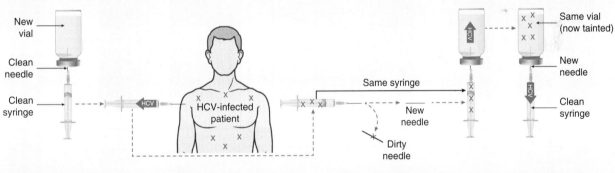

1. Clean needle and syringe are used to draw medication.

2. When used on an HCV-infected patient, backflow from the injection or removal of the needle contaminates the syringe.

3. When again used to draw medication, a contaminated syringe contaminates the medication vial.

4. If a contaminated vial is subsequently used for other patients, they can become infected with HCV.

Current safe injection practices include:[1]
- Never administer medications from the same syringe to multiple patients, even if the needle is changed.
- Never reuse a needle, or needleless access device, even on the same patient.
- Never refill a syringe once it has been used, even for the same patient.
- Never use infusion or intravenous administration sets on more than one patient.
- Never reuse a syringe or needle to withdraw medication from a multidose vial (MDV).
- Never re-enter a single-dose medication vial, ampule, or intravenous infusion bag.
- Syringes and needles are single-use items that must only be used once.

Image from Centers for Disease Control and Prevention (CDC). Acute Hepatitis C Virus Infections Attributed to Unsafe Injection Practices at an Endoscopy Clinic-Nevada, 2007. MMWR Morb Mortal Wkly Rep. 2008;57(19):513–517. https://www.cdc.gov/mmwr/preview/mmwrhtml/mm5719a2.htm.
[1] Safe Injection Guidelines for Needle and Syringe Use. Park Ridge, IL: American Association of Nurse Anesthetists; 2014.

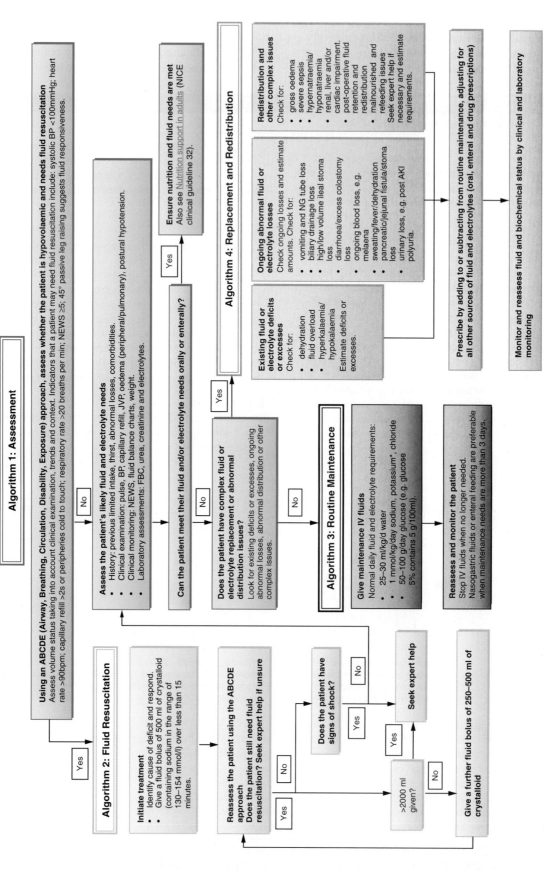

Fig. 9.8 Algorithms for IV fluid therapy in adults. (From National Institute for Health and Care Excellence. Intravenous fluid therapy for adults in hospital [clinical guideline 174]. www.nice.org.uk/CG174.)

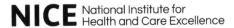

Algorithms for IV fluid therapy in adults

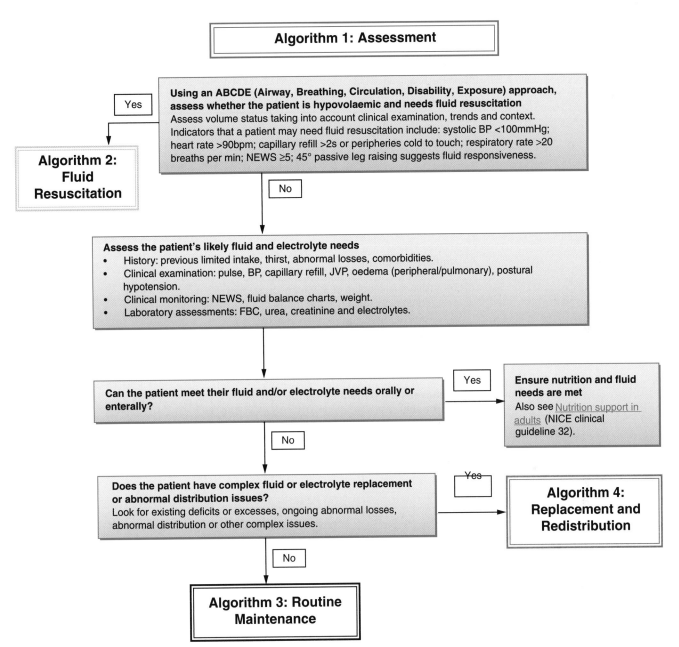

'Intravenous fluid therapy in adults in hospital', NICE clinical guideline 174 (December 2013. Last update December 2016)

© National Institute for Health and Care Excellence 2013. All rights reserved.

Fig. 9.8, **Cont'd**

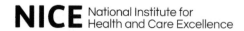

NICE National Institute for
Health and Care Excellence

Algorithms for IV fluid therapy in adults

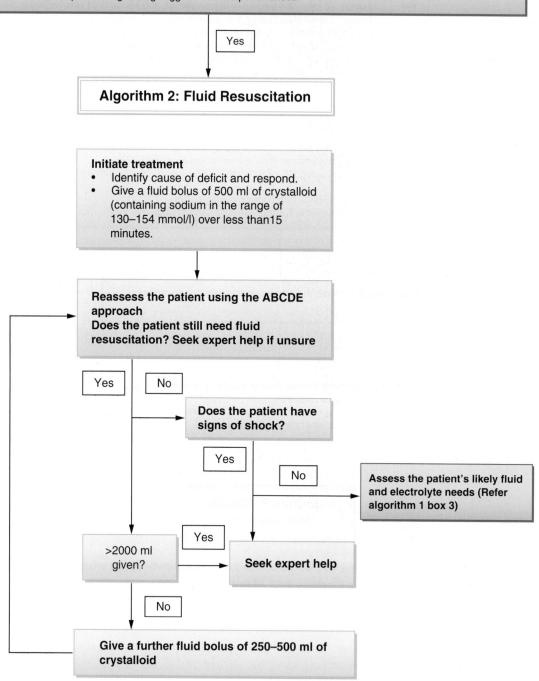

Using an ABCDE (Airway, Breathing, Circulation, Disability, Exposure) approach, assess whether the patient is hypovolaemic and needs fluid resuscitation
Assess volume status taking into account clinical examination, trends and context. Indicators that a patient may need fluid resuscitation include: systolic BP <100mmHg; heart rate >90bpm; capillary refill >2s or peripheries cold to touch; respiratory rate >20 breaths per min; NEWS ≥5; 45° passive leg raising suggests fluid responsiveness.

Yes

Algorithm 2: Fluid Resuscitation

Initiate treatment
- Identify cause of deficit and respond.
- Give a fluid bolus of 500 ml of crystalloid (containing sodium in the range of 130–154 mmol/l) over less than 15 minutes.

Reassess the patient using the ABCDE approach
Does the patient still need fluid resuscitation? Seek expert help if unsure

Yes   No

Does the patient have signs of shock?

Yes   No

Assess the patient's likely fluid and electrolyte needs (Refer algorithm 1 box 3)

>2000 ml given?   Yes → **Seek expert help**

No

Give a further fluid bolus of 250–500 ml of crystalloid

'Intravenous fluid therapy in adults in hospital', NICE clinical guideline 174 (December 2013. Last update December 2016)

Fig. 9.8, Cont'd

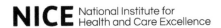

Algorithms for IV fluid therapy in adults

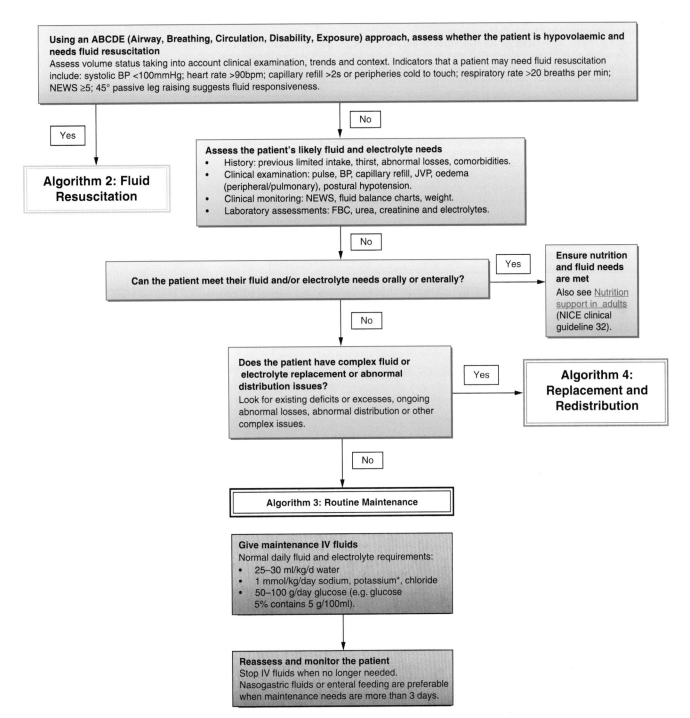

* Weight-based potassium prescriptions should be rounded to the nearest common fluids available (for example, a 67 kg person should have fluids containing 20 mmol and 40 mmol of potassium in a 24-hour period). Potassium should not be added to intravenous fluid bags as this is dangerous.

'Intravenous fluid therapy in adults in hospital', NICE clinical guideline 174 (December 2013. Last update December 2016)

Fig. 9.8, Cont'd

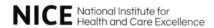

NICE National Institute for
Health and Care Excellence

Algorithms for IV fluid therapy in adults

Using an ABCDE (Airway, Breathing, Circulation, Disability, Exposure) approach, assess whether the patient is hypovolaemic and needs fluid resuscitation
Assess volume status taking into account clinical examination, trends and context. Indicators that a patient may need fluid resuscitation include: systolic BP <100mmHg; heart rate >90bpm; capillary refill >2s or peripheries cold to touch; respiratory rate >20 breaths per min; NEWS ≥5; 45° passive leg raising suggests fluid responsiveness.

No

Assess the patient's likely fluid and electrolyte needs
- History: previous limited intake, thirst, abnormal losses, comorbidities.
- Clinical examination: pulse, BP, capillary refill, JVP, oedema (peripheral/pulmonary), postural hypotension.
- Clinical monitoring: NEWS, fluid balance charts, weight.
- Laboratory assessments: FBC, urea, creatinine and electrolytes.

No

Can the patient meet their fluid and/or electrolyte needs orally or enterally?

Yes → **Ensure nutrition and fluid needs are met**
Also see Nutrition support in adults (NICE clinical guideline 32).

No

Does the patient have complex fluid or electrolyte replacement or abnormal distribution issues?
Look for existing deficits or excesses, ongoing abnormal losses, abnormal distribution or other complex issues.

Yes

Algorithm 4: Replacement and Redistribution

Existing fluid or electrolyte deficits or excesses
Check for:
- dehydration
- fluid overload
- hyperkalaemia/ hypokalaemia
Estimate deficits or excesses.

Ongoing abnormal fluid or electrolyte losses
Check ongoing losses and estimate amounts. Checks for:
- vomiting and NG tube loss
- biliary drainage loss
- high/low volume ileal stoma loss
- diarrhoea/excess colostomy loss
- ongoing blood loss, e.g. melaena
- sweating/fever/dehydration
- pancreatic/jejunal fistula/stoma loss
- urinary loss, e.g. post AKI polyuria.

Redistribution and other complex issues
Check for:
- gross oedema
- severe sepsis
- hypernatraemia/ hyponatraemia
- renal, liver and/or cardiac impairment.
- post-operative fluid retention and redistribution
- malnourished and refeeding issues
Seek expert help if necessary and estimate requirements.

Prescribe by adding to or subtracting from routine maintenance, adjusting for all other sources of fluid and electrolytes (oral, enteral and drug prescriptions)

Monitor and reassess fluid and biochemical status by clinical and laboratory monitoring

'Intravenous fluid therapy in adults in hospital', NICE clinical guideline 174 (December 2013. Last update December 2016)

Fig. 9.8, Cont'd

Our hospital Chief Quality Officer has approached our unit and stated that there were a significant number of our patient population citing IV site hematoma and bruising during their postprocedure patient surveys. Is there anything that can be done to reduce the incidence of these patient complaints?

Before discharge, sedation patients should have their IV catheter removed. Firm consistent pressure is applied until hemostasis is achieved. Patients taking, for example, blood thinners, aspirin, antiplatelet medications, or fish oils require prolonged pressure application to assure hemostasis. A 4 × 4- or 2 × 2-inch reinforcement dressing applied with tape provides additional pressure after discharge. This additional reinforcement may decrease the incidence of hematoma formation. Outpatients should be instructed to remove the gauze once they are at home and replace it with a Band-Aid. In-house patients or patients who require prolonged IV therapy require peripheral catheter care. Nursing documentation of patients with peripheral catheters should include the following:

- Identification of IV insertion site
- Catheter gauge
- Number of attempts
- IV volume infused
- Date and time of catheter insertion

SUMMARY

It is imperative that patients presenting for sedation services have adequate IV access. IV access provides a convenient mode of administration for IV medications while serving as a lifeline to the patient in the event of cardiopulmonary distress. Sedation providers must demonstrate competence in their ability to establish IV access. Complications associated with IV cannulation should be dealt with in a timely manner. Isotonic solutions are generally selected as the IV solution of choice for sedation procedures.

REFERENCES

1. Reddick AD, Ronald J, Morrison WG. Intravenous fluid resuscitation: Was Poiseuille right? *Emergency Medicine Journal.* 2011; 28:201–202.
2. Staples A, Dade J, Acomb C. Intravenous fluid therapy-what pharmacists need to monitor. *Hospital Pharmacy.* 2008; 15:277–282.
3. National Confidential Enquiry into Perioperative Deaths. Extremes of age: The 1999 report of the National Confidential Enquiry into Perioperative Deaths. www.ncepod.org.uk/1999report/99full.pdf
4. National Confidential Enquiry into Patient Outcome and Death. Knowing the risk: A review of the peri-operative care of surgical patients. www.ncepod.org.uk/2011report2/downloads/POC_fullreport.pdf
5. National Institute for Health and Care Excellence. *Intravenous fluid therapy for adults in hospital (clinical guideline 174).* www.nice.org.uk/CG174; 2013.

CHAPTER 9: REVIEW QUESTIONS

1. Intravenous cannulation for administration of fluids and medications provides _____.
   A. Delayed uptake of sedative and analgesic medications
   B. Delayed distribution of sedative and analgesic medications
   C. Immediate uptake of sedative and analgesic medications
   D. Random distribution of sedative and analgesic medications

2. Contraindications for vascular access in an affected extremity include all of the following except _____.
   A. Previous mastectomy
   B. Lymphoid dissection
   C. Presence of renal access graphs
   D. Minimal adipose tissue in the affected side

3. The largest vein with the straightest pathway in the upper arm includes which of the following?
   A. Basilic vein
   B. Median vein
   C. Accessory vein
   D. Median cubital vein

4. Warm cloths and rubbing of the extremity provides _____ for ease of IV cannula insertion.
   A. Vasoconstriction
   B. Vasodilation

   C. Reduced venous filling
   D. Peripheral edema

5. After appropriate localization via a small skin wheal of local anesthesia, the IV needle is advanced at a ____ à degree angle in the direction of the vein to be cannulated.
   A. 10–20
   B. 21–30
   C. 31–40
   D. >50

6. Inflammation along the course of a vein, which may occur in response to specific IV insertion techniques, types of medications infused, and catheter size, is termed which of the following?
   A. Infiltration
   B. Extravasation
   C. Phlebitis
   D. Hematoma formation

7. Infusion or seepage of IV fluid into extravascular tissue that is caused by partial or complete venous access dislodgement is termed which of the following?
   A. Infiltration
   B. Extravasation
   C. Phlebitis
   D. Hematoma formation

8. The presence of concomitant disease states (e.g., hypertension, dehydration, procedural fluid losses) and the patient's cardiovascular status are factors that have an impact on _____.
   A. Transcellular fluid replacement
   B. Intravascular fluid replacement
   C. Interstitial fluid replacement
   D. Iso-osmolar fluid replacement

9. Vein finding devices function on which of the following principles?
   A. Radiation emission
   B. Black light emission
   C. Infrared emission
   D. Ultrasound emission

10. Which of the following IV solutions are generally the crystalloid of choice for IV maintenance during the administration of sedation?
    A. Hypotonic solutions
    B. Isotonic solutions
    C. Hypertonic solutions
    D. Iso-osmolar solutions

11. Which of the following is the most effective mechanism to avoid hematoma formation when discontinuing a peripheral venous catheter?
    A. Apply a Steri-Strip and Tegaderm to the site.
    B. Directly apply a Band-Aid once the catheter is removed.
    C. Contact the physician to obtain coagulant orders.
    D. Apply direct pressure on the site followed by application of a pressure dressing.

12. Which IV catheter size is most appropriate for a healthy 36-year-old man presenting for a 10-minute moderate procedural sedation procedure?
    A. 12 gauge
    B. 14 gauge
    C. 16 gauge
    D. 20 gauge

Answers can be found in Appendix A.

Sedation Considerations for the Geriatric Patient

LEARNING OUTCOMES

At the completion of this chapter, the learner shall:
- Differentiate the terms *geriatric* and *gerontology.*
- Analyze the impact of cardiorespiratory, renal, hepatic, and central nervous system physiologic alterations that affect geriatric sedation patient care.
- Examine the pharmacodynamics and pharmacokinetic considerations associated with the aging process.
- Delineate the specific procedural considerations associated with administering benzodiazepines, opioids, and sedative-hypnotics to the geriatric patient population.

- Distinguish the airway management issues associated with caring for the older patient.
- Identify evidence-based nursing interventions to implement for the geriatric patient with postprocedure cognitive dysfunction.

COMPETENCY STATEMENT

The health care practitioner maintains homeostatic regulation through the assessment and management of physiologic care to minimize adverse events associated with the administration of moderate procedural sedation and analgesia to the geriatric patient population.

What particular challenges are associated with providing sedation care to the geriatric patient population?

All patients scheduled for moderate procedural sedation and analgesia require careful titration of medications and vigilant care. The geriatric patient population requires particular attention when presenting for sedation services. Their altered response to pharmacologic compounds occurs secondary to the physiologic alterations and pharmacokinetic and pharmacodynamic changes associated with the aging process. This competency module focuses on the special needs that the geriatric patient presents for sedation services.

What is meant by the term *geriatric syndrome*?

The phrase *geriatric syndrome* is often used collectively to refer to the many conditions associated with the aging process. These conditions include the following:
- Cognitive dysfunction
- Delirium
- Fatigue
- Malnutrition
- Sleep disorders
- Sensory and motor deficits
- Unstable gait

The clinician providing sedation care to the geriatric patient can identify many of these components during the presedation patient assessment. Cognitive dysfunction, delirium, malnutrition, and sleep disorders may require dosage reductions secondary to altered pharmacokinetics in the geriatric patient population. Sensory and motor deficits and unstable gait may affect postsedation patient care requiring delayed discharge from the procedure unit.

What is meant by the term *gerontology*?

Gerontology is the scientific study of the processes and problems of aging from all aspects—biologic, clinical, psychological, sociologic, legal, economic, and political. Geriatrics is the branch of medicine that deals with the diagnosis, management, and prevention of medical problems associated with senility and senescence.[1] Increased life expectancy and decreased mortality associated with the aging process in the United States have led to an explosion in the geriatric patient population. Between 2012 and 2050, the United States will have experienced considerable growth in its older population. In 2050, the population aged 65 years and over is projected to be 83.7 million, almost double its estimated population of 43.1 million in 2012. The "baby boomers" are largely responsible for this increase in the older population—they began turning 65 in 2011. By 2050, surviving baby boomers will be older than 85 years.[2] As identified in Fig. 10.1, older adults are projected to outnumber children by the year 2035 for the first time in US history.

What impact will these statistics have on the perioperative-sedation patient care environment?

From a perioperative perspective, these statistics indicate that 35% of surgeries in the United States are currently performed

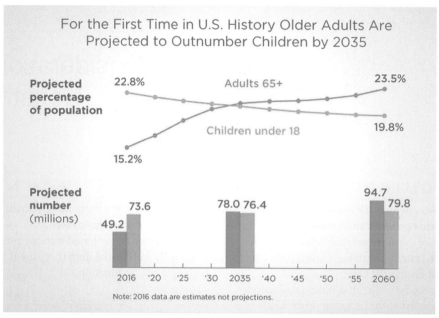

Fig. 10.1 An Aging Nation: Projected number of children and older adults, 2017. (From https://www.census.gov/library/visualizations/2018/comm/historic-first.html)

on patients older than 65 years. This figure equates to more than 16 million procedures annually. With statistics associated with geriatric patient care, the impact of the aging population and their specific clinical needs must be appreciated by the provider. Moving forward, it is apparent that a considerable percentage of sedation clinical practice will involve the geriatric patient population.

What is the medical definition of the term *geriatric*?

The aged population is arbitrarily defined as those patients who have reached the age of 65 years.[3] In 1907, the aged population was defined as 50 years or older. The definition of the term *aged* or *geriatric* has been continually changing. A currently accepted definition of the beginning of old age (geriatrics) is 65 years. However, an appreciation of the patient's functional age is far more important than is or her chronologic age. The biologic aging process affects all individuals and is accompanied by a wide variety of molecular and cellular damage. Over time, there is a continual decline in organ system function.[4,5] Progressive decline in organ function is responsible for the physiologic aging process. Aging is associated with progressive decreases (1%–1.5%/year) in the function of major organ systems after the age of 30 years.[6] Organ function eventually cannot compensate to restore the body to a homeostatic state. This reduction in functional capacity predisposes the body to additional stressors. Box 10.1 identifies the physiologic effects associated with the aging process. It is important that the sedation practitioner appreciates these specific needs of the geriatric patient and their impact on procedural care.

BOX 10.1 Physiologic Effects of the Aging Process

Body Composition
Increased proportion of body fat
Decreased skeletal muscle mass
Decreased intracellular fluid

Cardiovascular System
Myocardial hypertrophy
Myocardial stiffening
Diastolic dysfunction
Reduced beta receptor responsiveness
Conduction system abnormalities
Decreased tissue elasticity, resulting in increased blood pressure
Increased systolic blood pressure secondary to ventricular hypertrophy and decreased arterial wall compliance
Decreased baroreceptor activity
Dysrhythmias secondary to degenerative changes of the cardiac conduction system

Pulmonary System
Decreased total lung compliance
Decreased vital capacity
Decreased forced expiratory volume in 1 s (FEV_1)
Increased residual volume
Increased dead space
Decreased Pao_2
Increased small airway closure
Increased ventilation-perfusion mismatch
Decreased central and peripheral chemoreceptor sensitivity leading to hypoventilation, increased apnea, and decreased ventilator responses

Continued

BOX 10.1 Physiologic Effects of the Aging Process—cont'd

Neurologic System
Decreased cerebral blood flow
Decreased cerebral oxygen uptake
Increased sensitivity to central nervous system depressant drugs

Renal System
Decreased glomerular filtration rate (1%–1.5%/year)
Decreased creatinine clearance
Decreased tubular function

Hepatic System
Decreased hepatic blood flow
Decreased microsomal enzyme activity
Decreased albumin level—leads to decreased plasma protein binding, with resultant increased available free drug

Endocrine System
Decreased basal metabolic rate, 1%/year after the age of 30 years
Glucose intolerance

Airway
Decreased laryngeal and pharyngeal reflexes
Inadequate mask fit for positive pressure ventilation
Decreased neuronal function

What cardiovascular changes are associated with the aging process?

A variety of anatomic and physiologic changes occur in the cardiovascular and autonomic nervous system as people age. The most frequent cardiovascular diseases in the geriatric patient that the sedation provider will encounter on presedation assessment include the following:

- Hypertension
- Hyperlipidemia
- Coronary artery disease
- Ischemic heart disease
- Congestive heart failure

Diminished parasympathetic nervous system tone, a decline in beta receptor responsiveness, and stiffening of the vascular tree have serious consequences for the geriatric patient. Prolonged circulation time in the geriatric patient delays the onset of IV sedative and analgesic agents. Careful titration of medications is required secondary to this physiologic change. Myocardial tissue in the older patient population is less sensitive to the effects of beta-adrenergic modulation, manifesting as decreased heart rate and lower cardiac dilation at the end of diastole and systole. Table 10.1 features additional cardiovascular changes, clinical features, and sedation considerations associated with the geriatric patient.

What pulmonary changes are associated with the aging process?

The aging process reduces elasticity in the geriatric pulmonary system. This decreased elastic recoil, coupled with calcific changes, decreases lung compliance. As evidenced by loss of body height, the intervertebral spaces are diminished, causing a reduction in the thoracic curvature. This leads to changes in chest wall compliance. There is also an increase in anatomic and physiologic dead space secondary to the loss of gas-exchanging units. The normal aging process is associated with progressive loss and destruction of the alveolar septa, which leads to this increase in physiologic dead space. These changes eventually lead to reduction in tidal volume, increased air trapping, atelectasis, and shunting. A reduction in respiratory ciliary activity, reduction in airway reactivity, and protective reflexes predispose the geriatric patient to the development of gastric acid aspiration and pulmonary dysfunction.

These pulmonary anatomic and physiologic alterations reveal that the geriatric sedation patient has a limited pulmonary reserve, coupled with an inability to increase respiratory rate and volume in the presence of hypoventilation and hypoxia. The muscles of ventilation fatigue early secondary to the anatomic structural changes outlined in Table 10.2. In addition, the clinician providing sedation services to this sensitive patient population must recognize that procedural ventilatory inadequacy may occur. The mechanical, anatomic, and physiologic pulmonary changes associated with the aging process predispose the geriatric patient to pharmacologic sensitivity, which can lead to potential respiratory distress. Table 10.2 features additional pulmonary changes, clinical features, and sedation considerations associated with the geriatric patient.

What renal changes are associated with the aging process?

Loss of kidney mass, vascular changes, decreased renal blood flow, and a decreased glomerular filtration rate in the geriatric patient require decreased dosage requirements and the use of drugs with short half-lives and no active metabolites. As glomeruli become less functional and decrease in number, the glomerular filtration rate decreases. Renal blood flow also decreases with age. These factors lead to a 25% to 50% reduction in glomerular filtration rate, from 20 to 90 years of age. Therefore, the clearance of drugs primarily eliminated by the kidneys can be expected to be decreased in older patients.[7] Presedation patient assessment requires careful review of fluid and electrolyte status secondary to the geriatric patient's inability to conserve sodium, which may predispose to the development of hemodynamic instability.

What hepatic changes are associated with the aging process?

Liver blood flow at the age of 65 years is reduced to approximately 40% of the liver blood flow in patients at the age of 30 years. Hepatic microsomal enzymes, important in oxidizing drugs, are less active in older patients. The conversion by the liver of lipid-soluble drugs to water-soluble metabolites by conjugation is also hindered. This may also lead to increased duration of action for many lipid-soluble drugs, including some anesthetics and sedatives. The liver also produces key proteins (e.g., albumin, alpha-1-acid glycoprotein) that are

TABLE 10.1   Geriatric Cardiovascular Alterations

Anatomical/Physiologic Alteration	Clinical Feature	Sedation Considerations
Increased arterial rigidity Increased sympathetic nervous system activity	Left ventricle has to work harder to eject blood into a rigid aorta. Elevates systemic vascular resistance. Increased left ventricular strain may lead to the development of left ventricular hypertrophy.	Alterations in cardiovascular response to sedative, analgesic, and hypnotic medications. Vital signs may be labile secondary to left ventricular hypertrophy, increased afterload, and increased myocardial oxygen consumption associated with increased sympathetic nervous system activity and 'stiff' vessels
Vein stiffening	Decreased compliance of capacitance vessels	Reduces the body's ability to 'buffer' hemodynamic changes in intravascular tone Exaggerated hypotension
Left ventricular hypertrophy	Impaired diastolic filling	Reduction in end-diastolic function and coronary artery filling
Decreased peripheral nervous system tone	Tonic peripheral nervous system outflow declines	Inability to adjust cardiac output and blood pressure during sedation challenges (pain, anxiety, alterations in preload or afterload)
Decreased response to beta-adrenergic stimulation	Decreased inotropic and chronotropic response to beta stimulant medications	Decreased response to sympathetic nervous system stimulant medications. May result in profound bradycardia and hypotension which is refractory to pharmacologic treatment
Impaired chronotropic and inotropic responsiveness of the heart	Inability to respond to metabolic demands	Heart rate and ejection fraction may not be capable of maintaining cardiac output during periods of stress and anxiety
Altered baroreceptor response	Aortic arch and carotid sinus stretch receptor effectiveness is reduced secondary to arterial stiffening with resultant decrease in baroreflex	Increased susceptibility in geriatric patients to orthostatic hypotension and heart rate compensatory mechanisms
Decreased cardiac output	Reduced blood flow to major organ systems	Intravenously administered sedative, analgesic, and hypnotic medications take longer to reach their target receptor sites. Full pharmacologic effect be delayed in excess of 6-10 minutes depending on the patient's cardiac output. This delay in full pharmacologic effect frequently results in excessive doses of medication administration. *To avoid oversedation, hypercarbia, hypoxia, and airway obstruction allow ample time for the full pharmacologic effect of the medication to be appreciated prior to administering additional medication.*
Fibrotic changes in conduction system	SA node and pacemaker cells are accompanied by atrophy of conducting tissue	Conduction system anomalies may manifest as dysrhythmias, decreased conduction through the AV node, fascicular blocks and sick sinus syndrome

TABLE 10.2   Geriatric Pulmonary Alterations

Physiology Alteration	Clinical Feature	Sedation Considerations
Decreased chest wall compliance	Impaired gas exchange	Increased sensitivity to increased work of breathing Respiratory depressant effects associated with benzodiazepines, opioids, sedative-hypnotics
Decreased muscle strength	Increased work of breathing	Risk for respiratory failure Impaired airway reflexes Predisposition to apneic episodes
Decreased chemoreceptors	Decreased ventilatory response to hypoxemia and increased episodes of apnea	Provide continuous positive airway pressure (CPAP) or bilevel positive airway pressure (BiPAP) to obese or sleep apnea patients

responsible for plasma protein binding. Decreased plasma protein levels associated with the aging process predispose the patient to increased drug sensitivity secondary to an increase in free unbound drug in the plasma.

What central nervous system changes are associated with the aging process?

Among the important age-related changes in the geriatric patient is a consistent loss of neuronal density, beginning at the age of 30 years that progresses steadily for the next 6 decades.[8] Biochemical changes associated with the aging process includes a decrease in the following neurotransmitters:

- Acetylcholine
- Dopamine
- Tyrosine
- Serotonin
- Norepinephrine

The effects of aging on the central nervous system frequently result in an increased incidence of confusion, delirium, and sensitivity to pharmacologic agents.

Are geriatric patients at a higher risk for postoperative cognitive changes?

Postoperative cognitive impairment can affect patients of all ages, but it primarily affects geriatric patients. There are two types of cognitive changes that may affect the geriatric patient, postoperative delirium (POD) and postoperative cognitive dysfunction (POCD). There are two types of postoperative delirium:

- Emergence delirium (ED) occurs as the patient emerges from anesthesia. ED generally resolves shortly after emergence from anesthesia (minutes to hours) as the patient regains consciousness and reaches a more clear-headed state.
- Postoperative dysfunction is an acute organic brain syndrome that occurs within the first few postprocedure days.[9] Postoperative delirium affects approximately 15% of patients after elective procedures and is accompanied by a sudden onset of symptoms that occur throughout the day. Initial periods of the patient appearing lucid are followed by symptoms that may include the following:
  - Clouding of consciousness
  - Difficulty maintaining or shifting attention
  - Disorientation
  - Illusions
  - Hallucinations
  - Fluctuating levels of consciousness

The cause of POD is not well understood. It is postulated to be related to disturbances in the production, release, or inactivation of neurotransmitters.[10] Additional studies have noted that intraoperative oxidative stress is associated with POD.[11]

Are there specific recommendations associated with managing the older patient presenting for sedation services?

Recommendations for managing the older patient have been promulgated by the American Geriatric Society; they have given essential guidance on the prevention of POD in older patients at risk for delirium and on the treatment of older surgical patients with delirium.[12] The American Geriatric Society's Expert Panel on Postoperative Delirium in Older Adults Clinical Practice Guideline Summary is shown in Box 10.2. Their clinical practice guidelines provide the sedation practitioner with eight strong recommendations on

---

BOX 10.2 American Geriatric Society Expert Panel on Postoperative Delirium in Older Adults: Clinical Practice Guideline Summary

This clinical practice guideline provides eight strong recommendation statements. For these recommendations, the panel weighed the evidence for each intervention and determined that the benefits clearly outweighed the risks or that the risks clearly outweighed the benefits.

- Multicomponent nonpharmacologic interventions delivered by an interdisciplinary team should be administered to at-risk older adults to prevent delirium.
- Ongoing educational programs regarding delirium should be provided for health care professionals.
- A medical evaluation should be performed to identify and manage underlying contributors to delirium.
- Pain management (preferably with nonopioid medications) should be optimized to prevent postoperative delirium.
- Medications with high risk for precipitating delirium should be avoided.
- Cholinesterase inhibitors should not be newly prescribed to prevent or treat postoperative delirium.
- Benzodiazepines should not be used as first-line treatment of agitation associated with delirium.
- Antipsychotics and benzodiazepines should be avoided for the treatment of hypoactive delirium.

This clinical practice guideline provides an additional three weak recommendation statements. The panel judged the evidence to be in favor of these interventions, but the current level of evidence or potential risks of the treatment did not support a strong recommendation.

- Multicomponent nonpharmacologic interventions implemented by an interdisciplinary team may be considered when an older adult is diagnosed with postoperative delirium to improve clinical outcomes.
- The injection of regional anesthetic at the time of surgery and postoperatively to improve pain control with the goal of preventing delirium may be considered.
- The use of antipsychotics (e.g., haloperidol, risperidone, olanzapine, quetiapine, ziprasidone) at the lowest effective dose for the shortest possible duration may be considered to treat delirious patients who are severely agitated or distressed or who are threatening substantial harm to self and/or others.

This clinical practice guideline also provides one insufficient evidence recommendation statement. The panel wanted to provide a recommendation statement for this intervention to be considered, but the current level of evidence or potential risks of the treatment did not support a strong or weak recommendation.

Continued

BOX 10.2   American Geriatric Society Expert Panel on Postoperative Delirium in Older Adults: Clinical Practice Guideline Summary—cont'd

- Use of processed electroencephalographic monitors of anesthetic depth during IV sedation or general anesthesia may be used to prevent delirium.

  Finally, the panel concluded that there was insufficient evidence to recommend either for or against the following:
- Prophylactic use of antipsychotic medications to prevent delirium.
- Specialized hospital units for the inpatient care of older adults with postoperative delirium.

From American Geriatrics Society Expert Panel on Postoperative Delirium in Older Adults. American Geriatrics Society abstracted clinical practice guideline for postoperative delirium in older adults. J Am Geriatr Soc. 2015;63(1):142–150.

BOX 10.3   Mini-Cog Cognitive Assessment Examination for the Older Patient

1. Get the patient's attention, then say:
   - "I am going to say three words that I want you to remember now and later. The words are banana, sunrise, chair. Please say them for me now."
   - Give the patient three tries to repeat the words. If unable after three tries, go to the next item.
2. Say all the following phrases in the order indicated:
   - "Please draw a clock in the space below. Start by drawing a large circle. Put all the numbers in the circle and set the hands to show 11:10 (10 past 11)."
   - If the patient has not finished the clock drawing in 3 minutes, discontinue and ask for recall items.
3. Say: "What were the three words I asked you to remember?"

In Chow WB, Rosenthal RA, Merkow RP, et al.; American College of Surgeons National Surgical Quality Improvement Program, American Geriatrics Society. Optimal preoperative assessment of the geriatric surgical patient: a best practices guideline from the American College of Surgeons National Surgical Quality Improvement Program and the American Geriatrics Society. J Am Coll Surg. 2012;215(4):453–466.

managing the older patient who is presenting for sedation or anesthesia care.

Is a cognitive assessment prescreening tool recommended for use in the older patient population?

It is important to assess the patient's decision-making capability prior to the procedure. Patients signing their informed consent must be competent to understand the planned procedure, risks, and complications associated with the planned procedure. A preprocedure neuropsychiatric assessment clearly establishes a baseline in the event of postprocedure cognitive dysfunction. There are a number of neurocognitive screening examinations that are available for preprocedure assessment of the older patient.[13-15] The Mini-Cog neurologic assessment tool is highly sensitive and can be administered in a brief and timely fashion prior to the procedure; the Mini-Cog Cognitive Assessment featuring three recall items and a clock drawing is presented in Box 10.3.

⚡ PATIENT SAFETY SBAR FOCUS

Sedation Considerations for the Geriatric Patient: The Combative Patient

Situation
A 68-year-old male patient presented to our interventional radiology suite. The patient was scheduled for a renal biopsy. Although he had multiple surgical procedures in the past, he arrived in the preprocedure area agitated. Ultimately, he refused to go into the interventional suite for the procedure.

Background
The patient was seen in the interventional radiologist's office three weeks prior to the procedure. The patient was identified in the office by both the physician and the nurse practitioner to be at high risk for belligerent behavior. A consult was placed with the hospital for preprocedure evaluation. Diagnostic testing was ordered and a consult was requested with the facilities gerontologist for presedation patient evaluation.

Assessment
A hostile and combative patient is characterized as uncooperative with medical and nursing staff. Hostile patients may be a danger to self as well as hospital staff. There are many causes of uncooperative patient behavior. Causes of hostile patient behavior include anxiety, phobias, medication over/undersedation, alcohol abuse, alcohol withdrawal, hypoxia, psychotic disorders, pain, and sociopathic behavior. If the patient had an adequate preprocedural gerontologic evaluation, patient procedural refusal may have been averted.

Recommendations
A thorough presedation assessment coupled with a consult with a gerontologist may have prevented the cancellation of the procedure. Presedation patient assessment also helps to allay patient fears and allows adequate time for patient questions to be addressed. Consult with a gerontology specialist can help identify behaviors that can be modified prior to the procedure and lead to procedural acceptance. Attempts to modify uncooperative patient behavior can occur through scripted conversations, education, and persuasion. Additionally, presedation patient assessment allows the clinician the ability to assess the need for premedication. Oral benzodiazepines (diazepam, lorazepam) provide an effective option to help manage the potential combative patient *when ordered by a physician and administered to the patient prior to the procedure.* Fortunately, empathy, kindness, and common sense frequently are effective modalities when dealing with the combative patient. However, failure to effectively psychologically prepare a previously identified combative or belligerent patient prior to the planned procedure may ultimately lead to procedure cancellation.

At our facility, we do some very prolonged procedures and, at times, have difficulty maintaining the patient's body temperature. How does hypothermia affect the older sedation patient population?

Although patients presenting for sedation are generally not exposed to the wide temperature fluctuations or environmental extremes of the general operating room population, the geriatric patient does not regulate body temperature as efficiently as the young adult. Geriatric patients in the sedation setting should be kept warm during all procedures to prevent the development of shivering. Shivering can increase oxygen consumption by 300% to 500%, contributing to a potentially significant oxygen demand mismatch that can lead to myocardial ischemia in susceptible patients.[16] This increase in oxygen consumption increases myocardial strain and may result in the development of tissue hypoxia. Pharmacologic considerations associated with hypothermia include decreased clearance of medications, with resultant pronounced and prolonged pharmacologic effects.

Are there specific pharmacokinetic or pharmacodynamic considerations in the older patient population?

Physiologic changes associated with the aging process affect the geriatric patient's response to pharmacologic compounds. Additional considerations associated with the older patient population include the following:

- Decreased plasma protein binding
- Body composition changes

Plasma protein binding is often decreased in the geriatric patient population due to a reduced amount of circulating protein. Plasma proteins bind pharmacologic compounds, with the bound portion of the drug inactive secondary to its inability to penetrate cell membranes and exert a pharmacologic effect. The remaining free fraction of the drug exerts pharmacologic effects. This decrease in plasma protein binding is one of the important reasons that geriatric patients frequently exhibit an exaggerated response and side effects associated with the administration of sedatives, hypnotics, and opioid medications.

Additionally, age-related changes in body composition include a loss of skeletal muscle (lean body mass) and an increase in the percentage of body fat. This increased adipose content, coupled with a 20% to 30% reduction in blood volume, occurs with the aging process. Therefore, injection of anesthetic drugs will initially be dispersed into a contracted blood volume in the older patient, producing a higher than expected initial plasma drug concentration.[17] Furthermore, many anesthetic drugs are then redistributed to the fat tissue, leading to prolonged somnolence in the geriatric patient. Table 10.3 features the impact of many of these changes on the half-lives of commonly used sedation medications. To avoid adverse central nervous system effects, geriatric patients require a dosage reduction of 30% to 50%, use of small incremental doses of sedative and analgesic agents, and longer time between doses to assess their full pharmacologic effect.

TABLE 10.3 Elimination Half-Lives of Common Sedation Medications

Medication	Young Adult	Older Patient	Sedation Considerations
Morphine	2.9 h	4.5 h	Increased brain sensitivity; profound physiologic effects; slower onset and delayed recovery; consider route of metabolism and metabolites
Fentanyl	250 min	925 min	As identified above
Midazolam	2.8 h	4.3 h	Increased brain sensitivity

What are the pharmacologic effects of the benzodiazepines specific to the older patient population?

Geriatric patients are particularly vulnerable to sedative effects associated with the administration of benzodiazepines.[18,19] Dosage reduction of 30% to 50% may be required when benzodiazepines are administered to the geriatric patient. The sedative effects of benzodiazepines are enhanced by decreased hepatic microsomal enzyme activity and renal clearance. Considerations regarding the administration of benzodiazepines include careful titration, decreased total dose, and the use of benzodiazepines with inactive metabolites (e.g., midazolam).

What are the pharmacologic effects of opioids specific to the older patient population?

Decreased protein binding and reduced pharmacologic clearance, coupled with an increased volume of distribution, may result in a prolonged duration of action and an enhanced pharmacologic effect. These variations also result in significant respiratory and cardiovascular depression in the geriatric patient population. The addition of opioids in the presence of benzodiazepines produces a pronounced synergistic effect. Respiratory depression is a common complication associated with the combination of benzodiazepines and opioids.

What are the pharmacologic effects of benzodiazepines specific to the older patient population?

Decreased total dosage of all central nervous system depressant medications is required in the geriatric patient population. Reduced clearance, coupled with altered pharmacokinetics, requires careful titration of all sedative and opioid medications. Specific gerontologic considerations include a reduced total dose (30%–50%), titrated slowly to clinical effect. Reduced cardiac output in the geriatric patient population requires the sedation practitioner to wait several minutes after the administration of each medication dose to allow sufficient circulation time to assess the pharmacologic effect fully.

Are there any special considerations related to the older patient population when completing their airway evaluation prior to administering sedation?

During sedation procedures, management of the geriatric patient's airway may prove particularly challenging. Redundant oropharyngeal tissue in the edentulous patient may result in premature airway collapse and upper airway obstruction. Arthritis in this patient population frequently results in limited range of motion and the potential for a difficult airway. Limited range of motion must be appreciated by sedation clinicians to avoid deep sedative states. Arthritic patients' limited range of motion predisposes them to potential difficult airway management if an emergency situation occurs. Loss of bony jaw structure in the older patient distorts the face, which may make it difficult to resuscitate the patient or deliver positive pressure ventilation. An oropharyngeal or nasopharyngeal airway may be required to function as a mechanical conduit to maintain airflow.

SUMMARY

Administration of sedation to the geriatric patient must focus on proper presedation preparation strategies (see Chapter 2) to identify the presence of concomitant disease, prescribed treatment protocol, and effectiveness of therapy. A careful review of the cardiopulmonary system is required to identify the presence of coronary artery disease, hypertension, prior myocardial infarction, and/or chronic obstructive pulmonary disease. Careful titration with reduced doses of medications is required to avoid the development of deep sedation states, prolonged recovery time, and cardiovascular depression. Decreased gastroesophageal sphincter tone, decreased laryngeal reflexes, and the physiologic changes associated with the aging process, listed in Table 10.1, increase the potential for morbidity and mortality in the geriatric patient.

It is also important to consider the psychologic well-being of the geriatric patient when providing sedation services. Many geriatric patients are acclimated to a specific daily routine. Administration of sedation for diagnostic, therapeutic, or minor surgical procedure removes patients from their specific pattern of daily behavior. Physical limitations (e.g., hearing, vision loss) and lack of autonomy may lead to increased levels of frustration and feelings of confusion. The practitioner engaged in the care of this patient population should use slow diction, assess specific patient needs, and provide information as needed. It is important for the sedation practitioner to appreciate that older patients do not respond well to fast-paced, disorganized practice settings. A controlled environment is required for the geriatric patient that is sensitive to his or her social and clinical needs.

REFERENCES

1. National Research Council Committee on Chemical Toxicology and Aging. *Aging in Today's Environment.* Washington DC: National Academies Press; 1987.
2. Ortman JM, Velkoff VA, Hogan H. *An Aging Nation: The Older Population in the United States, Current Population Reports.* Washington, DC: US Census Bureau; 2014.
3. World Health Organization. *Proposed working definition of an older person in Africa for the MDS project.* http://www.who.int/healthinfo/survey/ageingdefnolder/en/; 2002.
4. Steves CJ, Spector TD, Jackson SH. Ageing, genes, environment and epigenetics: What twin studies tell us now, and in the future. *Age Ageing.* 2012; 41:581–586.
5. Vasto S, Scapagnini G, Bulati M, et al. Biomarks of aging. *Frontiers in Bioscience.* 2010; 1:392–402.
6. Evans TI. The physiological basis of geriatric anesthesia. *Anesthesia and Intensive Care Journal.* 1973; 1:319–328.
7. Rivera R, Antognini JF. Perioperative drug therapy in older patients. *Anesthesiology.* 2009; 110:1176–1181.
8. Peters R. Aging and the brain. *Postgraduate Medical Journal.* 2006; 82:84–88.
9. Saczynski J, Marcantonio ER, Quach L, et al. Cognitive trajectories after postoperative delirium. *New England Journal of Medicine.* 2012; 367:30–39.
10. Tune LE. Serum anticholinergic activity levels and delirium in the elderly. *Seminars in Clinical Neuropsychiatry.* 2000; 5:149–153.
11. Rosenthal T. *Intraoperative oxidative stress associated with postoperative delirium.* https://www.anesthesiologynews.com/Clinical-Anesthesiology/Article/04-17/Intraoperative-Oxidative-Stress-Associated-With-Postoperative-Delirium/40903; 2017.
12. American Geriatrics Society. American Geriatrics Society abstracted clinical practice guideline for postoperative delirium in older adults. *Journal of the American Geriatrics Society.* 2015; 63:142–150.
13. Cordell CB, Borson S, Boustani M, et al. Alzheimer's Association recommendations for operationalizing the detection of cognitive impairment during the Medicare annual wellness visit in a primary care setting. *Alzheimers & Dementia.* 2013; 9:141–150.
14. Brodaty H, Pond D, Kemp NA, et al. The GPCOG: A new screening test for dementia designed for general practice. *Journal of the American Geriatric Society.* 2002; 50:530–534.
15. Tsoi KK, Chan JY, Hirai HW, et al. Cognitive tests to detect dementia: A systemic review and meta-analysis. *Journal of the American Medical Association Internal Medicine.* 2015; 175:1450–1458.
16. Reed AP, Yudkowitz FS. *Clinical Cases in Anesthesia.* 4th ed. Philadelphia: Elsevier; 2014.
17. McLeskey C. Pharmacokinetic and pharmacodynamic differences in the elderly. In: *American Society of Anesthesiologists Committee on Geriatric Anesthesiology. Syllabus on Geriatric Anesthesiology.* Park Ridge, IL: American Society of Anesthesiologists; 2002:1–39.
18. Schoeler SG, Schafer DF, Potter JF. The effect of age on the relative potency of midazolam and diazepam sedation in upper gastrointestinal endoscopy. *Journal of Clinical Gastroenterology.* 1990; 12:145–147.
19. McLeskey C. *Geriatric Anesthesiology.* Baltimore: Williams & Wilkins; 1997:134.

CHAPTER 10: REVIEW QUESTIONS

1. What is the term for the study of the effects of time on human development and study of aging?
   A. Internal medicine
   B. Radiology
   C. Pediatrics
   D. Gerontology

2. The geriatric population is defined as those patients older than ___ years of age.
   A. 50
   B. 55
   C. 60
   D. 65

3. After the age of 30 years, aging is associated with progressive decreases in major organ system function of approximately ____ per year.
   A. 1%–1.5%
   B. 2%–2.5%
   C. 3%–3.5%
   D. 4%–4.5%

4. Cardiovascular system changes associated with the geriatric patient include which of the the following?
   A. Enhanced parasympathetic nervous system tone
   B. Diminished parasympathetic nervous system tone
   C. Enhanced beta receptor responsiveness
   D. Relaxation of the vascular tree

5. Hepatic microsomal enzyme activity is _____ in the geriatric patient.
   A. Decreased
   B. Not affected
   C. Increased
   D. Nonexistent

6. Among the important age-related changes in the geriatric patient is a consistent loss of neuronal density beginning at the age of 30 years that progresses steadily for the next 6 decades.
   A. True
   B. False

7. To avoid adverse central nervous system effects, geriatric patients generally require how much of a drug dosage reduction?
   A. 10%–20%
   B. 30%–50%

C. 60%–70%
D. 80%

8. Plasma protein binding is decreased in the geriatric patient, resulting in an excess _____ portion of sedative medications, with resultant exaggerated pharmacologic effects.
   A. Bound
   B. Unbound
   C. Nonreactive
   D. Reactive

9. Anesthetic drugs will initially be injected into a _____ blood volume in the older patient, producing a higher than expected initial plasma drug concentration.
   A. Diluted
   B. Contracted
   C. Hyperthermic
   D. Hypothermic

10. Which of the following conditions predisposes the geriatric patient to potential difficult airway management?
    A. Stiffening of peripheral blood vessels
    B. Increased beta receptor responsiveness
    C. Polycythemia
    D. Arthritis

11. The Postoperative Delirium Clinical Practice Guideline for Older Adults is promulgated by which professional organization?
    A. American Society of Anesthesiologists
    B. American Association of Nurse Anesthetists
    C. American Geriatric Society
    D. American Academy of Medicine

12. Hypothermia in the moderate procedural sedation and analgesia patient predisposes to shivering, which increases oxygen consumption by _____.
    A. 50%–100%
    B. 125%–200%
    C. 300%–500%
    D. 600%–1000%

Answers can be found in Appendix A.

Sedation Considerations for the Pediatric Patient

Robert W. Simon

LEARNING OUTCOMES

At the completion of this chapter, the learner shall:

- Articulate the goals of pediatric procedural sedation in the clinical setting.
- Identify the most recent sedation guidelines of the American Academy of Pediatrics.
- Examine the role of parents or primary caregivers of children receiving procedural sedation.
- Categorize the developmental subsets of pediatrics, and state examples of appropriate support.
- State the role of parents or primary caregivers of children receiving procedural sedation.
- Appraise the infant's physiologic response to pain.
- List three characteristics of the infant central nervous system.
- State the relationship of the parasympathetic versus the sympathetic nervous system in children younger than 1 year.
- List significant differences between the cardiovascular system of a small child versus an adult.
- Describe the primary cause of bradycardia in infants.

- List three distinct features of the infant's upper airway.
- List three distinct features of the infant's lower airway.
- Describe the natural breathing pattern of infants.
- Explain the significance of subglottic edema in children.
- State one method to determine the appropriate-sized pediatric endotracheal tube.
- List three airway maneuvers that may improve ventilation in a sedated pediatric patient.
- List the physiologic response of infants and young children to hypothermia.
- Describe methods to decrease heat loss in sedated pediatric patients.
- State the method of determining hourly fluid requirements in pediatric patients.
- Discuss the importance of current NPO guidelines for pediatric patients prior to sedation.
- Describe the importance of medication titration in pediatric patients.
- List at least four criteria that should be met prior to pediatric patient discharge after procedural sedation.

COMPETENCY STATEMENT

The health care practitioner maintains homeostatic regulation through assessment and management of physiologic care to minimize adverse events associated with the administration of moderate procedural sedation and analgesia to the pediatric patient population.

How does pediatric sedation practice differ from adult moderate procedural patient care?

The anatomy, physiology, and developmental needs of a child are significantly different than those of an adult. The need for procedural sedation may also differ, depending on the patient and the procedure.[1] Sedation in the pediatric population is administered to alleviate pain and anxiety, or to achieve immobility.[1] This competency module provides a broad overview of the emotional needs, physiologic variations, monitoring parameters, and pharmacologic techniques to provide safe pediatric procedural sedation.

What are the goals of pediatric sedation and procedural care?

The goals of pediatric procedural sedation include the following:
- Minimization of physical pain and discomfort
- Control of behavioral movement to promote patient safety
- Management of anxiety
- Limiting psychological trauma[1]

Diagnostic and therapeutic procedures performed on pediatric patients have a greater success rate when children are stationary and their pain and anxiety are effectively managed.[2]

Children younger than 6 years of age and those with developmental delays may require deeper levels of sedation.[1-3] Children younger than 6 months of age are also at greater risk for an adverse event.[1-7] Interventions aimed at pediatric procedural sedation must include consideration of the child's age, developmental level, and clinical condition.[1-7] Practitioners engaged in pediatric sedation should never treat the child as a small adult. Treating a child as a small adult ultimately compromises patient safety, leading to errors in drug dosage, fluid administration, and airway management. Each sedation plan should be customized to the individual child's clinical situation, age, and psychosocial needs, when appropriate.[1]

What are the indications for pediatric procedural sedation?

Numerous indications exist for pediatric procedural sedation.[1-7] Sedation has been used successfully for diagnostic studies (e.g., MRI, CT scans), minor surgical procedures (e.g., suturing skin lacerations), and invasive procedures (e.g., endoscopies, lumbar punctures).[1,5] Some procedures may be completed successfully without the administration of sedative medication. Typically, distraction techniques, including guided imagery, parental presence, and use of local anesthetics (numbing medicine), can be a successful alternative and adjunct to sedation.

Are all pediatric sedation techniques the same?

Not all sedation techniques are the same. Some diagnostic and therapeutic procedures require limited patient movement, whereas others may require a substantial amount of analgesia. Procedural sedation is a dynamic practice used by a variety of practitioners in a multitude of clinical settings.[1-12] Many children also receive procedural sedation in nonhospital settings.[1,4-12] In these environments, skilled pediatric rescue teams may be least accessible.[1,4-12] Therefore, adverse events that occur during non–hospital-based sedation procedures are more likely to be fatal than those that occur in a hospital or hospital-like setting.[1,13-23] Sedation regimens are broad and wide ranging, based on procedural needs, patient specific requirements, and physician preferences. Consequently, there is no "one size fits all" approach to pediatric sedation techniques.

What is meant by the term *pediatric population*?

The term *pediatric population* has been defined by the American Academy of Pediatrics (AAP) as any patient younger than 21 years.[24-26] Table 11.1 identifies the pediatric patient population by subset age.

The diverse pediatric population consists of numerous age-related physical, intellectual, and psychological differences.[1,3] Classic research studies related to adverse outcomes in pediatric anesthesia have suggested that neonates are at a higher risk than older infants for adverse complications.[13,14,16] Also, older infants are at greater risk for adverse outcomes when compared to pediatric patients older than 2 years.[13-23] Distinction of the pediatric patient population by subset age group is endorsed secondary to the numerous anatomic, physiologic, and psychological differences that exist among the various pediatric age groups.[1,3,13,14,24-27]

⚡ PATIENT SAFETY SBAR FOCUS

Sedation Considerations for the Pediatric Patient

Situation

There has been a recent increase in the amount of pediatric patients with "behavioral issues" in our dental office. Many of our dentists are unsure of the best sedation protocol needed to manage these challenging patients. In an effort to enhance patient cooperation and to get the children to remain stationary during the procedure, one dentist often administers a second dose of midazolam.

Background

One of our pediatric dentists, who is licensed in providing moderate sedation, devised a specific sedation protocol for our pediatric patients with "behavioral issues." In the waiting room, 15 mg of oral midazolam is administered to each patient regardless of age. Local anesthetic solutions are also administered for extraction cases. Patients are then brought to the dental chair, and 50% nitrous oxide mixed with 50% oxygen is administered via mask. A dental assistant is in charge of monitoring the patient's sedation during the procedure. If the patient is not tolerating the procedure, a second dose of oral midazolam is administered. Since initiating this new protocol, patients arrive in our postsedation area obtunded, hypoxic (decreased oxygen saturation), and with altered levels of consciousness. This protocol recently resulted in the death of a 5-year-old patient.

Assessment

Early childhood dental caries is the most common chronic childhood condition in the United States.[1] To aid in the treatment of this disease, pediatric patients frequently are given moderate or deep sedation. Despite updated pediatric sedation guidelines, concerns remain related to inaccurate dosing of sedative medications, lack of adequate presedation assessment, and the inability of practitioners to recognize the onset of adverse events.

Recommendation

There currently is no mandatory reporting system, nor is there a standard mechanism for reporting adverse outcomes related to sedation in dental offices.[2] Therefore, the incidence of complications and adverse events reported is most likely grossly underestimated.[2] Based on recent sedation guidelines, sedation administered in the office or clinic setting should not exceed the level of moderate sedation.[2] Medications that may induce deep levels of sedation, possess active metabolites, or demonstrate longer duration of action must be administered judiciously. Proper training of sedation providers and strict adherence to the guidelines developed by the American Academy of Pediatrics, the American College of Emergency Physicians, and the American Society of Anesthesiologists are paramount to insuring patient safety.

1. Dye BA, Tan S, Smith V, Lewis BG, Barker LK, Thorton-Evans G, et al. Trends in oral health status: United States, 1988-1994 and 1999-2004. National Center for Health Statistics. Vital Health Stat 11(248). 2007.
2. Lee, Helen, et al. "Ethics rounds: death after pediatric dental anesthesia: an avoidable tragedy?" *Pediatrics* (2017): e20172370.

TABLE 11.1 Pediatric Population Classified by Subset Age

Classification	Subset Age
Premature infant	<37 weeks' gestation
Full term	37–42 weeks' gestation
Post term	Born after 42 weeks' gestation
Newborn	<1 day old
Neonate	Birth–1 month
Infants	1 month–2 years
Developing children	2–12 years
Adolescent	12–17 years
Young adult	17–21 years

Modified from the US Food and Drug Administration. Guidance for Industry: General Considerations for Pediatric Pharmacokinetic Studies for Drugs and Biological Products. Rockville, MD: FDA Center for Drug Evaluation and Research; 1998.

What are some of the psychological needs of the pediatric patient that need to be appreciated as a sedation provider?

Medical and diagnostic procedures can be psychologically distressing to the pediatric patient.[24,26,28] Children must cope with a variety of stressful factors that include the unfamiliar sedation environment, separation anxiety, and the potential for postprocedure pain.[1,28] Practitioners should attempt to alleviate some of the child's anxiety by creating a child-friendly environment and communicating at an age-appropriate level. Appropriate developmental mechanisms of pediatric patient rapport include the following[17]:

Trust Versus Mistrust (Birth to 1 Year)
- Familiarity and trust with the primary caregiver(s) are vital.
- Separation (especially after 6 months of age) may result in a screaming, clinging infant.
  - Consider parental involvement.
  - Consider premedication with midazolam to address separation anxiety.

Autonomy Versus Shame and Doubt (1–3 Years)
- Children are determined to maintain control of themselves and their surrounding environment.
- Fears of abandonment and separation anxiety are present.
  - Allow objects of security (stuffed animal, blanket).
  - Clearly delineate end of procedure ("all done," "no more").

Initiative Versus Guilt (3–5 Years)
- Children are striving for a sense of independence.
- The have fears of bodily harm and mutilation.
  - Use simple, concise information, and directions should be relayed.
  - Use positive reinforcement because it is well received.

Industry Versus Inferiority (6–12 Years)
- School and after-school activities are good topics for conversation.
- Making choices is crucial to this age group.

- Participation and completion of tasks can decrease stress.
- Example is a patient helping push a stretcher to the procedure room.

Identity Versus Role Confusion (12–18 Years)
- Self-consciousness and modesty are important to this age group.
  - Providing privacy is imperative.
- Peer relationships are valued.
  - Conversing in a welcoming, calm, informational manner is helpful to the patient.
  - Music or other forms of entertainment media may be useful.

Should a patient's family member or legal guardian be present when I sedate a child?

Parents and surrogate caregivers are becoming increasingly involved in their children's medical care and may expect to be present during the initiation of procedural sedation. Studies continue to demonstrate that parental presence during the induction of general anesthesia is beneficial for children older than 4 years of age when both the parent and child are relatively calm prior to the procedure.[26,28-30]

Children tend to look to their parents for behavior modeling in times of crisis. Parental anxiety can be transmitted to the patient, further distressing an already anxious child. Prior to the procedure, any parental and patient concerns should be addressed in a caring, considerate manner by the practitioner to relieve any potential anxiety.[25-28,30] An open and honest dialogue with the parent, along with a clear concise description of the sedation process, is recommended.[26,28-30] Ultimately, the practitioner must decide if parental presence is in the best interest of the patient based on the anxiety level of the patient and parent and the requirements of the procedure.

What are the most current guidelines for monitoring and managing the pediatric sedation patient?

In 2016, the AAP released their report on guidelines for sedating pediatric patients for diagnostic and therapeutic procedures.[1] The purpose of the AAP's most recent update was to amalgamate sedation guidelines used by medical and dental practitioners, clarify recommended monitoring modalities, inform the practitioner, and recommend additional safety and quality improvement methods.[1] The AAP guidelines recommend the following:
- A systematic approach should always be used when preparing for, administering, and recovering from sedation, especially regarding the pediatric patient.
- Sedative or anxiolytic medications should not be administered without proper medical or dental supervision and guidance.
- A focused presedation evaluation and examination is paramount in ensuring patient safety. The evaluation should take into consideration the child's age, developmental status, fasting times, and any underlying medical or surgical

conditions, including but not limited to, any airway abnormalities.

- The practitioner administering the sedation should have a strong understanding of the medications' pharmacokinetic and pharmacodynamic properties, as well as any potential drug-drug interactions.
- It is required that at least one individual must be present who is trained in, and capable of, providing pediatric basic life support, if not pediatric advanced life support. The practitioner should be skilled in airway management and cardiopulmonary resuscitation potentially to "rescue" the pediatric patient, when needed.
- It is critical that age-appropriate airway management equipment, resuscitation equipment, and resuscitation medications be immediately available.
- Patient- and procedure-specific physiologic monitoring, in conjunction with continuous observation by the sedation practitioner, can often allow for precise and rapid diagnosis of complications.
- The use of expired carbon dioxide monitoring devices (ETCO$_2$ devices) is now mandated (with limited exceptions) for all deeply sedated children, especially when other methods of assessing adequate ventilation are inadequate.
- Regardless of location (e.g., hospital, physician's office, outpatient area), the facility should have a properly equipped and staffed recovery area. Based on a careful and documented review of the patient's medical history, physical examination, and proposed procedure, a practitioner may determine that a hospital is the only appropriate venue for administering sedation.
- The goal of recovering a patient from sedation should focus on restoration of the patient's presedation level of consciousness.

What are the key components of a thorough presedation assessment focusing on the central nervous system?

A focused presedation evaluation and examination is paramount in ensuring patient safety.[1,3,31,32,33] A systematic assessment of the following systems is critical to identify any potential physiologic or pathophysiologic contraindications prior to administering procedural sedation. The infant's central nervous system is relatively immature when compared to that of older children and adults. This immaturity predisposes newborns to dangers such as seizures, increased intracranial pressure, and subsequent intraventricular hemorrhages.[1,26,32,34,35] Even though the infant's central nervous system continues to develop until the end of the first year of life, it has been established that newborns and infants experience pain similar to that of adults, resulting in tachycardia, increased blood pressure, and increased intracranial pressure.[35-42]

Research studies have also suggested that the neuroendocrine response exhibited by infants in reaction to painful procedures may surpass that of the adult.[35-42] An infant's behavior and short-term development may be adversely affected following procedures completed without adequate analgesia.[38] Therefore, appropriate analgesia should be considered and administered to infants with the same care and consideration that would be provided to an adult.

Anatomically, the infant's skull is more compliant than the adult's. The presence of expandable fontanelles allows for the accommodation to increases in cerebral volume and pressure. Palpation of the fontanelles can provide the practitioner with valuable information regarding infant intracranial pressure and fluid volume status.[43-45] Studies have confirmed that infants born with baseline hydrocephalus due to increased cerebral pressure are at a greater risk for developing airway management complications secondary to their large occiput.[44-46] Sedation is often contraindicated in this patient population secondary to the risk of hypoventilation, hypercapnia, and possible brain herniation.[45,46] Sedation procedures for patients with known elevated intracranial pressure should be performed in a hospital setting, with appropriate personnel, equipment, and medications available to treat a neurologic, medical, or surgical emergency.

An increase in intracranial pressure, coupled with the delicate cerebral capillary network, can predispose the newborn infant to intraventricular hemorrhage (IVH), which is a leading cause of mortality and morbidity in this patient population.[44-49] Box 11.1 identifies factors that contribute to IVH in newborns. Invasive procedures in awake patients without adequate analgesia are notable contributors to increased intracranial pressure.[44,45,47-49] Sedation for neurologic procedures should focus on achieving optimal levels of analgesia, limiting increases in intracranial pressure, and maintaining adequate cerebral perfusion.[47-49]

What are the key components of a thorough presedation assessment focusing on the cardiac and pulmonary systems?

The diversity of the pediatric patient population requires the sedation provider to be knowledgeable of age-appropriate vital signs. Table 11.2 identifies normal cardiovascular and respiratory parameters for the pediatric patient population. Table 11.3 identifies cardiovascular variations between adults and children. When providing sedation to the pediatric patient it is important to remember that "one size does not fit all," and blood pressure devices must be properly sized for each subset of the pediatric patient population.[1,50]

The infant myocardium is pointedly less compliant than the adult heart and results in a relatively fixed infant stroke

---

BOX 11.1   Potential Sources of Increased Intracranial Pressure in Infants During Procedural Sedation

Hypoxia
Hypercarbia
Fluctuations in blood pressure
Low hematocrit
Hypertonic fluid administration

Data from Newfield P, Cottrell JE, eds. Pediatric neuroanesthesia. Handbook of Neuroanesthesia. 5th ed. Philadelphia: Lippincott Williams & Wilkins; 2012, 207–218.

TABLE 11.2 Summary of Expected Age-Appropriate Vital Signs

Age	Awake (min–max)	Resting (min–max)	SBP (mm Hg; min–max)	DBP (mm Hg; min–max)	MAP (mm Hg; min–max)	RR (breaths/min; min–max)
Neonate (<30 days)	100–205	90–160	67–84	35–53	45–60	30–60
Infant (1 month–1 year)	100–190	90–160	67–84	35–53	50–62	30–60
Toddler (1–2 years)	60–140	80–120	86–106	42–63	49–62	24–40
Preschool (3–5 years)	60–140	65–100	89–112	46–72	58–69	20–34
School age (6–11 years)	60–100	60–90	97–115	57–76	66–72	18–30
Adolescents (13–18 years)	60–100	50–90	110–131	64–83	73–84	12–20

DBP, Diastolic blood pressure; *MAP*, mean arterial pressure; *RR*, respiratory rate; *SBP*, systolic blood pressure.
Adapted from de Caen AR, Berg MD, Chameides L, et al. Part 12: Pediatric Advanced Life Support: 2015 American Heart Association Guidelines Update for Cardiopulmonary Resuscitation and Emergency Cardiovascular Care. Circulation. 2015;132(18 Suppl 2):S526-S542; and Berg MD, Schexnayder SM, Chameides L, et al. Part 13: pediatric basic life support: 2010 American Heart Association Guidelines for Cardiopulmonary Resuscitation and Emergency Cardiovascular Care. Circulation. 2010;122(18, Suppl 3):S862–S875.

TABLE 11.3 Cardiovascular Variations Between Infants and Adults

Cardiac Parameter	Neonates	Adults
Cardiac output	Heart rate (HR) dependent	Increased by stroke volume, preload changes, HR
Starling response	Limited due to decreased compliance	Normal
Contractility	Decreased	Normal
Compliance	Decreased	Normal
Catecholamine responses	Diminished	Normal

Modified from Lake CL, Booker P: Pediatric Cardiac Anesthesia. 4th ed. Philadelphia: Lippincott Williams & Wilkins; 2005.

volume.[50] This physiologic principle accounts for the fact that the infant's heart rate is the principal factor responsible for changes in pediatric cardiac output.[50-54] Physiologically, bradycardia is not well tolerated in the infant population. Hypotension and oxygen desaturation frequently accompany episodes of bradycardia. Hypoxemia in the presence of bradycardia decreases cardiac output and increases systemic acidosis and pulmonary vasoconstriction. Airway obstruction is a major cause of hypoxemia. To prevent respiratory obstruction, the pediatric patient's airway must be reassessed frequently in the sedation setting to prevent the development of a hypoxic state.

The parasympathetic nervous system is predominantly active in young pediatric patients, whereas the sympathetic nervous system is underdeveloped in children younger than 1 year of age.[55] Hypoxia, airway obstruction, deep sedation, and painful procedures stimulate the parasympathetic nervous system, resulting in unopposed bradycardia.[55,56] When left untreated, bradycardia can progress to cardiovascular decompensation. Because the sympathetic nervous system is immature in children younger than 1 year of age, adrenergic receptor activity, circulating catecholamine levels, and the physiologic response to exogenous catecholamine administration are diminished in the pediatric patient population.

Is it important to remove all air bubbles from intravenous lines used in infants and small children?

The foramen ovale, the fetal connection between the right and left atria, undergoes functional closure shortly after birth.[51,52] Anatomic closure of the foramen ovale tends to occur 4 to 6 weeks after birth, but can be delayed up to 1 year.[51,52] A patent foramen ovale is present in up to 20% to 30% of adults.[52] The ductus arteriosus, the fetal connection between the pulmonary artery and aorta, constricts after birth in response to increased PaO_2 with ventilation. The presence of hypoxemia contributes to the reopening of the ductus arteriosus that shunts deoxygenated blood from the pulmonary to the systemic system.[51,52]

Atrial or ventricular septal defects allow for direct access to the cerebral circulation, often bypassing the lungs.[51,52] These defects remove the safety net that is the pulmonary vascular bed. The vascular bed functions as a reservoir that absorbs small air emboli prior to entering the systemic and cerebral circulation.[55] Because of these anatomic variations, it is recommended that all intravenous stopcocks and injection ports be manually expunged of any air to avoid potential life-threatening air emboli. Box 11.2 identifies provider safety measures to prevent the inadvertent administration of air through an intravenous line.

BOX 11.2   Safety Measures to Prevent the Development of Intravascular Air Bubbles

- Inspect the IV line before the child enters the sedation suite or procedure room.
- Remove all air from the IV line, stopcocks, and fluid connections.
- Reinspect the tubing prior to patient arrival.
- Always have a free flow of both tubing and cannula (blood) prior to connecting fluid-filled tubing to IV cannulas.
- Flush a small amount of drug from the IV syringe to clear air from the syringe and needle hub prior to administration.
- Avoid injecting the last millimeter of syringe contents because there might be microbubbles on the plunger.
- If available, use air traps on IV lines.
- Never leave IV and central lines open to air.
- Never inject air into a central or IV line.
- Use vigilance throughout the procedure to ensure that the fluid lines do not run dry.

BOX 11.3   Pediatric Syndromes Associated with Cardiac Anomalies

- DiGeorge syndrome
- Down syndrome (trisomy 21)
- Goldenhar syndrome
- Marfan syndrome
- Noonan syndrome
- Polysplenia
- Sebaceous nevi syndrome
- VATER syndrome
- Williams syndrome

Syndromes Associated with Cardiomyopathy
- Duchenne muscular dystrophy
- Hunter syndrome
- Hurler syndrome
- Stevens-Johnson syndrome

Adapted from Krane JK, Davis PJ, Smith RM. Preoperative preparation. In Motoyama EK, Davis PJ (eds). *Smith's Anesthesia for Infants and Children.* 6th ed. St. Louis: Mosby; 1996:219.

What if my patient has been diagnosed with a congenital heart defect?

Patients with congenital heart defects or anomalies present a variety of medical management issues during the administration of procedural sedation. This patient population is frequently referred to a hospital setting with a pediatric anesthesia team prepared to assess and treat the hemodynamic consequences of sedation thoroughly in patients with congenital heart defects. Pediatric syndromes associated with cardiac anomalies are identified in Box 11.3.

What are the respiratory physiology and airway management considerations for the pediatric procedural sedation patient?

Given the immaturity of the infant respiratory center, the breathing patterns of the full-term newborn can be classified as irregular. During quiet sleep, periods of regular breathing are interrupted with 5 to 10 seconds of apnea.[55-57] This pattern diminishes over time as the respiratory center matures. Thus, episodic breathing is rarely present at 12 months of age.

The muscles associated with ventilation in the newborn are predisposed to quick fatigue due to a decreased type I muscle fiber distribution.[55,57] Children, therefore, have an increased metabolic rate that results in higher oxygen consumption, identified by the following[55,57]:

- Metabolic rate of oxygen consumption in an adult—6 to 8 mL/kg per minute
- Metabolic rate of oxygen consumption in a pediatric patient—3 to 4 mL/kg per minute

Due to this increased oxygen demand, alveolar ventilation also increases.[55,57-59] As a result of the higher rate of oxygen consumption and alveolar ventilation, apneic infants will become hypoxic within 30 seconds.[55,57-59] In the parasympathetic-predominant child, this hypoxemia swiftly progresses to bradycardia. Given these physiologic considerations, sedative, hypnotic, and analgesic agents must be administered judiciously in a fully monitored patient care area.

What is meant by the phrase *central apnea*?

The term *central apnea* of infancy is defined as a breathing pause greater than 15 to 20 seconds. This phenomenon is generally associated with bradycardia, cyanosis, and/or pallor.[59] Young infants who have received sedation or general anesthesia are at greater risk for developing apnea and subsequent bradycardia in the first 12 hours postprocedure. Those infants most at risk include postconceptual age less than 45 weeks.[59] It is advised that infants younger than 45 weeks' postconceptual age are observed in a hospital setting to evaluate the postprocedure respiratory depressant effects of sedation or general anesthesia fully.

Health care practitioners sedating infants younger than 45 weeks' postconceptual age or a full-term baby younger than 5 to 9 weeks must also consider the postsedation risks of apnea and bradycardia secondary to sedative agents administered during the procedure. Extended monitoring, prolonged postprocedure care, and parent education are also required for this patient population.

What airway skills should the health care provider administering procedural sedation to the pediatric patient possess?

The intention of pediatric procedural sedation is for children to maintain their own airway, with minimal support from the practitioner. However, at times, airway obstruction and respiratory depression may unintentionally occur. Practitioners engaged in pediatric sedation must be proficient in pediatric airway assessment and management. Airway skills mandate skilled bag-valve-mask management, proficient placement of oral or nasal airway devices, and endotracheal intubation competency in the event of apneic episodes that do not resolve during the diagnostic or therapeutic procedure.[1,57-60] During moderate sedation procedures, pediatric patients should be able to maintain their own airway, with minimal support from the practitioner. Careful drug administration, coupled with vigilant monitoring, provides the health care practitioner the ability to achieve this goal in most sedation cases.

Because airway obstruction is a leading cause of hypoxemia in children, the patient's airway should be reassessed frequently for signs of obstruction. Upper airway obstruction results in hypoxemia, bradycardia, decreased cardiac output, increased systemic acidosis, and pulmonary vasoconstriction. If needed, 100% oxygen should be administered when the heart rate decreases, because rapid intervention is essential to avoid a quick physiologic descent toward cardiac arrest. Pediatric rescue medications must be available during all sedation cases. The most common recommended pediatric emergency medications are identified in Table 11.4.

What are some of the differences between infant and adult airways?

There are many differences between the infant's and adult's upper and lower airways. The infant upper airway is characterized by the following distinct anatomic features[1,46,57,59]:

- Large occiput
- Large tongue
- Short neck

TABLE 11.4   Emergency Pediatric Advanced Life Support (PALS) Drug Dosages

Drug	Use	Dose	Notes
Adenosine	SVT PSVT Wide QRS tachycardia	**First dose:** 0.1 mg/kg IV push (max, 6 mg) **Second dose:** 0.2 mg/kg IV push (max, 12 mg)	Give as bolus, followed by flush Can cause bronchospasm Chest tightness, flushing are common
Amiodarone	Pulseless VT V-fib Recurrent hemodynamically unstable ventricular tachycardia Hypertrophic cardiomyopathy Supraventricular tachyarrhythmias	**Pulseless VT, V-fib:** 5-mg/kg bolus (max dose, 300 mg) **VT, SVT:** 5 mg/kg over 20–60 min (max dose, 300 mg)	Rapid infusion can result in hypotension Avoid administration with any drug that may prolong QT interval.
Atropine	Symptomatic bradycardia	0.02 mg/kg IV (repeat every 3–5 min; max single dose, 0.5 mg)	No minimum recommended dose Dose < 0.1 mg can cause paradoxic bradycardia. Max dose total: 1 mg for a child, 3 mg for an adolescent
Dopamine	Bradycardia Hypotension	2–20 µg/kg per min infusion	Titrate based on clinical response with slow on-off taper Adequate volume resuscitation required prior to dopamine therapy initiation Use with caution with peripheral IV access because extravasation can occur.
Epinephrine	Cardiac arrest Symptomatic bradycardia Severe hypotension Anaphylaxis Severe allergic reactions	0.01 mg/kg, IV, IO (0.1 mL of 1:10,000 solution) Repeat every 3–5 min, with IV fluid flush following each dose	Higher doses often needed in case of beta blocker or calcium channel blocker overdose High dose does not improve survival, neurologic outcome High dose cause myocardial dysfunction in postresuscitation period.
Glucose	Hypoglycemia	0.5–1 g/kg IV, IO	**<30 days**: $D_{10}W$, 5–10 mL/kg, IV, IO **30 days–2 years**: $D_{25}W$, 2–4 mL/kg, IV, IO **>2 years**: $D_{50}W$, 1–2 mL/kg, IV, IO
Lidocaine	Cardiac arrest from VT, VF; VT; VF	1 mg/kg, IV, IO bolus Maintenance infusion: 20–50 µg/kg per min	Can be used for stable polymorphic ventricular tachycardia with normal baseline QT and torsades de pointes Decrease maintenance doses in patients with left ventricular dysfunction and/or impaired liver function Not used prophylactically after myocardial infarction

Continued

TABLE 11.4   Emergency Pediatric Advanced Life Support (PALS) Drug Dosages—cont'd

Drug	Use	Dose	Notes
Magnesium	Torsades de pointes Hypomagnesemia Digitalis toxicity	**Initial dose**: 25–50 mg/kg IV, IO over 15 + 30 min in 10 mg/mL D_5W (max, 2 g)	Rapid administration may drop blood pressure High doses can cause respiratory distress (**calcium is antidote**) Use with caution for patients with renal failure.
Naloxone	Opioid reversal	0.01–0.1 mg/kg (max single dose, 2 mg)	
Procainamide	Ventricular arrhythmias SVT	**Loading dose**: 15 mg/kg IV/IO **Give over at least 30 min**	Serious reactions can result in hemolytic anemia Other common reactions include hypertension, bradycardia, angioedema, flushing, and urticaria.
Sodium bicarbonate	Metabolic acidosis	1 mEq/kg, IV, IO (give slowly; max, 50 mEq)	Ensure adequate ventilation before administering Prevent or correct respiratory acidosis Monitor pH via ABG results

ABG, Arterial blood gas; D_5W, dextrose 5% in water; $D_{10}W$, dextrose 10% in water; $D_{25}W$, dextrose 25% in water; $D_{50}W$, dextrose 50% in water; *IO*, intraosseous; *PSVT*, paroxysmal supraventricular tachycardia; *SVT*, supraventricular tachycardia; *VF*, *V-fib*, ventricular fibrillation; *VT*, ventricular tachycardia.

- Small mandible
- Narrow nasal passages

In the presence of a deep sedative state and general anesthesia, these anatomic features may predispose the infant to difficult airway management.[46,57,49]

What technique is recommended when selecting an oral airway for a pediatric patient?

The appropriate length of an oral airway can be estimated by selecting an airway that is the same length as the distance from the mouth to the angle of the mandible.[60,61] Additional external facial measurements are also recommended as reference points for estimating approximate oropharyngeal airway size; these include the following[61]:

- Measuring the distance between the maxillary incisors to the angle of the mandible
- Measuring the distance from the corner of the mouth to the angle of the mandible
- Holding the airway next to the side of the child's face and comparing the mouth to mandibular distance against the length of the plastic oral airway.

When should an oral airway be placed?

Oral airways should only be placed in deeply sedated patients requiring bag-mask ventilation. An oral airway placed in lightly sedated or awake patients may elicit a gag response, vomiting, and vagally mediated bradycardia.[61] Fig. 11.1 depicts the range of oral airway sizing available for the sedation provider. Correct oral airway placement during mask ventilation of the obstructed pediatric sedation patient is identified in Fig. 11.2. After successful oral airway placement, bag-valve-mask ventilation requires that the practitioner's fingers remain on the bony mandible. Pressure on the soft tissue below the mandible may result in further airway obstruction by pushing the tongue forward. Proper pediatric mask management technique is identified in Fig. 11.3.

When is it appropriate to select a nasal airway to manage airway obstruction in the pediatric sedation patient?

Because narrow nasal passages are easily obstructed with secretions, nasal trumpets (soft nasal airways) have been deemed to be more appropriate for the mild or moderately sedated patient.[62,63] Placement of an appropriately sized nasal trumpet

Size 0, **infant**, 50 mm
Size 1, **small child**, 60 mm
Size 2, **child**, 70 mm
Size 3, **small adult**, 80 mm
Size 4, **medium adult**, 90 mm
Size 5, **large adult**, 100 mm

Traditional

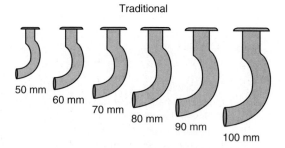

Color coded

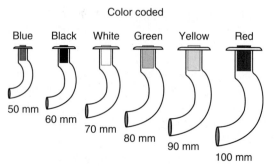

Fig. 11.1 Oral airway sizing.

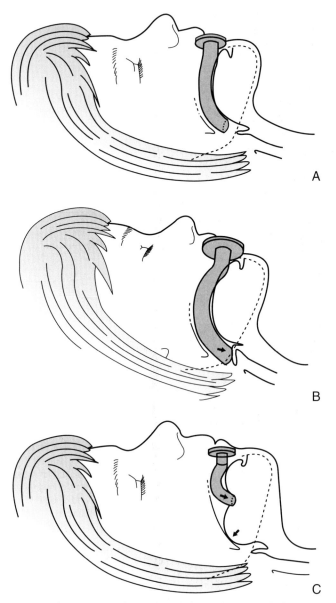

Fig. 11.2 Correct versus incorrect oral airway placement during mask ventilation of the obstructed pediatric sedation patient. An artificial airway of proper size should relieve airway obstruction secondary to the tongue without damaging laryngeal structures. The appropriate size can be estimated by holding the airway against the child's face. (A) The tip of the oral airway should end just cephalad to the angle of the mandible, resulting in proper alignment with the glottic opening. (B) If too large an oral airway is inserted, the tip lines up posterior to the angle of the mandible and mechanically obstructs the glottic opening with the epiglottis. (C) If too small an oral airway is inserted, the tip lines up well above the angle of the mandible and exacerbates airway obstruction by kinking the tongue against the roof of the mouth. (Redrawn from Coté CJ, Anderson BJ, Lerman J: *A Practice of Anesthesia for Infants and Children.* 6th ed. Philadelphia: Elsevier; 2019.)

reestablishes ventilation by physically displacing the tongue obstruction and decreasing the resistance of breathing. Nasal airways must be well lubricated to avoid trauma to the adenoidal tissue.[63] Nasal trumpets are better tolerated by the pediatric patient while decreasing vagally mediated bradycardia.

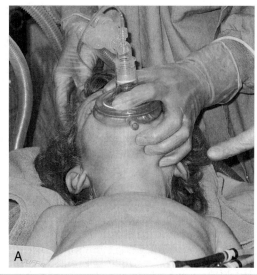

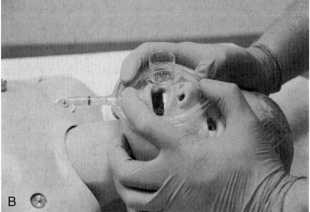

Fig. 11.3 Proper pediatric mask management. (A) E-C clamp method of ventilating pediatric patient with a bag-valve mask. Notice the provider is lifting jaw into mask. (B) Proper area of the face for face mask application. Note that no pressure is applied to the eyes. Two-handed method for securing a mask and giving a jaw thrust. An additional rescuer will need to attached the bag-device (not pictured) and squeeze the bag to give ventilations. (A from Santillanes G, Gausche-Hill M. Pediatric Airway Management. Emergency Medicine Clinics of North America 26(4): 961–975, 2008; B from Janeczek M, et al. Pediatric Resuscitation Guidelines. Disease-a-Month 59(5):182–195, 2013.)

When is intubation indicated in the pediatric sedation patient?

There are a variety of scenarios in which the pediatric patient may lose the ability to ventilate spontaneously or develop airway obstruction. Several airway maneuvers must be considered prior to intubation. These interventions may include the following:

- Maintenance of the head in a neutral position to align the oral-pharyngeal-tracheal axis (removing extreme flexion)[57,59]
- Gentle jaw lift
- Nasopharyngeal airway placement (lubricated nasal trumpet)
- Oral airway if patient deeply sedated (placed with tongue blade)
- Positive pressure ventilation with Ambu bag and 100% oxygen

When these maneuvers prove unsuccessful, and pharmacologic reversal of sedative and analgesic medications do not restore effective ventilation, immediate intubation must be considered.

What anatomic considerations must be appreciated by the procedural sedation health care provider regarding pediatric intubation?

If the need for intubation occurs, it is important to appreciate several anatomic variations between the adult and pediatric airway. As identified in Fig. 11.4, successful intubation requires proper alignment of the pharyngeal, laryngeal, and oral axes.[46,57] However, the short neck, small mandible, and large occiput in the infant frequently prevent proper alignment, which increases the incidence and severity of airway obstruction in the sedated child. Proper positioning of the pediatric patient to the so-called sniffing position is detailed in Fig. 11.5. Extreme neck flexion in an obstructed apneic pediatric patient increases airway obstruction.[60-64] Proper positioning, demonstrated in Fig. 11.5, frequently alleviates airway obstruction by helping keep the head neutral or slightly flexed.[60]

The infant's larynx lies more cephalad in the neck of the pediatric patient (C3-4) when compared to the adult (C4-5), which makes the pediatric airway slightly more anterior. The stiff omega or U-shaped infant epiglottis frequently obscures visualization of the glottic opening during laryngoscopy.[46,60-64] Manipulation of the extremely sensitive pseudostratified, ciliated epithelium lining of the infant cricoid cartilage may result in significant swelling and edema.[64]

What is the narrowest part of the infant's airway?

Contemporary studies have demonstrated that the glottic opening is smaller than the cricoid opening. However, the expansion of glottic tissues and the relatively stiff cricoid cartilage contribute to the conclusion that the cricoid cartilage is still functionally referred to as the narrowest portion of the

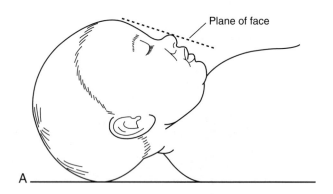

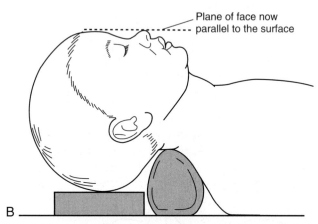

Fig. 11.5 Proper head position and axis alignment for the pediatric patient. (A) Flexion of the neck, producing airway obstruction. This position interrupts the alignment of the oral, pharyngeal, and laryngeal axes necessary for an adequate view of the vocal cords during laryngoscopy. (B) Proper positioning of the infant neck and shoulder roll demonstrates proper alignment for endotracheal intubation.

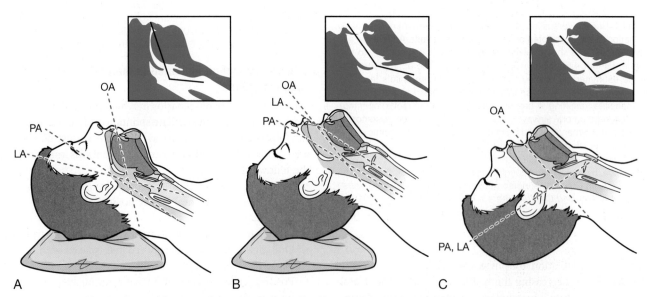

Fig. 11.4 Proper alignment of the oral, pharyngeal and laryngeal axes are required for endotracheal intubation. (A) Head in neutral position, (B) Head in 'sniffing' position, which has been postulated to align all three axes. (C) Head on bed, head extended on neck.

pediatric airway.[57,65] The clinical significance of these anatomic attributes remains; when an endotracheal tube with an excessively large external diameter is placed in a child, edema in this subglottic space occurs. This subglottic edema narrows the circumference of the patient's airway, resulting in increased resistance and respiratory effort.

Intubation is required in the procedural sedation suite for a pediatric patient. How do I determine the proper size of the endotracheal tube?

Stridor and respiratory distress develop rapidly when pediatric patients are intubated with an incorrectly sized endotracheal tube (ETT). Table 11.5 serves as a reference for patient age and appropriate endotracheal tube sizing. Pediatricians and anesthesia providers frequently use the equation listed below also to select the appropriate size uncuffed endotracheal tubes for children younger than 10 years.[60] The equation is as follows:

$$(16 + age\ in\ years)/4 = ETT\ size$$

Premature infants and those requiring prolonged mechanical ventilation are at risk for developing subglottic stenosis. These children frequently require smaller than normal endotracheal tube sizing. Uncuffed endotracheal tubes have generally been used in children younger than 8 years due to the anatomically narrower cricoid cartilage when compared to adults. Recent studies, however, have demonstrated that the use of cuffed tubes in children may offer some benefit over uncuffed endotracheal tubes.[57,65] An inflatable cuff allows for easier creation of the glottic airway seal and reduces the requirement for repeated intubation attempts required to place a properly fitting endotracheal tube in the pediatric patient. When a cuffed endotracheal tube is selected for a pediatric patient, the health care provider is required to select at least one full size smaller endotracheal tube prior to placement.[65]

Once placed, how do I determine if the endotracheal tube is fitted properly?

Once endotracheal tube placement is secured, a leak test determines if the endotracheal tube is properly placed. Properly seated endotracheal tubes demonstrate a leak that is heard when the practitioner applies positive pressure (15–25 cm of water pressure) with a bag-valve-mask. An audible leak at less than 10 cm H_2O pressure indicates that the endotracheal tube is too small, inhibiting the ability to generate adequate positive pressure ventilation when needed. An audible leak that is not discernible until 30 cm H_2O pressure or higher indicates that the endotracheal tube is too large and may contribute to the development of subglottic edema and resulting stridor.[57,66,67]

We frequently do prolonged procedures within our interventional platform. What types of heat loss do children experience during these procedures?

There are four primary types of heat loss in children[74-77]:
- Conductive
- Evaporative
- Radiation
- Convection

Conduction is the transfer of heat between two objects that are in contact with each other. Evaporation refers to heat loss from skin, respiratory, bowel, and wound surfaces. Evaporation accounts for roughly 10% to 20% of all temperature loss in the operating room environment; however, diagnostic and therapeutic procedures requiring procedural sedation generally have minimal evaporative heat loss during the procedure. Radiation heat loss occurs when two objects of a different temperature come into contact.[68,69] Convective loss occurs when heat is lost from the patient to the environment. Contributing factors that increase convective heat loss include the following:
- Temperature gradient in the procedure room
- Decreased temperature
- Uncovered patients

A summary of the types of heat loss is shown in Fig. 11.6.

What methods are available to minimize heat loss in the pediatric sedation environment?

A variety of methods are available to decrease temperature loss in the pediatric sedation environment. The simplest maneuver includes warming the environment (procedure room) to 75° to 80°F. The use of warmed blankets and hats during the procedure can also significantly reduce heat loss.

What fluid management calculations does the health care provider administering sedation need to consider for the pediatric patient population?

Infants have a greater total body water composition than adults.[70-73] As identified in Table 11.6, body composition varies with the pediatric patient population.[70-73] Prolonged fasting times in the pediatric patient population are not well tolerated. Sedation in a dehydrated pediatric patient can lead to decreased cardiac output, thereby worsening the hypovolemic state.[70-73]

To prevent the development of a hypovolemic state, pediatric fluid calculations are available to aid the health care provider. The infant's glomerular filtration rate and tubular function are considered to be immature until 6 to 12 months of age.[70-73] Because of this immaturity, the infant is prone to sodium loss in the urine. For this reason, all intravenous solutions given to infants should contain sodium.[74] The hourly fluid maintenance calculations featured in Table 11.7 may

TABLE 11.5	Endotracheal Tube Sizes
Age	**Size (mm internal diameter [ID])**
Preterm	
1000 g	2.5
1000–2500 g	3
Neonate–6 months	3.0–3.5
6 months–1 year	3.5–4.0
1–2 years	4.0–5.0
>2 years	(Age in years + 16)/4

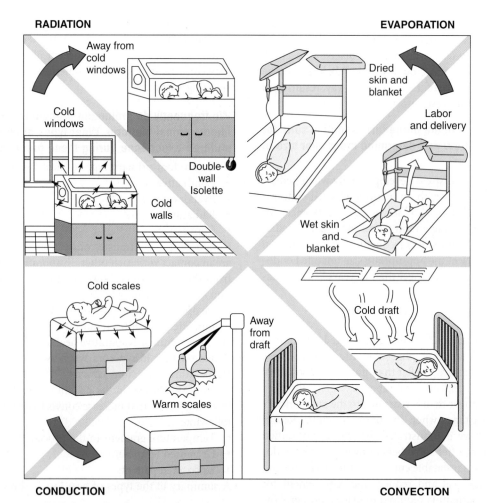

RADIATION

Away from cold windows

Cold windows

Double-wall Isolette

Cold walls

Cold scales

Warm scales

CONDUCTION

EVAPORATION

Dried skin and blanket

Labor and delivery

Wet skin and blanket

Cold draft

Away from draft

CONVECTION

Fig. 11.6 Radiation, or heat loss in the form of electromagnetic photons, occurs from warm skin surfaces to a cooler object not in contact with the newborn (e.g., inside the incubator wall, nursery wall, window). Radiant heat loss is independent of ambient air temperature and is the main source of heat loss because of the infant's large exposed body surface area. Conduction is the loss of heat to a cooler object in direct contact with the newborn (e.g., cold scale, unwarmed bed, stethoscope, examiner's hand). Convection is the loss of heat to moving air at the skin surface and depends on the air's velocity and temperature. Evaporation of water from the skin and mucous membranes also causes heat loss, especially in the delivery room. (Courtesy Lynn Jones, RN.)

be administered with a balanced salt solution, such as lactated Ringer's, (0.9%), or half-normal saline (0.45%). Dextrose 5% to 10% may also be included for intravenous supplementation, but one should check the patient's glucose level and medical history prior to the administration of a glucose-containing solution.[74,75]

The use of an infusion pump with free flow protection for accurate fluid volume administration is recommended for

TABLE 11.6 Body Composition of Pediatric Patients

Component	Infant	Child	Adult
Total body water	75%	70%	55%–60%
Extracellular fluid	40%	30%	20%
Intracellular fluid	35%	40%	40%

TABLE 11.7 Hourly Fluid Maintenance Calculations

Weight	Hourly Fluid Rate	Example
0–10 kg	4 mL/kg/hr	7 kg × 4 = 28 mL/hr
0–20 kg	4 mL/kg/hr for the first 10 kg	10 kg × 4 = 40 mL/hr
	2 mL/kg/hr for remaining kg	5 kg × 2 = 10 mL/hr 15 kg maintenance = 50 mL/hr
>20 kg	4 mL/kg/hr for first 10 kg	10 kg × 4 = 40 mL/hr
	2 mL/kg/hr for next 20 kg	10 kg × 2 = 20 mL/hr
	1 mL/kg/hr for remaining kg	6 kg × 1 = 6 mL/kg/hr 26 kg maintenance = 66 mL/hr

pediatric patients because it provides an accurate infusion rate, information on volumes administered, and warning if infusion patency becomes obstructed.[76,77] Newer infusion pumps are equipped with drug infusion libraries and air detector sensors to increase patient safety. Table 11.7 demonstrates how to calculate hourly pediatric fluid requirements appropriately.[73]

Should I be concerned with glucose replacement in children?

Compared with adults, pediatric patients have a decreased tolerance for fasting and can become hypoglycemic.[75] Glucose monitoring is recommended for infants who have experienced a long fasting time and have not received any glucose supplementation because severe hypoglycemia has been shown to cause cerebral ischemia and acidosis, resulting in irreversible brain damage.[75,78]

Recommendations have suggested that maintenance fluids containing 2.5% dextrose, as opposed to 5% dextrose, should be administered because replacement with 5% dextrose solutions has been associated with hyperglycemia.[70-75] Hyperglycemia can result in osmolar diuresis, which would further exacerbate the patient's hypovolemic state.[79] Appropriate maintenance fluids for pediatric patients include any of the following:

- 2.5% dextrose and lactated Ringer's
- 2.5% dextrose and half-normal saline
- Dextrose 5% with sodium (if 2.5% dextrose is not available)

An infusion rate of 4 to 6 mg/kg per minute is suggested to maintain normal glucose concentrations of 50 to 90 mg/dL in newborns.[70,72,73]

Why must my patient remain NPO prior to sedation?

Sedative medications have the potential to impair a patient's own protective airway reflexes, especially those medications administered for the goal of achieving a deep level of sedation. If the child's protective airway reflexes are not preserved, there is a chance, although rare, that the child may vomit his or her stomach contents. This increases the potential for pulmonary aspiration.[1] Thus, the practitioner should evaluate and inquire about the patient's previous fluid and food intake before administering any sedation medications.[1]

How long should a pediatric patient be NPO prior to procedural sedation?

Little is known regarding the absolute risks of aspiration during procedural sedation.[1,80,81] As a result, the AAP observes the same NPO guidelines established by the American Society of Anesthesiologists (ASA). These guidelines should be observed, especially in relation to solid food, because research has revealed an increased chance of pulmonary injury in the presence of particulate matter aspiration.[1,80] Procedural sedation NPO guidelines are given in Table 11.8. Small children and infants who arrive after a lengthy fasting period (>10–12 hours) may need to be rescheduled.

TABLE 11.8   Recommended NPO Times

Ingested Material	Minimum Fasting Time (hours)
Clear liquid (e.g., water, black coffee, clear tea, fruit juice without pulp, carbonated beverage)	2
Breast milk	4
Infant formula	6
Nonhuman milk	6
Light meal (clear liquid and toast)	6
Meat, fried foods, fatty food (any solid not considered a light meal)	8

Adapted from American Society of Anesthesiologists: Practice guidelines for preoperative fasting and the use of pharmacologic agents to reduce the risk of pulmonary aspiration: an updated report. Anesthesiology 2011;114:495–511.

What is the best strategy to initiate intravenous access in the pediatric population?

Intravenous placement may be particularly challenging in young children and infants secondary to fear, anxiety, movement, and lack of developmental cooperation A 24- or 22-gauge intravenous catheter is generally adequate for most sedation cases in small infants and children.[82,83] The best intravenous catheter insertion sites include the following[82]:

- The dorsum of the hand
- The lateral aspect of the foot
- The medial aspect of the ankle

Regardless of the size of the intravenous catheter, studies have reported that children rank needle sticks as their most feared medical event.[83-85] The acute pain and anxiety associated with intravenous insertion can negatively affect children and their parents.[83-85]

Are there any medications available to localize the intravenous insertion site?

Any measure aimed at alleviating the stress and pain associated with intravenous placement has been shown to benefit the child. For procedures that require an intravenous catheter, a eutectic mixture of local anesthetics (EMLA cream, Astra Pharmaceuticals) is available for use. EMLA cream should be applied at least 30 to 60 minutes prior to the intravenous insertion attempt.[84-86] EMLA cream is an emulsified (melts into oil below room temperature) mixture of lidocaine 2.5% and prilocaine 2.5% that provides dermal analgesia up to 5 mm deep[84-86]

EMLA cream should be applied to the dry intact skin surrounding a potential intravenous insertion site. This site should then be covered with an occlusive dressing and left for 1 hour after the cream has been placed. As with any medication, EMLA should be used with caution in infants because of the risk of methemoglobinemia.[84-86] Table 11.9 identifies guidelines for proper EMLA cream administration.[84-86]

An additional medication that may be administered to localize an intravenous insertion site is Gebauer's Ethyl

TABLE 11.9	Current EMLA Dosing Guidelines		
Age and Body Weight Requirements	Maximum EMLA Total Dose (g)	Maximum Application Area (cm²)	Maximum Application Time (hours)
0–3 months or <5 kg	1	10	1
3–12 months and >5 kg	2	20	4
1–6 years and >10 kg	10	100	4
7–12 years and >20 kg	20	200	4

EMLA, Eutectic mixture of local anesthetics.
Adapted from EMLA Cream: Physician's Desk Reference (PDR). Montvale, NJ: Thompson PDR; 2003:600.

BOX 11.4   American Society of Anesthesiologists Physical Status (PS)[a]

PS 1—a normal, healthy patient

PS 2—a patient with mild systemic disease that does not limit activities, such as controlled asthma or controlled diabetes without target organ damage

PS 3—a patient with severe systemic disease that does limit activities, such as severe heart failure or poorly controlled asthma

PS 4—a patient with sever systemic disease that is a constant threat to life, such as severe heart failure or end-stage renal disease

PS 5—a moribund patient who is not expected to survive without the operation or other intervention

PS 6—a patient declared brain dead whose organs are being removed for donation

[a]If the procedure is an emergency, the physical status classification is followed by an E (PS 2E).
From American Society of Anesthesiologists. Physical classification system. http://asahg.org/clinical/physicalstatus.html.

Chloride instant topical anesthetic skin refrigerant (vapocoolant), which does not have the risks of adverse side effects associated with EMLA administration.[87] A popular nonpharmacologic device that may be used to localize the intravenous insertion site includes the Buzzy, which is a vibrating, palm-sized device that combines ice and vibration to block sharp sensations on the arm. Multiple studies have demonstrated its efficacy and have reported similar, if not better, results in alleviating the pain associated with IV catheter placements, as compared to EMLA or other pharmacologic interventions.[88]

What is the most efficient method to classify patient physical status prior to the administration of procedural sedation?

In 1941, the ASA asked a committee of three physicians to devise a system to record the overall health status of a patient prior to surgery. In 1963, the ASA proposed the subjective physical status classification system identified in Box 11.4. Pediatric patients classified as ASA I or II are often considered to be ideal candidates for procedural sedation.[1,89] Children with an ASA classification of III or greater, special needs patients, and the presence of tonsillar hypertrophy or anatomic airway anomalies should be referred to the appropriate subspecialty consultant for further evaluation.

Additionally, a focused presedation assessment must focus on identifying conditions involving major organ systems and previous problems with sedation or anesthesia. The current medication history (including herbal preparations and over-the-counter products), allergies, and NPO times must also be obtained from the parents. The child's medications should be evaluated carefully. Teenagers should be asked about alcohol, tobacco, and drug use in the absence of their parents. A urine pregnancy test should be administered to pubescent girls to avoid administering drugs to the fetus inadvertently, because the administration of benzodiazepines has been associated with cleft lip and palate malformations.[90,91] Additionally, most sedation and analgesia agents are highly lipid-soluble and have a low molecular weight, meaning that they can cross the placenta easily and potentially harm the fetus.[92]

What patient care considerations must be afforded for the pediatric patient presenting with a developmental delay or mental impairment?

Patients with a developmental delay or mental impairment may have an unpredictable response to the sedative and analgesic effects administered.[93] Cerebral palsy patients also have difficulty managing oral secretions, and gastroesophageal reflux is common, making them more prone to gastric acid aspiration. Antiseizure medications can also interfere with the pharmacokinetics and pharmacodynamics of sedative medications. Prior to the administration of procedural sedation, it is important to document the frequency, type, and last witnessed seizure as part of the presedation evaluation.[93]

Children with developmental delays, mental impairment, and cerebral palsy may present to the sedation setting with a wide range in intellect and demonstrated ability to communicate. Preprocedure parental inquiry by the sedation provider must establish baseline neurologic status and the patient's preferred method of communication. The sedation provider must be cautioned that a decrease in the ability to communicate should not be regarded as decreased pain sensation.

What patient care considerations must be afforded for the pediatric patient presenting with a cardiac history?

Presedation evaluation of patients with known or suspected cardiac disease should include cardiac consultation and presedation testing, including electrocardiography and other detailed cardiac diagnostic tests. Careful auscultation of the pediatric patient's heart may reveal a murmur not detected previously by other health care practitioners. If this is detected, cardiology should be contacted.[94]

Potential signs of cardiac disease in children include the following:

- Failure to thrive symptoms
- Tachypnea
- Cyanosis
- Diaphoresis

Pediatric patients with cardiac anomalies should be treated individually and referred to a pediatric cardiac anesthesia team, if appropriate.

What components of the pediatric airway assessment should be documented prior to the procedure?

The AAP guidelines for sedating pediatric patients for diagnostic and therapeutic procedures state that all patients undergo a documented presedation medical evaluation, including a focused airway examination.[1,46] This examination should be performed by a practitioner or medical provider with expertise in pediatric tracheal intubation because proper airway evaluation is particularly important if a deep level of sedation is inadvertently reached and respiratory or airway support is required.

A systematic approach to pediatric airway evaluation is important. One method of focused evaluation includes stepwise evaluation of the following criteria[46,60]:

- Mouth and tongue
- Extent of mouth opening
- Thyromental distance relative to associated structures
- Degree of neck extension
- Mallampati classification; more valuable in older children and teenagers

Most untoward airway events are associated with failure to anticipate and identify the potential for difficult airway management correctly.[64,66,95,96] Many objective measures have been evaluated in the attempt to define particular features associated with difficult bag-valve-mask ventilation. The Mallampati airway classification system identified in Fig. 7.6 (Chapter 7) provides an airway assessment method that evaluates the extent to which the base of the tongue obscures the view of pharyngeal structures.[46]

Although correlation has been established in adult patients between the Mallampati score and the degree of difficulty when exposing vocal cords during direct laryngoscopy, the large tongue structure inherent to the pediatric airway frequently leads to poor correlation with the use of this system in evaluating children younger than 10 years.

Are there any medical conditions or physical airway anomalies that suggest the potential for difficult airway management during the sedation procedure?

Some medical conditions and their respective physical abnormalities predispose the patient to the potential for difficult procedural airway management. The presence of micrognathia (small submandibular space) can indicate the potential for difficult airway management secondary to the mandibular anatomic proportion. This limited submandibular space may prohibit proper placement of an oral airway and inhibit visibility of the vocal cords if laryngoscopy is needed.[95-97]

Asking patients to open their mouth as wide as they can helps aid in the acquisition of the Mallampati score and can identify any potential loose, chipped, or missing teeth. It also may identify the presence of temporomandibular joint (TMJ) problems. Maxillary and mandibular joint stiffness will inhibit the ability of the patient to open the mouth fully. Patients with other types of TMJ problems will experience variations in this examination.[46,98] The atlantooccipital joint should also be assessed if there are no contraindications, such as trisomy 21 or other known patient factors associated with laxity or fusion of the joint. This assessment identifies any potential limitations when placing an older child in the sniffing position to alleviate airway obstruction or to assist with vocal cord visualization if tracheal intubation is indicated. A complete review of each airway evaluation maneuver is featured in Chapter 7.

Some pediatric patients presenting for sedation have coexisting disease that will affect airway management. Patients with trisomy 21 (Down syndrome) have large tongues, short mandibles, small oral and nasal passages, and pharyngeal hypotonia. As a result, trisomy 21 patients are at a greater risk for obstruction when sedated. Care must be taken while managing the airway because approximately 20% of Down syndrome patients have ligamentous laxity of the atlantoaxial joint that predisposes to C1-2 subluxation. This subluxation can lead to permanent spinal cord injury, ranging from loss of sensation to paralysis.[99,100]

From age 6 through adolescence, children lose deciduous teeth and should be questioned about and examined for any loose teeth prior to starting the sedation procedure. Airway maneuvers and manipulations can dislodge a loose tooth and further jeopardize airway management and patient status. Orthodontia generally does not interfere with airway manipulation or management; however, metal palate expanders may make intubation slightly more difficult due to pharyngeal spatial restrictions.

Patients presenting with wired jaws will not be able to open their mouths. If these patients are to be sedated, wire clippers must be present in the procedural area.[101,102] Anesthesia should be consulted for patients presenting with fractured jaws that are in the process of healing. Pediatric syndromes associated with airway management difficulty are identified in Box 11.5.

When should procedural sedation procedures be cancelled due to patient illness?

On average, a child has three to eight colds or upper respiratory tract infections (URIs)/year.[103] Symptoms of upper respiratory infection include congestion, fever, cough, and general malaise. Presenting must be evaluated during the presedation assessment and before administering any sedative agent, which could further obstruct breathing in an already compromised patient airway. The patient presenting with significant nasal congestion may be difficult to sedate without simultaneously affecting spontaneous ventilation. Elective sedation

BOX 11.5 Pediatric Syndromes Associated with Difficult Airway Management

Congenital anomalies associated with difficult airway and intubation problems include the following:
- Encephalocele
- Cleft palate
- Micrognathia or Pierre Robin syndrome
- Craniofacial deformity (Crouzon, Apert syndromes)
- Mandibular hypoplasia (Treacher Collins, Goldenhar syndromes)
- Hurler syndrome

From Cladis FP, Davis PJ: *Smith's Anesthesia for Infants and Children.* 9th ed. Philadelphia,: Elsevier; 2017.

cases should be postponed and rescheduled if any of the following are present[103,104]:
- Croupy cough
- Rectal temperature above 38°C (plus any other significant sign of a URI)
- Malaise or decreased appetite
- Evidence of recent lower respiratory infection (e.g., rales, wheezing, productive cough)

Children with hypertrophied tonsils or adenoids tend to have airway obstruction while sleeping that manifests as snoring. These patients are at a greater risk of hypoxemia, even during procedures not involving the airway.[74]

What are the important aspects of obtaining consent in the pediatric patient population?

The patient's parents or legal guardian must provide informed consent for the procedure and sedation services. It is equally important that children be informed about the procedure in a manner consistent with their developmental age. If required, placement of an intravenous catheter should occur after the initial assessment, physical examination, and consent forms are completed.

What are the American Academy of Pediatrics guidelines regarding emergency drug and airway equipment availability in the sedation setting?

Recommendations by the AAP regarding emergency drug and equipment availability for pediatric sedation facilities are featured in Boxes 11.6 and 11.7.[1,3] A variety of age-appropriate airway management and sedation equipment and an emergency cart containing appropriate drugs and equipment

BOX 11.6 Suggested Resuscitation Drugs for Pediatric Sedation

Oxygen
Glucose (50%)
Atropine
Epinephrine (1:1000, 1:10,000)
Phenylephrine
Dopamine
Diazepam
Diphenhydramine hydrochloride

BOX 11.6 Suggested Resuscitation Drugs for Pediatric Sedation—cont'd

Hydrocortisone
Calcium chloride or calcium gluconate
Methylprednisolone
Succinylcholine
Aminophylline
Racemic epinephrine
Albuterol by inhalation
Ammonia spirits
Naloxone hydrochloride
Hydrocortisone
Isoproterenol
Sodium bicarbonate

NOTE: The choice of emergency drugs may vary according to individual need.

BOX 11.7 Suggested Emergency Equipment for Pediatric Sedation

Intravenous Equipment
IV catheters
  24, 22, 20, 18, and 16 gauge
Tourniquets
Alcohol wipes
Adhesive tape
Assorted syringes
  1, 3, 6, and 12 mL
IV tubing
  pediatric drip (60 drops/mL)
  pediatric burette type
  adult drip (10 drops/mL)
  extension tubing
IV fluid
  lactated Ringer's solution
  normal saline
Three-way stopcocks
Pediatric IV boards
Assorted IV needles
  22, 20, and 18 gauge
Intraosseous bone marrow needle
Sterile gauze pads

Airway Management Equipment
Face masks
  infant, child, small adult, medium adult, large adult
Breathing bag and valve set
Oral airways
  infant, child, small adult, medium adult, large adult
Nasal airways
  small, medium, large
Laryngoscope handles
Laryngoscope blades
  straight (Miller) No. 1, 2, 3
  curved (Macintosh) No. 2, 3
Endotracheal tubes
  2.5, 3.0, 3.5, 4.0, 4.5, 5.0, 5.5, 6.0 uncuffed
  5.0, 5.5, 6.0, 7.0, 8.0 cuffed

> ## BOX 11.8 Preparation for Sedation Procedures: SOAP ME Mnemonic
>
> **S**—suction; make sure appropriately sized catheters are available.
>
> **O**—oxygen; ensure adequate O_2 supply.
>
> **A**—airway equipment; inspect and check airway equipment such as oral and nasal airways, bag-valve-mask, laryngeal mask airway (LMA), laryngoscope blades, and endotracheal tubes.
>
> **P**—pharmacology; make sure rescue drugs are not expired and are readily available.
>
> **M**—monitors; all should be inspected to make sure they function; electrocardiogram (ECG), blood pressure (BP), and pulse oximetry required; $ETco_2$ recommended; precordial stethoscope recommended.
>
> **E**—equipment; any special equipment needed, such as a defibrillator.

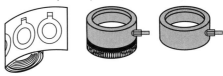

Chestpieces/precordial stethoscopes

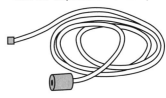

Soft ear disposable monoscope

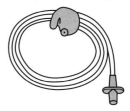

Monoscope reusable ear pieces

Fig. 11.7 Precordial stethoscope.

to rescue a sedation patient in respiratory distress must be immediately available. In the event of patient decompensation, contents of the emergency cart must provide the sedation provider with the medication and supplies necessary for providing continuous life support while the patient is being transported to another area within the medical facility.

How often should I check the emergency drug and airway equipment?

Age- and size-appropriate equipment and medications to sustain life must be checked before every sedation case.

Are there any tips regarding planning and preparation for a sedation procedure?

Yes. The AAP has devised a mnemonic that is useful for planning and preparing for sedation cases. The modified SOAP ME—*s*uction, *o*xygen, *a*irway, *p*harmacy, *m*onitors, *e*quipment—mnemonic is detailed in Box 11.8.[1]

What monitoring requirements should be implemented for the pediatric patient undergoing sedation?

Requirements for monitoring pediatric patients undergoing procedural sedation parallel those for monitoring a patient receiving general anesthesia. During deep sedation procedures, one person must constantly observe the patient's airway, adequacy of ventilation, and vital signs; vital signs should be recorded at least every 10 minutes in a time-based record.[105,106]

Precordial or amplified pretracheal stethoscopes are useful adjuncts for the pediatric sedation provider and are strongly recommended. The use of a precordial stethoscope allows the sedation provider the ability to monitor changes in heart rate and respiratory status continually and can lead to the detection of subtle changes in both before the monitor perceives it.

The precordial stethoscope disc (Fig. 11.7) is placed over the child's left sternal border at the second to fourth intercostal space.[106,107] This location allows the practitioner to hear breath sounds, heart rate, and heart tones clearly during the procedure. Double-stick adhesive (3M, St. Paul. MN) maintains contact of the bell of the stethoscope to the skin.

The opposite end of the stethoscope is attached by disposable lightweight tubing to a soft foam compressible ear piece (Kalayjian Enterprises, Chapel Hill, NC).[107]

All patients sedated for a procedure must also be continuously monitored with a pulse oximeter.[3] Pulse oximetry is a noninvasive mean of continuously measuring the arterial oxygen saturation of hemoglobin.[106] Studies have suggested that the pulse oximeter provides a more reliable warning of hypoxemia in children relative to the capnograph and changes in clinical signs.[106,108-111] Detrimental outcomes have been associated with the practitioner's failure to respond to pulse oximeter changes.[108] The AAP requires it for every case.

The AAP strongly endorses the use of capnography, when feasible. Capnography monitors exhaled carbon dioxide ($ETco_2$). Exhaled carbon dioxide creates a visible waveform on the monitor and is used to detect changes in ventilatory status.[109-113] Capnography waveforms can alert the practitioner to potential hypoventilation, respiratory depression, and hypoperfusion situations.[109-113]

Are there any specific monitoring requirements for the pediatric sedation patient undergoing a MRI scan?

Yes. AAP guidelines for monitoring the MRI patient state the following[1,3,114,115]:

The special technologic problems associated with monitoring patients in a magnetic resonance imaging scanner—specifically, the powerful magnetic field and the generation of radiofrequency—necessitates the use of special equipment to provide continuous patient monitoring throughout the scanning procedure. Pulse oximeters capable of continuous function, even during scanning, are now available and should be used in any sedated or restrained pediatric patient. Thermal injuries can result if appropriate precautions are not taken; avoid coiling the oximeter wire and place the probe as far from the magnetic coil as possible to diminish the possibility of injury. Electrocardiogram monitoring during magnetic resonance imaging has been associated with thermal injury, and it should be used with caution in this setting.

What, if any, standards exist regarding pain assessment and management in the pediatric patient population?

In 2001, The Joint Commission updated its standards requiring health care providers to be knowledgeable about pain assessment and management techniques. As a result, facilities are expected to develop policies and procedures supporting the appropriate assessment of pain and the proper use of analgesics. Pain assessment documentation must reflect a standardized age-appropriate pain scale, such as the Wong-Baker FACES Sedation Scale identified in Fig. 11.8.[116-118] Preverbal infants may be assessed using the Neonatal and Infant Pain Scale (Box 11.9).[116-118]

Is there a standardized pediatric sedation scale?

A standardized sedation scale should be used to evaluate and document the pediatric patient's level of sedation during the procedure.[116-118] The Ramsay Sedation Scale, featured in

Chapter 2, identifies the key components used to assess the patient's level of sedation during the procedure objectively. Also, the Observer's Assessment of Alertness and Sedation Scale, also featured in Chapter 2, can be used to evaluate the degree of alertness in patients.[116-118] Most sedation scales are relatively easy to use, but some may not detect subtle changes in sedation level.[66]

What is the optimal medication administration technique for the pediatric sedation population?

The pharmacology of pediatric sedation is as complex as the patients presenting for sedation services. Prior to selecting a drug regimen, the practitioner must recognize and establish the goals for procedural sedation, which frequently include the following:
- Cooperation
- Immobility
- Analgesia
- Sedation
- Amnesia

Currently, there is no one drug that can achieve all these goals. Therefore, as identified in Table 11.10, sedative medications are selected based on their demonstrated advantages and disadvantages. Depending on their desired clinical effects, sedatives and analgesics are often used in combination to achieve an optimal effect. Synergistically, these combinations

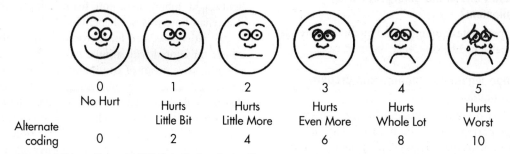

	0 No Hurt	1 Hurts Little Bit	2 Hurts Little More	3 Hurts Even More	4 Hurts Whole Lot	5 Hurts Worst
Alternate coding	0	2	4	6	8	10

Fig. 11.8 Wong–Baker FACES Pain Rating Scale. (From Hockenberry MJ, Wilson D, Rodgers CC: Wong's Nursing Care of Infants and Children. 11th ed. 11, St. Louis: Elsevier; 2019.)

BOX 11.9   Neonatal and Infant Pain Scale (NIPS)[a]

Pain Assessment

Facial Expression
0—relaxed muscles, restful face, neutral expression
1—grimace, tight facial muscles; furrowed brow, chin, jaw, (negative facial expression—nose, mouth and brow)

Cry
0—no cry, quiet, not crying
1—whimper, mild moaning, intermittent
2—vigorous cry, loud scream; rising, shrill, continuous
NOTE: Silent cry may be scored if baby is intubated, as evidenced by obvious mouth and facial movements.

Breathing Patterns
0—relaxed, usual patterns for this infant
1—change in breathing, indrawing, irregular, faster than usual; gagging; breath holding

Arms
0—relaxed, restrained, no muscular rigidity; occasional random movements of arms
1—flexed, extended tense, straight arms; rigid and/or rapid extension, flexion

Legs
0—relaxed, restrained, no muscular rigidity; occasional random leg movement
1—flexed, extended tense, straight legs; rigid and/or rapid extension, flexion

State of Arousal
0—sleeping, awake, quiet, peaceful sleeping or alert random leg movement
1—fussy alert, restless, and thrashing

[a]Recommended for children < 1 year old. A score > 3 indicates pain.
Adapted from Lawrence, J. et al. The development of a tool to assess neonatal pain. Neonatal Network. 1993;12:59–66.

TABLE 11.10 Advantages and Precautions Associated with Pediatric Sedative Agents

Drug	Advantages	Precautions and Comments
Ketamine	• Rapid onset • Fairly short duration of action (IV) • Minimal CV, CNS effects • Airway reflexes preserved	• Raised intracranial pressure • Laryngospasm • Tachycardia, hypertension • Exacerbation of psychosis • Hypertonicity, clonus • hypersalivation • Consider addition of atropine
Midazolam	• Rapid onset • Short duration of action • Can be reversed with flumazenil	• Respiratory, CNS depression • Paradoxic excitement • Hypotension • Side effects may arise when in combination with opiate
Fentanyl	• Rapid onset • Short duration of action • Can be reversed with naloxone	• Respiratory, CNS depression • Nausea, vomiting • Chest wall rigidity (high doses, rapid administration)
Morphine	• Longer duration of action, 2–4 hours • Can be reversed with naloxone	• Nausea, vomiting, respiratory depression, hypotension, sedation, pruritus • Use with caution in patients with asthma, preexisting respiratory compromise, or obstructive sleep apnea • Dose may be decreased to half the recommended dose in these patients
Etomidate	• Rapid onset • Short duration of action • Minimal cardiovascular effects • Minimal histamine release	• Injection site pain • Transient myoclonus • Hemodynamic changes with large doses • Respiratory depression • Caution in patients with history of focal seizures and those who are critically ill (inhibits cortisol production)
Propofol	• Rapid onset • Short duration of action • Quick recovery	• Rapid deepening of sedation to that of general anesthesia • Respiratory, CNS depression • Hypotension • Avoid in those with egg or soy allergies • Caution in critically ill patients ("propofol infusion" syndrome)
Nitrous oxide (N$_2$O)	• Short duration of action • Mild side effect profile	• Nausea, vomiting • Lightheadedness, dizziness • Not to be administered without oxygen • Postprocedure, administer 100% oxygen for 3–5 minutes to prevent diffusion hypoxia CAUTION IN CHILDREN WITH: • Increased risk of airway loss • Increased intracranial pressure • Pulmonary hypertension • Risk of expansion of air-filled closed space, such as pneumothorax, bowel obstruction • Recent neurosurgical interventions within the last 7 days
Chloral hydrate	• Effective for painless procedures • Mild side effect profile	• Gastrointestinal irritation, nausea, vomiting, diarrhea • Cardiac arrhythmias, hypotension (large doses) • Caution in neonates and children with preexisting cardiac conditions: cardiac monitoring important • Beware of residual sedative effects up to 24 hours • Effects unreliable if age > 2 years

CNS, Central nervous system; CVS, cardiovascular system.
Adapted from Tham LP, Lee KP. Procedural sedation and analgesia in children: perspectives from paediatric emergency physicians. Proc Singapore Health Care 2010;19(2):137.

of medications work together to maximize sedative and analgesic effect while minimizing the total dose of each drug administered to the patient. Table 11.11 identifies a pediatric sedation summary that may be used in an institution.

Studies have demonstrated that the administration of multiple sedation medications (three or more) is frequently associated with adverse outcomes.[119,120] The "sedate and wait" approach is often prudent to avoid the oversedation

TABLE 11.11 Pediatric Sedation Regimen

Class	Drug (Example)	Dosage and Administration[a]	Advantages	Cautions[b]
Opioid	Fentanyl	0.5–1 µg/kg IV over 2 min until appropriate analgesia reached	Short-acting analgesic; reversal agent (naloxone) available	May cause apnea, respiratory depression, bradycardia, dysphoria, muscle rigidity, nausea, and vomiting; hypotension described but is uncommon when used as a single agent; use lower aliquots and/or longer dosing intervals for older people or those with renal or hepatic dysfunction[9]
	Morphine	50–100 µg/kg IV, then 0.8–1 mg/hr IV as needed	Reversal agent (naloxone) available; prolonged analgesic properties (longer duration of action than fentanyl, alfentanil, sufentanil, and remifentanil)	Uncommon first-line agent for procedural analgesia; slow onset, peak effect time, and less reliable than fentanyl, alfentanil, sufentanil, and remifentanil
	Remifentanil	0.025–0.1 µg/kg/min IV	Ultra–short-acting drug; no solid organ involved in metabolic clearance	Difficult to use without an infusion pump
Benzodiazepine	Midazolam	Small IV doses of 0.02–0.03 mg/kg until clinical effect ("sleepy," ptosis, dizziness, slurred speech) achieved; repeat dosing of 0.5–1 mg for 3–5 min, with total dose < 5 mg	Familiar emergency drug; minimal effect on respiration; reversal agent (flumazenil) available	No analgesic effect; may cause hypotension, particularly when given rapidly or combined with opioids (may need to decrease midazolam dose); paradoxic excitation can occur (uncommon)
Volatile agent	Nitrous oxide	50% nitrous oxide–50% oxygen mixture delivered by physician or patient holding mask over mouth and nose	Rapid onset and recovery; cardiovascular and respiratory stability; few contraindications	Acute tolerance may develop; specialized equipment needed; for prolonged use, requires a well ventilated space, possibly with scavenging system of waste gases
Propofol	Propofol	Intermittent bolus of 0.1–0.3 mg/kg IV over 1–5 min or continuous infusion of 100 µg/kg per min for 3–5 min; then reduce to ~50 µg/kg per min titrated to effect	Rapid onset; short-acting drug; anticonvulsant properties	May cause rapidly deepening sedation, airway obstruction, apnea, hypotension secondary to myocardial depression; consider reducing dosage (by 50%, or more) in older patients or those with reduced physiologic reserve
Phencyclidine	Ketamine	0.2–0.5 mg/kg IV over 2–3 min; 2–4 mg/kg intramuscularly	Rapid onset; short-acting drug; potent analgesic even at low doses; cardiovascular stability; bronchodilator; synergy with propofol; few contraindications	Avoid in patients with history of psychosis because it may (re-)activate psychiatric disease; may cause nausea and vomiting; emergence reactions common,[c] but midazolam, 0.03 mg/kg IV, may attenuate or eliminate these reactions,[9,13] and quiet spaces for recovery may also help[17]; consider adding an antisialagogue, such as glycopyrrolate

TABLE 11.11   Pediatric Sedation Regimen—cont'd

Class	Drug (Example)	Dosage and Administration	Advantages	Cautions
Etomidate	Etomidate	0.1–0.15 mg/kg, slow (30–60 s) IV injection; may readminister every 3–5 min	Rapid onset; short-acting drug; cardiovascular stability in nonhypovolemic patients; respiratory depression rare[6,9]	May cause myoclonus, pain on injection, nausea, vomiting, lower seizure threshold (caution when using in patients with seizure disorders, epilepsy—may induce seizures),[6] and adrenal suppression (importance unclear in trauma[7,9]); recommended IV dose lasts 5–15 min

[a]Dosing regimens and protocols should be verified for each individual institution before starting any procedural sedation technique. The doses given are suggestions only, and doses and injection intervals may need to be adjusted on the basis of individual clinical presentation and comorbidities.
[b]Combinations of sedatives and analgesic drugs—synergistic combinations of these agents can augment their depressive effects on respiration and slow the patient's return to consciousness compared with the use of each drug alone.[4] Dosages should therefore be appropriately reduced when multiple agents are used. Certain combinations have better safety profiles. For example, before propofol-induced deep sedation, low-dose ketamine (at subdissociative levels) seems to be a safer analgesic than fentanyl; a small prospective trial for this indication has shown that ketamine is associated with fewer significant intrasedative adverse events (47%; 95% CI, 31%–64%) versus 84% (67%–93%)).[18]
[c]Emergence reactions are undesirable psychological reactions that can occur during recovery from sedative regimens when ketamine is a key component. They can vary in severity and composition but commonly involve vivid dreaming, a sensation of floating or leaving one's body, and misinterpretations of true sensory stimuli (illusions). These are often associated with excitement, confusion, euphoria, and fear.[19]
Adapted from Atkinson P. Procedural sedation and analgesia for adults in the emergency department. *BMJ* 2014;348:g2965.

associated with administering multiple drug regimens to the pediatric patient. Additionally, intravenous medications should always be administered in incremental doses, and adequate time should be permitted to assess their sedative or analgesic effect(s). Nonparenteral drugs also must be allowed adequate time for full absorption to evaluate their full sedative effect.[119,120] Vigilance, coupled with a repeated assessment of vital signs and level of consciousness, should be recorded while titrating medications to reduce the risk of oversedation.[1,119,120]

SUMMARY

The anatomic, physiologic, and developmental needs of children vary greatly when compared with the adult population. Sedation providers administering moderate procedural sedation and analgesia to the pediatric patient must recognize these variations and customize their sedation plan accordingly. Vigilance, coupled with proper physiologic monitoring, level of consciousness assessment, and continuous airway assessment, helps promote safety and mitigates the increased risks associated with pediatric patient sedation care.

REFERENCES

1. Cote CJ, Wilson S. American Academy of Pediatrics; American Academy of Pediatric Dentistry. Guidelines for Monitoring and Management of Pediatric Patients During and After Sedation for Diagnostic and Therapeutic Procedures: Update 2016. *Pediatrics. Jpeds.* 2016;138.
2. Bhatt M, Kennedy RM, Osmond MH, et al. Consensus-based recommendations for standardizing terminology and reporting adverse events for emergency department procedural sedation and analgesia in children. *Ann Emerg Med.* 2009;53:426.
3. American Academy of Pediatrics. Guidelines for Monitoring and Management of Pediatric Patients During and After Sedation for Diagnostic and Therapeutic Procedures (addendum). *Pediatrics.* 2002;110(4):836–838.
4. Flood RG, Krauss B. Procedural sedation and analgesia for children in the emergency department. *Emerg Med Clin North Am.* 2003;21(1):121–139.
5. Krauss B, Green SM. Procedural sedation and analgesia in children. *Lancet.* 2006;367:766.
6. Milnes AR. Intravenous procedural sedation: an alternative to general anesthesia in the treatment of early childhood caries. *J Can Dent Assoc.* 2003;69:298–302.
7. Jaggar SI, Haxby E. Sedation, anaesthesia and monitoring for bronchoscopy. *Pediatric Respiratory Rev.* 2002;3(4):321–327.
8. Mason KP, Michna E, DiNardo JA, et al. Evolution of a protocol for ketamine-induced sedation as an alternative to general anesthesia for interventional radiologic procedures in pediatric patients. *Radiology.* 2002;225(2):457–465.
9. Houpt M. Project USAP 2000—use of sedative agents by pediatric dentists: a 15-year follow-up survey. *Pediatr Dent.* 2002;24(4):289–294.
10. Ljungman G, Gordh T, Sörensen S, Kreuger A. Lumbar puncture in pediatric oncology: conscious sedation vs. general anesthesia. *Med Pediatr Oncol.* 2001;36(3):372–379.
11. Hopkins KL, Davis PC, Sanders CL, Churchill LH. Sedation for pediatric imaging studies. *Neuroimaging Clin N Am.* 1999;9(1):1–10.
12. Bauman LA, Kish I, Baumann RC, Politis GD. Pediatric sedation with analgesia. *Am J Emerg Med.* 1999;17(1):1–3.
13. Cravero JP, Beach ML, Blike GT, et al. Pediatric Sedation Research Consortium. The incidence and nature of adverse events during pediatric sedation/anesthesia with propofol for procedures outside the operating room: a report from the Pediatric Sedation Research Consortium. *Anesth Analg.* 2009;108(3):795–804.

14. Cote CJ, Notterman DA, Karl HW, et al. Adverse sedation events in pediatrics: a critical incident analysis of contributing factors. *Pediatrics.* 2000;105:805–814.

15. Olsson GL, Hallen B. Cardiac arrest during anesthesia: a computerized study. *Acta Anaesthesiol Scand.* 1988;32:653–664.

16. Tiret L, Nivoche Y, Hatton F, et al. Complications related to anaesthesia in infants and children. *Br J Anaesthesiol.* 1988;61:263–269.

17. Campling EA, Devlin HB, Lunn JN. *The Report of the National Confidential Enquiry into Perioperative Deaths (NCEPOD) 1989.* London: Royal College of Surgeons of England; 1990.

18. Cohen MM, Cameron CB, Duncan PG. Pediatric anesthesia morbidity and mortality in the perioperative period. *Anesth Analg.* 1990;70:160–167.

19. Morray JP, Geiduschek JM, Caplan RA, et al. A comparison of pediatric and adult anesthesia closed malpractice claims. *Anesthesiology.* 1993;78:461–467.

20. Holzman RS. Morbidity and mortality in pediatric anesthesia. *Pediatr Clin North Am.* 1994;41:239–256.

21. Geiduschek JM. Registry offers insight on preventing cardiac arrests in children. *Newslett Am Soc Anesthesiol.* 1998;62:6.

22. Joint Commission on Accreditation of Health Care Organizations. *Sentinel Event Alert.* Nov 30, 2000;15.

23. Green SM, Kuppermann N, Rothrock SG, et al. Predictors of adverse events with intramuscular ketamine sedation in children. *Ann Emerg Med.* 2000;35(1):35–42.

24. American Academy of Pediatrics. Guidelines for the pediatric perioperative anesthesia environment (RE9820). 1999;103 (2):512–515.

25. Steward DJ, Lerman J. *Manual of Pediatric Anesthesia.* Philadelphia: Churchill Livingstone; 2001:3–5.

26. Kost M. *Manual of Conscious Sedation.* WB Saunders: Philadelphia; 1998.

27. O'Donnell JM, Bragg K, Sell S. Procedural sedation: Safely navigating the twilight zone. *Nursing.* 2003;33(4):36–45.

28. Zeev N, Mayes L, Caraminco L, et al. Parental presence during induction of anesthesia: a randomized controlled trial. *Anesthesiology.* 1996;84:1060–1067.

29. Rackow H, Salanitre E. Modern concepts in pediatric anesthesiology. *Anesthesiology.* 1969;30:208–234.

30. Poe SS, Nolan MT, Dang D, et al. Ensuring safety of patients receiving sedation for procedures: evaluation of clinical practice guidelines. *Jt Comm J Qual Improv.* 2001;27 (1):28–41.

31. Practice Guidelines for Moderate Procedural Sedation and Analgesia 2018: A Report by the American Society of Anesthesiologists Task Force on Moderate Procedural Sedation and Analgesia, the American Association of Oral and Maxillofacial Surgeons, American College of Radiology, American Dental Association, American Society of Dentist Anesthesiologists, and Society of Interventional Radiology. *Anesthesiology* 2018;128(3):437–479

32. Hamid RK, Newfield P. Pediatric Neuroanesthesia. In: *Handbook of Neuroanesthesia.* Philadelphia: Lippincott Williams & Wilkins; 1994:270–284.

33. Maxwell LG, Zuckerberg AL, Motoyamo EK, et al. Systemic disorders in pediatric anesthesia. In: Motoyama EK, Davis PJ, Eds. Smith's Anesthesia for Infants and Children. 6th ed St. Louis; Mosby: 867–868.

34. Noble Y, Boyd R. Neonatal assessments for the preterm infant up to 4 months corrected age: a systematic review. *Dev Med Child Neurol.* 2012;54(2):129–139.

35. Pang LM. Physiologic considerations. In: Krauss B, Brustowicz RN, eds. *Pediatric Procedural Sedation and Analgesia.* Philadelphia: Lippincott Williams & Wilkins; 1999:11–16.

36. Fitzgerald M. Development of pain pathways and mechanisms. In: Anand KJS, McGrath PJ, eds. *Pain in Neonates.* Amsterdam: Elsevier; 1993:19–37.

37. Fazzi E, Farinotti L, Scelsa B, et al. Response to pain in a group of healthy term newborns: behavioral and physiological aspects. *Funct Neurol.* 1996;11(1):35–43.

38. Pembrook L. Studies reveal pediatric pain inadequately managed after ambulatory surgery. *Anesthesiology News Nov.* 2002;28(11):7–11.

39. Deshpande JK, Tobias JD. *The Pediatric Pain Handbook.* St. Louis: Mosby; 1996.

40. Ferrari L, ed. *Anesthesia and Pain Management for the Pediatrician.* Baltimore: John Hopkins University Press; 1999.

41. Malvyia S. *Sedation Analgesia for Diagnostic and Therapeutic Procedures.* Totowa, NJ: Humana Press; 2001.

42. Yaster M, Krane EJ, Kaplan RF, et al. *Pediatric Pain Management and Sedation Handbook.* St. Louis: Mosby-Year Book; 1997.

43. Vender JS, Gilbert HC. Monitoring the anesthetized patient. In: Barash PG, Cullen BF, Stoelting RK, eds. *Clinical Anesthesia.* 3rd ed. Philadelphia: Lippincott-Raven; 1997:621–641.

44. Berry FA. Neonatal anesthesia. In: Barash PG, Cullen BF, Stoelting RK, eds. *Clinical Anesthesia.* 3rd ed. Philadelphia: Lippincott-Raven; 1997:1091–1114.

45. Kaiser AM, Whitelaw AG. Intracranial pressure estimation by palpation of the anterior fontanelle. *Archives of disease in childhood.* 1987;62(5):516–517.

46. Mallampati SR, Gatt SP, Gugino LD, et al. A clinical sign to predict difficult tracheal intubation: A prospective study. *Can Anaesth Soc J.* 1985;32:429.

47. McPherson C, Haslam M, Pineda R, Rogers C, Neil J, et al. Brain injury and development in preterm infants exposed to fentanyl. *Annals of Pharmacotherapy.* 2015;49 (12):1291–1297.

48. Tutiven JL, Sundararaman LV, Sarah G. Anatomy and physiology: Brain, fontanelles, cranial sutures, and spinal cord. In: Kaye A, Fox C, Diaz J, eds., *Essentials of Pediatric Anesthesiology.* Cambridge: Cambridge University Press; 2014; 268–295 [Chapter 9].

49. Lyvonne NT. The nursing management of children with severe traumatic brain injury and raised ICP. *British Journal of Neuroscience Nursing.* 2007;3(10):461–467.

50. Howlin F, Brenner M. Cardiovascular assessment in children: Assessing pulse and blood pressure. *Paediatric Nursing.* 2009;22(1):25–35.

51. Levi M, Bharati S. Embryology of the heart and great vessels. In: Arcinieges E, ed. *Pediatric Cardiac Surgery.* Chicago: Year Book Medical; 1985:1–12.

52. Hagen PT, Scholtz DG, Edwards WD. Incidence and size of patent foramen ovale during the first 10 decades of life on autopsy study of 965 normal hearts. *Mayo Clin Proc.* 1984;59:17–20.

53. Jain R, Petrillo-Albarano T, Parks WJ, et al. Efficacy and safety of deep sedation by non-anesthesiologists for cardiac MRI in children. *Pediatr Radiol.* 2013;43(5):605–611.

54. Krauss B, Green SM. Sedation and analgesia for procedures in children. *N Engl J Med.* 2000;342(13):938–945.

55. Krauss B, Brustowicz RN, eds. Airway and respiratory control. In: *Pediatric Procedural Sedation and Analgesia.* Philadelphia: Lippincott Williams & Wilkins; 1999:3–10.

56. Steward DJ, Lerman J. *Manual of Pediatric Anesthesia.* Philadelphia Churchill Livingstone. 2001;15–25.
57. Harless J, Ramaiah R, Bhananker SM. Pediatric airway management. *International Journal of Critical Illness and Injury Science.* 2014;4(1):65–70.
58. Keidan I, Fine G, Kagawa T, et al. Work of breathing during spontaneous ventilation in anesthetized children: A comparative study among the face mask, laryngeal mask, and endotracheal tube. *Anes Analg.* 2000;91:1381–1388.
59. Litman RS, Berkowitz RJ, Ward DS. Levels of consciousness and ventilatory parameters in young children during sedation with oral midazolam and nitrous oxide. *Arch Pediatr Adolesc Med.* 1996 Jul;150(7):671–675.
60. Fincane BT, Santora AH. *Evaluation of the Airway Prior to Intubation: Principles of Airway Management.* Philadelphia: FA Morris; 1969.
61. Kim HJ, Kim SH, Min NH, Park WK. Determination of the appropriate sizes of oropharyngeal airways in adults: correlation with external facial measurements: A randomised crossover study. *Eur J Anaesthesiol.* 2016;33(12):936–942.
62. Holm-Knudsen R, Eriksen Kirsten, Rasmussen Lars S. Using a nasopharyngeal airway during fiberoptic intubation in small children with a difficult airway. *Pediatric Anesthesia.* 2005;15(10):839–845.
63. Zwank Michael. Middle turbinectomy as a complication of nasopharyngeal airway placement. *The American Journal of Emergency Medicine.* 2009;27(4):513.e3–513.e4.
64. Samsoon GLT, Young JRB. Difficult tracheal intubation: A retrospective study. *Anaesthesia.* 1987;42:487.
65. Wani T, Bissonette B, Hayes D, Rafiq M. Age-based analysis of pediatric upper airway dimensions using computed tomography imaging. *Pediatric pulmonology.* 2016;51(3):267–271.
66. King TA, Adams AP. Failed intubation. *Br J Anaesth.* 1990;65:400.
67. Shukry M, Hanson RD, Koveleskie JR, Ramadhyani U. Management of the difficult pediatric airway with Shikani Optical Stylet. *Pediatric Anesthesia.* 2005;15(4):342–345.
68. Bissionette B, Davis PJ. Thermal regulation—physiology and perioperative management in infants and children. In: Motoyama EK, Davis PJ, Eds. *Smith's Anesthesia for Infants and Children.* 6th ed. St. Louis: Mosby, 139–158.
69. Nilsson K. Maintenance and monitoring of body temperature in infants and children. *Pediatr Anaesth.* 1991;(1):13–20.
70. Fluid, electrolytes, and transfusion therapy. In: Bell C, Kain ZN, Eds. *The Pediatric Anesthesia Handbook.* 2nd ed. St. Louis: Mosby; 1997;71–96.
71. Tommasino C. Fluid management. In: Newfield P, Cottrell J. *Handbook of Neuroanesthesia.* Philadelphia: Lippincott Williams & Wilkins; 2012;412.
72. Cohen IT, Motoyama EK. Intraoperative and postoperative management. In: Motoyama EK, Davis PJ, Eds. *Smith's Anesthesia for Infants and Children.* 6th ed. St. Louis: Mosby; 313–345.
73. Dabbagh S, Demetrius E, Gruskin AB. Regulation of fluids and electrolytes in infants and children. In: Motoyama EK, Davis PJ, Eds. *Smith's Anesthesia for Infants and Children.* 6th ed. St. Louis: Mosby, 105–137.
74. Yung Michael, Keeley Steve. Randomised controlled trial of intravenous maintenance fluids. *Journal of paediatrics and child health.* 2009;45(1-2):9–14.
75. Welborn LG, McGill WA, Hannallah RS, et al. Perioperative blood glucose concentrations in pediatric outpatients. *Anesthesiology.* 1986;65:543.
76. Kim BG, Ayoub A, Sokolsky O, et al. Safety-Assured Development of the GPCA Infusion Pump Software, International Conference on Embedded Software (EMSOFT 2011); 2011; 155–164.
77. Committee on Standards and Practice Parameters. Standards for Basic Anesthetic Monitoring. Chicago: American Society of Anesthesiologists; 2011.
78. Axelin A, Salanterä S, Kirjavainen J, Lehtonen L. Oral glucose and parental holding preferable to opioid in pain management in preterm infants. *The Clinical journal of pain.* 2009;25(2):138–145.
79. Smith EO, Sunehag AL. Hyperglycemia is a risk factor for early death and morbidity in extremely low birth-weight infants. *Pediatrics.* 2006;118(5):1811–1818.
80. American Society of Anesthesiologists. Practice guidelines for preoperative fasting and the use of pharmacologic agents to reduce the risk of pulmonary aspiration: application to healthy patients undergoing elective procedures: an updated report. *Anesthesiology.* 2017;126(3):376–393.
81. Cravero JP, Blike GT. Review of pediatric sedation. *Anesth Analg.* 2004;99(5):1355–1364.
82. Cravero JP, Blike GT. Pediatric sedation. *Curr Opin Anaesthesiol.* 2004;17(3):247–251.
83. Shavit I, Keidan I, Augarten A. The practice of pediatric procedural sedation and analgesia in the emergency department. *Eur J Emerg Med.* 2006;13(5):270–275.
84. Physician's Desk Reference (PDR). *EMLA cream.* Montvale, NJ: Thompson PDR; 2003:599–602.
85. Ehrenstrom-Reiz GM, Reiz SL, Stockman O. Topical anesthesia with EMLA, a new lidocaine-prilocaine cream and the CUSUM technique for detection of minimal application time. *Acta Anaesthesiol Scand.* 1983;27:510.
86. Bjerring P, Anderson PH, Arendt-Nielsen L. Vascular response of human skin after analgesia with EMLA cream. *Br J Anaesth.* 1989;63:655–660.
87. Potts DA, Davis KF, Elci OU, Fein JA. A vibrating cold device to reduce pain in the pediatric emergency department. *Pediatr Emerg Care.* 2017;1.
88. Moadad N, Kozman K, Shahine R, et al. Distraction using the BUZZY for children during an IV insertion. *J Pediatr Nurs.* 2016;31(1):64–72.
89. Doyle DJ, Garmon EH. American Society of Anesthesiologists Classification (ASA Class) [Updated 2019 Jan 19]. In: StatPearls [Internet]. Treasure Island (FL): StatPearls Publishing; 2018. Available from: https://www.ncbi.nlm.nih.gov/books/NBK441940/.
90. Motoyama EK, Davis PJ, Eds. *Smith's Anesthesia for Infants and Children.* 6th Ed. St. Louis: Mosby, 229–279.
91. Monroe KK, Beach M, Reindel R, et al. Analysis of procedural sedation provided by pediatricians. *Pediatr Int.* 2013;55(1):17–23.
92. Resek J. Conscious sedation. *Anesthesia Today.* 2000;11(2):4–10.
93. Anderson BJ. My child is unique: the pharmacokinetics are universal. *Paediatr Anaesth.* 2012;22(6):530–538.
94. Hoffman Julien IE, Kaplan Samuel. The incidence of congenital heart disease. *Journal of the American college of cardiology.* 2002;39(12):1890–1900.

95. Apfelbaum JL, Hagberg CA, Caplan RA, et al. American Society of Anesthesiologists Task Force on Management of the Difficult Airway. Practice guidelines for management of the difficult airway: an updated report by the American Society of Anesthesiologists Task Force on Management of the Difficult Airway. *Anesthesiology 118*. 2013;2:251–270.

96. Weiss M, Engelhardt T. Proposal for the management of the unexpected difficult pediatric airway. *Pediatric Anesthesia*. 2010;20(5):454–464.

97. Walker Robert WM. Management of the difficult airway in children. *J R Soc Med*. 2001;94(7):341–344.

98. Kopp VJ, Bailey A, Valley R, et al. Utility of the Mallampati classification for predicting difficult intubation in pediatric patients. *Anesthesiology*. 1995;3(3):91–116.

99. Jacobs Ian N, Gray Robert F, Wendell Todd N. Upper airway obstruction in children with Down syndrome. *Archives of Otolaryngology–Head & Neck Surgery*. 1996;122(9):945–950.

100. Shott Sally R. Down syndrome: analysis of airway size and a guide for appropriate intubation. *The Laryngoscope*. 2000;110(4):585–592.

101. Hartman RA, Castro Jr T, Matson M, Fox DJ. Rapid orotracheal intubation in the clenched-jaw patients: A modification of the lightwand technique. *Journal of Clinical Anesthesia*. 1992;4(3):245–246.

102. Barkett PA. Obstructed airway with wired jaws. *Nursing*. 1991;21(12):33.

103. Wald Ellen R, Guerra Nancy, Byers Carol. Upper respiratory tract infections in young children: duration of and frequency of complications. *Pediatrics*. 1991;87(2):129–133.

104. Metzner J, Domino KB. Risks of anesthesia or sedation outside the operating room: the role of the anesthesia care provider. *Curr Opin Anaesthesiol*. 2010;23(4):523–531.

105. Langhan ML, Mallory M, Hertzog J, et al. Pediatric Sedation Research Consortium. Physiologic monitoring practices during pediatric procedural sedation: a report from the Pediatric Sedation Research Consortium. *Arch Pediatr Adolesc Med*. 2012;166(11):990–998.

106. Bell C, Kain Zeev N, eds. Equipment and monitoring. In: *The Pediatric Anesthesia Handbook*. 2nd ed. St. Louis: Mosby; 1997:35–69.

107. Prielipp Richard C, Kelly Jeffrey S, Roy Raymond C. Use of esophageal or precordial stethoscopes by anesthesia providers: are we listening to our patients. *Journal of Clinical Anesthesia*. 1995;7(5):367–372.

108. Grunwell Jocelyn R, McCracken Courtney, Fortenberry James, et al. Risk factors leading to failed procedural sedation in children outside the operating room. *Pediatric Emergency Care*. 2014;30(6):381–387.

109. Tobias JD, Cravero JP. *Procedural Sedation for Infants, Children, and Adolescents*. Elk Grove Village, IL: American Academy of Pediatrics; 2015; 234.

110. Sammartino M, Volpe B, Sbaraglia F, Garra R, D'Addessi A. Capnography and the bispectral index-their role in pediatric sedation: a brief review. International journal of pediatrics 2010;828347.

111. Yarchi D, Cohen A, Umansky T, et al. Assessment of end-tidal carbon dioxide during pediatric and adult sedation for endoscopic procedures. *Gastrointest Endosc*. 2009;69(4):877–882.

112. Lightdale JR, Goldmann DA, Feldman HA, et al. Microstream capnography improves patient monitoring during moderate sedation: a randomized, controlled trial. *Pediatrics*. 2006;117(6):e1170–e1178.

113. Yldzdaş D, Yapcoglu H, Ylmaz HL. The value of capnography during sedation or sedation/analgesia in pediatric minor procedures. *Pediatr Emerg Care*. 2004;20(3):162–165.

114. Slovis TL. Sedation and anesthesia issues in pediatric imaging. *Pediatr Radiol*. 2011;41(Suppl 2):514–516.

115. Emrath ET, Stockwell JA, McCracken CE, et al. Provision of deep procedural sedation by a pediatric sedation team at a freestanding imaging center. *Pediatr Radiol*. 2014;44(8):1020–1025.

116. Franck Linda Sturla, Greenberg Cindy Smith, Stevens Bonnie. Pain assessment in infants and children. *Pediatric Clinics*. 2000;47(3):487–512.

117. Committee on Psychosocial Aspects of Child and Family Health. Task Force on Pain in Infants, Children, and Adolescents. The assessment and management of acute pain in infants, children, and adolescents. *Pediatrics*. 2001;108(3):793–797.

118. Merkel Sandra, Voepel-Lewis Terri, Malviya Shobha. Pain assessment in infants and young children: The FLACC scale: A behavioral tool to measure pain in young children. *AJN The American Journal of Nursing*. 2002;102(10):55–58.

119. Meredith JR, O'Keefe KP, Galwankar S. Pediatric procedural sedation and analgesia. *J Emerg Trauma Shock*. 2008;1(2):88–96.

120. Dial S, Silver P, Bock K, Sagy M. Pediatric sedation for procedures titrated to a desired degree of immobility results in unpredictable depth of sedation. *Pediatr Emerg Care*. 2001;17(6):414–420.

CHAPTER 11: REVIEW QUESTIONS

1. Which of the following is not a goal of pediatric procedural sedation?
   A. Analgesia
   B. Amnesia
   C. Behavior modification
   D. Inability to maintain patient safety at all times

2. Adverse pediatric procedural sedation events that occur in the _____ setting are more likely to be fatal.
   A. Hospital
   B. Outpatient clinic attached to a hospital
   C. Physician's or dentist's office
   D. Intensive care unit

3. The term *neonate* is defined as which of the following?
   A. An infant 30 days old or younger
   B. An infant 1 to 12 months old
   C. An infant younger than 12 months
   D. Exclusively, an infant 1 day old or younger

4. Infants born with hydrocephalus can have _____ due to _____.
   A. Difficult airways; large occiputs
   B. Small occiputs; increased cerebral pressure
   C. Difficult airways; small occiputs
   D. Small occiputs; difficult airways

5. _____ is the primary cause of brady-cardia in infants.
   A. Hypoglycemia
   B. Hypovolemia
   C. Hypoxia
   D. Hyponatremia

6. Hard plastic oral airways are most appropriate _____.
   A. In mildly sedated toddlers
   B. In deeply sedated children with upper airway obstruction
   C. In wide awake infants
   D. In cooperative adolescents

7. The infant breathing pattern of pauses longer than 15 to 20 seconds associated with bradycardia, cyanosis, and pallor is termed _____.
   A. Central apnea of infancy
   B. Sleep apnea of childhood
   C. Irregular apnea
   D. Infantile obstructive sleep apnea

8. The underdeveloped premature and newborn kidney loses which electrolyte via the urine?
   A. Glucose
   B. Sodium
   C. Magnesium
   D. Dextrose

9. The ASA generally recommends pediatric procedural sedation only be performed by nonanesthesiologists in which of the following patient populations?
   A. ASA III and IV patients only
   B. Any ASA status
   C. ASA I and II only
   D. None of the above

10. Trisomy 21 (Down syndrome) patients have the following characteristics:
    A. Large tongues
    B. Short mandibles
    C. Small oral and nasal passages
    D. All of the above

11. Children have on average _____ colds or upper respiratory infections (URI) a year.
    A. One or two
    B. Two to four
    C. 10–12
    D. Three to eight

12. The pediatric environment, as defined by the American Academy of Pediatrics, includes _____.
    A. Pediatric-appropriate equipment
    B. Pediatric-appropriate drugs
    C. Personnel comfortable with and knowledgeable about children
    D. All of the above

Answers can be found in Appendix A.

Postsedation Patient Care

LEARNING OUTCOMES

At the completion of this chapter, the learner shall:
- Identify characteristics associated with phase I and phase II perianesthesia nursing practice.
- Describe the recommended patient care equipment that should be maintained in a postsedation patient care area.
- Differentiate the components of a postsedation patient care report.
- Demonstrate the mechanism to assign a postsedation Aldrete score based on ten objective scoring criteria.
- Delineate the objective scoring subset parameters that comprise the postsedation Aldrete scoring mechanism.
- Analyze appropriate discharge scoring criteria for the inpatient and outpatient patient populations.

COMPETENCY STATEMENT

The moderate sedation health care practitioner will provide direct supervision of the patient's postsedation care and will not discharge patients until specific discharge readiness criteria are met.

When does the postsedation period start?

The postsedation phase of care begins as soon as the procedure is completed and ends when the patient is returned to her or his presedation physiologic state.

Are there any parameters associated with the administration of moderate procedural sedation and analgesia that affect the level of required postsedation care?

The length of postsedation recovery and patient monitoring after a sedation procedure is dependent on the following considerations:
- Diagnostic, therapeutic, or surgical procedure performed
- Length of procedure
- Presedation patient's physiologic condition
- Presence of procedural complications
- Sedative, hypnotic, and analgesic medications administered
- Quantity of medication administered
- Pharmacologic reversal agents being administered

What is the purpose of postsedation monitoring?

The purpose of postsedation is to ensure the return of physiologic function prior to discharge or return to the inpatient setting. Patient monitoring and care should continue until the patient achieves the presedation level of consciousness and normalization of respiration. Additional goals include an opportunity for the health care practitioner to increase patient satisfaction, optimize quality patient care, educate patients, and manage patient complications proficiently. The postsedation period provides time to assess, diagnose, and treat complications associated with the administration of sedation and analgesia. Postsedation monitoring and discharge policies are required by accrediting bodies and recommended by professional practice organizations.[1-3] Ultimately, the postsedation period provides a time period for the patient to meet institutionally approved discharge criteria.

What is meant by the phases of postsedation patient care?

The success of any sedation program depends on providing quality presedation and procedural patient care. However, it must also embrace adequate postsedation monitoring and proper discharge planning. To avoid allegations of premature patient discharge or abandonment, mechanisms must be in place to assess home readiness or ability to return to the inpatient setting. Nurses engaged in the postsedation management of patients receiving moderate procedural sedation and analgesia participate in phases I and II aspects of postsedation care. The distinct phases of postsedation care are rooted in the characteristics or phases defined by the American Society of Perianesthesia Care Nurses. These include the following.

Phase I. During phase I postsedation care, the patient is closely monitored and continuously assessed on return to presedation physiologic status. Phase I postsedation patients should never be left unattended. Nursing care remains focused on ensuring that the patient maintains a patent airway, demonstrates hemodynamic stability, recovers with manageable pain levels, and successfully returns to a presedation cognitive level.

Phase II. Phase II postsedation care focuses on preparing the patient for additional inpatient care, discharge to self-care, or care to be provided by another caregiver.

What equipment should be available in the postsedation setting?

Postsedation monitoring may be provided in a variety of settings. Patients may remain monitored in the treatment area or can be transferred to a designated postsedation recovery area. The recovery area should be physically conducive to meeting the needs of the patient and caregiver. Postsedation recovery areas must be well lighted and located in a central area, with appropriate monitoring and emergency resuscitative equipment available.

Who should transport the patient to the postsedation setting?

Facility policies and procedures should clearly outline requirements for transfer to and from the postsedation area. If the health care provider who administered moderate procedural sedation and analgesia does not monitor the patient after the procedure, the patient must be safely transported to a postsedation recovery area. It is important to ensure that the patient has a patent and stable airway prior to transport. Oxygen should be available for transport to the postsedation area. The health care provider who administered sedation to the patient should accompany the patient to the postsedation care area. On arrival to the postsedation unit, the accompanying health care provider should immediately reevaluate the patient's status and provide a handoff report only when the postsedation provider is prepared to assume responsibility for the patient.

Why are accurate handoff reports so critical in health care?

The act of transferring information from one provider to another is termed *handoff* or *sign out*. Inadequate handoff communication is a contributing factor to adverse events, including many types of sentinel events.[4] A study by the Risk Management Foundation of Harvard Medical Institution estimated that communication failures in US hospitals and medical practices were responsible for at least 30% of all malpractice claims, which resulted in 1744 deaths and 1.7 billion dollars in malpractice costs over a 5-year period.[5] Handoff communication that is incomplete, not timely, misinterpreted, or inaccurate can directly lead to patient harm.

What contributing factors lead to inaccurate handoffs?

A number of factors contribute to ineffective or inadequate handoff processes, including the following:
- Insufficient information between sender and receiver
- Poor handoff timing
- Unit and workload production pressure
- Lack of standardized institutional handoff policy
- Inadequate staffing patterns
- Distractions during handoff process
- Increased frequency of handoff process
- Lack of formality or professional presentation of handoff process

Which patient care components should be incorporated for an effective handoff process to occur?

The critical components that must occur between the sender and receiver during the handoff process include the following:
- Sender contact information
- Illness assessment
  - Including severity
- Patient summary
  - Events leading up to illness or admission
  - Hospital course—ongoing assessment
  - Plan of care
- To do (action) list
- Contingency plans
  - Allergy list
  - Code status
  - Medication list
  - Dated laboratory tests
  - Dated vital signs

Are there any tools available that provide a formal structure to guide the handoff process?

Improved handoffs incorporating a variety of evidence-based mnemonics, tools, forms, and checklists are available for incorporation into the moderate procedural sedation setting.[6-12] I PASS (THE) BATON, featured in Table 12.1, was

TABLE 12.1   I PASS (THE) BATON Mnemonic for Effective Patient Handoff

Letter	Stands for:	Components
I	Introduction	Introduce yourself and your role or job (include patient)
P	Patient	Give name, identifiers, age, gender, and location
A	Assessment	Present chief complaint, vital signs, symptoms, and diagnosis
S	Situation	Current status or circumstances, including code status, level of (un)certainty, recent changes, and response to treatment
S	Safety concerns	Critical laboratory values or reports, socioeconomic factors, allergies, and alerts (e.g., falls, isolation)
THE		
B	Background	Comorbidities, previous episodes, current medications, and family history
A	Actions	What actions were taken or are required? Provide a brief rationale
T	Timing	Level of urgency and explicit timing and prioritization of actions
O	Ownership	Who is responsible (person or team), including patient or family?
N	Next	What will happen next? Are there anticipated changes? What is the plan? Are there contingency plans?

Modified from Agency for Healthcare Research and Quality. TeamSTEPPS: national implementation. https://www.ahrq.gov/teamstepps/index.html.

developed by the Agency for Healthcare Research and Quality and the US Department of Defense as part of its TeamSTEPPS program. TeamSTEPPS (Team **S**trategies and **T**ools to **E**nhance **P**erformance and **P**atient **S**afety) is an evidence-based framework to optimize team performance across the health care delivery system.[13,14] The core of the TeamSTEPPS framework is comprised of five key skills:

- Team structure
- Communication
- Leadership
- Situation monitoring
- Mutual support

In 2015, Moon et al.[15] introduced the I PUT PATIENTS FIRST mnemonic (Box 12.1) to serve as a guideline to

---

BOX 12.1 Mnemonic: I PUT PATIENTS FIRST

I
- Identify yourself and role
  - Obtain nurse's name

P
- Patient's past medical history
  - Surgical and social factors

U
- Underlying diagnosis and procedure

T
- Technique of anesthesia or sedation

P
- Peripheral IVs, arterial lines, central lines, drains

A
- Allergies

T
- Therapeutic interventions
  - Pain
  - Medications
  - Antibiotics

I
- Intubation
  - Very difficult
  - Moderately difficult
  - Easy

E
- Extubation likelihood
  - Already extubated
  - Very likely
  - Unlikely
  - Definitely no extubation planned

N
- Need for drips
  - Epinephrine
  - Vasopressin
  - Norepinephrine
  - Insulin
  - Propofol

T
- Treatment plan for postoperative care
  - Blood pressure goals
  - Ventilator settings

Continued

BOX 12.1 Mnemonic: I PUT PATIENTS FIRST—cont'd

S
- Signs
  - Vital signs (during case, most recent)

F
- Fluids
  - Ins
  - Outs
  - Blood products

I
- Intraoperative events

R
- Recent laboratory tests

S
- Suggestions for immediate postoperative care
  - Special positioning
  - Pain control
  - Need for pumps

T
- Timing
  - Expected time for arrival in admitting unit

C
- Concluding remarks

---

improve the effectiveness of the handover process from the operating room to the intensive care unit. I PUT PATIENTS FIRST standardizes the handoff process while serving as an educational tool for all health care providers.

As an ensign in the US Navy on a nuclear submarine, Bonacum had to brief the captain of the ship following his nighttime shift, reporting about potentially dangerous situations that might emerge. In his report, he described the "situation, background, assessment, and recommendation." The implementation of the SBAR communication (Box 12.2) temporarily flattened the hierarchy between the ensign and the ship's captain.[16-18] Bonacum further developed SBAR strategies to facilitate effective communication between obstetricians and nurses while serving at Kaiser Permanente Health.[19]

What specific information should be incorporated into a handoff mnemonic specific to moderate procedural sedation and analgesia practice?

Components of the handoff or sign out process that are specific to the sedation setting are included in Box 12.3.

Our facility currently does not use, and our nurse manager recently reiterated, that our moderate procedural sedation unit has no plans in the near future to implement such strategies. Are strategies for handoff communication tools mandatory?

The Joint Commission requires a standardized approach to patient handoffs; it is one of the National Patient Safety Goals (2006 National Patient Safety Goal 2E). In 2010, the requirement became a Provision of Care standard (PC.02.02.01), element of performance (EP) 2. The element of performance

BOX 12.2 SBAR: A Standard Mnemonic to Improve Clinical Communication

S: Situation
- What is happening at the present time
- Identifies why the notification is taking place and allows statement of the problem

B: Background
- What circumstances led up to the situation
- Summarizes information relevant to the current problem or concern, including medications, laboratory results, diagnostic tests or diagnostic or therapeutic procedure

A: Assessment
- Identifies the problem or situation of concern
- Summarizes relevant information gathered, what has changed, provider's interpretation of the situation
- Describes what was found on examination of the patient, including an ABC assessment or early warning score

R: Recommendation
- Allows the provider placing the inquiry to ask for what he or she would like to happen without hinting or hoping for the right action; determines time for mutual agreement on a clearly defined action plan

BOX 12.3 Components of Postsedation Report

- Patient's name
- Age
- Diagnostic, therapeutic, or surgical procedure
- Past medical history
- Prescribed, over-the-counter medications, and herbal and homeopathic preparations
- Allergies
- Presedation and procedural vital signs
- Level of consciousness
- Airway status
- Sedative, analgesic, hypnotic medications administered
  - Total dose and frequency of administration
  - Antagonist administered (time)
- Response and reaction to medications
- Adverse response and reaction
  - ECG, blood pressure, Sao_2, respirations
  - Complications
  - Treatment
- Fluid balance
  - Site and size of IV catheters
  - IV solution infused and amount
  - Blood loss
- Postsedation concerns or considerations
  - Review of medical orders
- Location of responsible physician

requires that the organization's process for handoff communication provides for the opportunity for discussion between the giver and receiver of patient information.[1]

Once these requirements have been understood by the nurse manager, establishing a multidisciplinary team to

review mnemonics that would be effective for implementation in your sedation unit is advisable. The Joint Commission's "8 Tips for High Quality Hand-Offs," identified in Fig. 12.1, can provide any multidisciplinary sedation team with the structure to create an effective handoff protocol for your unit.[20]

What is the best practice for rolling out a newly adopted postsedation handoff process?

Once the evidence-based postsedation process has been properly created and supported by the multidisciplinary team and hospital administration, assigning sedation team members (or "champions") to support its implementation is essential. To avoid some of the more common mistakes when adopting a newly created initiative, practitioners should do the following[21]:

- Communication steps of the mnemonic should not be removed arbitrarily to fit their practice.
- The mnemonic should not be a catch-all tool that is beyond the scope of the original work of the multidisciplinary team that created the tool.
- The practitioner should not wait to engage physicians.
- The weight of one-on-one conversations should not be underestimated.
- Allow for time to provide robust mnemonic education delineating the importance of an accurate handoff process.
- Beta-test the newly created handoff process prior to initiating full unit implementation.
- Continue to coach teams on enhancing the handoff process while consistently investigating methods to improve the process.
- Do not focus on those who argue against a formalized handoff process.

We are in the process of successfully implementing a formalized handoff process, but one barrier to effective implementation continues to be constant interruptions by other health care providers during the sign out process. What strategies are available to discourage these interruptions during the sign out process?

Distractions, including irrelevant case communication, continue to correlate negatively with patient safety initiatives, including the completion of simple checklists.[22] Distractions and interruptions during the handoff process need to be limited to ensure that accurate information is conveyed to the provider responsible for accepting responsibility for the patient. Comparisons have often been made between safety management in aviation and health care.[23,24] In 1981, a federal aviation regulation, "The Sterile Cockpit Rule," was implemented after a series of accidents that occurred when pilots became distracted during critical phases of their flight.[25] Since this ruling was implemented, all nonessential conversation is prohibited during critical phases of a flight. Applying this airline industry analogy to the health care setting, creating what is called a *no-interruption zone* during critical phases of a procedure includes the following:

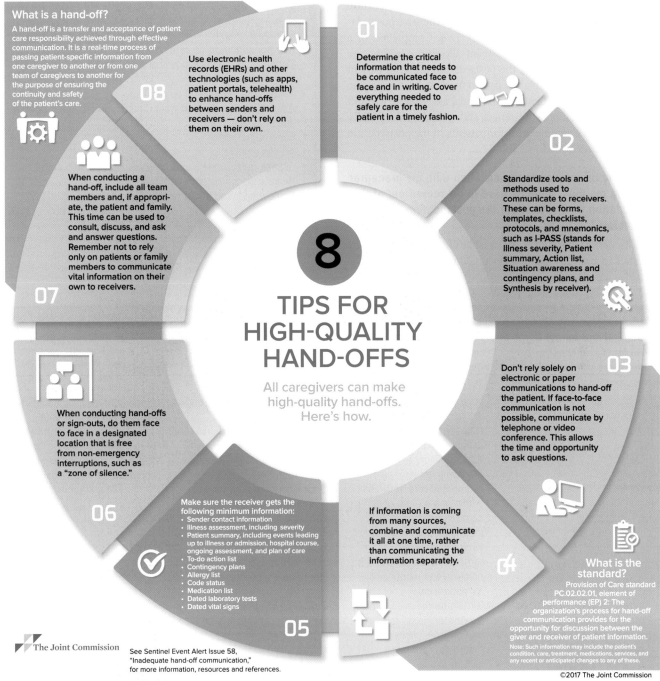

Fig. 12.1 Eight tips for high-quality handoffs. (From https://www.jointcommission.org/sentinel_event_alert_58_inadequate_handoff_communications.)

- Flight takeoff
  - Induction of anesthesia
  - Establishing patient's airway
  - Establishing initial sedation levels for all patients
- Landing
  - Completion of the procedure
  - Initial phases of postsedation recovery
  - Handoff communication process

Individuals who fail to adhere to this sterile cockpit rule need to be reminded that preparations for the next patient, the difficulty of the daily schedule, or discussing favorite sports teams comprises essential communication. Staff must be instructed to stop their discussion immediately until all handoff and sign out activities are completed, and the individual health care provider accepting responsibility for the patient has had all questions answered satisfactorily.

What components are included in a comprehensive postsedation patient assessment once the handoff process is completed?

The health care provider assuming responsibility after the handoff process is completed must perform a complete systems assessment during the first few minutes of the postsedation admission process. Components of a comprehensive postsedation assessment are identified in Box 12.4. Completion of a comprehensive admission assessment allows the health care provider the ability to plan the postsedation phase of patient care appropriately. The plan of care in the postsedation setting is derived from the patient history, initial assessment, handoff report, use of situational awareness, and critical thinking skills. Sample patient outcome grids for patients in the postsedation care area are identified in Table 12.2.

During my orientation to the sedation unit, my preceptor informed me that "patients have to be scored out of the postsedation unit." What are the postsedation scoring parameters?

A postsedation scoring system must be clearly understood by the staff to provide accurate documentation and ensure the

---

BOX 12.4   Components of Postsedation Patient Assessment

- Monitor and improve cardiorespiratory function
- Continue to maintain physical and emotional comfort and provide privacy
- Assess procedural and surgical site
- Assess, document, and treat data observed during postsedation assessment
- Encourage fluids
- Advise ambulation as tolerated
- Assess genitourinary status and patient voiding status
- Review discharge plan with family or responsible adult
- Review sedation and procedural discharge instructions
- Provide follow-up as outlined by hospital policy and procedure

---

TABLE 12.2   Postsedation Patient Outcome Grids: Phase II

Potential and Actual Problems and Nursing Diagnoses	Outcome Goals: Patient Will Be Able To:	Nursing Interventions	Resources
Altered thought processes and/or memory loss R/T sedation/anesthesia	Display, verbalize appropriate orientation to surroundings and situations Respond lucidly to questions Avoid self-injury R/T altered thought patterns Assume self-care activities within parameters of surgical restrictions Rely on RA who understands nature of patient's temporarily altered thought patterns and responsibility for patient care	Provide frequent affirmations of orientation to time, place, and events Assess patient's orientation Monitor and oversee patient care while patient is vulnerable to environment Provide adequate time for drug clearance before patient discharge Administer medications with caution to avoid further sedation that would greatly alter patient's mental status	Comprehensive report from prior caregivers regarding sedative medications, prior mental status Predetermined discharge criteria that include assessment of mental status and availability of RA to drive and provide home support ASPAN Standards of Perianesthesia Nursing Practice
Ineffective airway clearance Potential for aspiration Ineffective breathing patterns, respiratory depression R/T sedation, anesthesia, positioning, pain, increased respiratory secretions, vomiting, or untoward reactions to medications or local anesthetics	Maintain normal respiratory parameters (e.g., rate, depth, ease, clarity of breath sounds) Maintain a clear airway Avoid aspiration Maintain adequate oxygenation of tissues Avoid symptoms of hypoxia Perform effective cough and deep breathing exercises	Know about of effects of anesthetics, analgesics, sedatives, and muscle relaxants and associated drug interactions Use airway maintenance techniques, including suctioning and bag-valve-mask resuscitative techniques as needed Apply stir-up regimen Administer oxygen per protocols Continuous assessment of respiratory status Give timely report of untoward symptoms to anesthesiologist and surgeon Provide adequate hydration and safe positioning Identify preexisting respiratory	Physiologic monitoring equipment, oxygen, suction and emergency equipment available in unit Crash cart, resuscitator bag, ventilator, airway maintenance supplies, drugs Adequate staffing patterns to ensure proper nurse-to-patient ratio Immediate access to anesthesia provider Comprehensive anesthesia and/ or nursing report before transfer of patient care ASPAN Standards of Perianesthesia Nursing Practice Facility policies regarding interventions for cardiovascular and respiratory problems

TABLE 12.2 Postsedation Patient Outcome Grids: Phase II—cont'd

Potential and Actual Problems and Nursing Diagnoses	Outcome Goals: Patient Will Be Able To:	Nursing Interventions	Resources
		disease and individualize care appropriately	IV fluids and venipuncture supplies Spirits of ammonia available, especially in bathrooms Emergency call bell system functional
Potential alteration in tissue perfusion Cardiovascular instability	Maintain normal cardiovascular parameters, avoiding hypertension and hypotension Demonstrate expected postoperative arousal and mental status Demonstrate normal parameters of peripheral circulation Ambulate without faintness or hypotension	Assess all parameters of vital signs in ongoing fashion, including heart rate and rhythm and blood pressure Assess mental status and progression Assist patient in progressive ambulation within individual patient's abilities Check peripheral pulses, color, and sensory adequacy in ongoing fashion Give timely report of untoward symptoms to anesthesiologist and surgeon Maintain adequate fluid balance and hydration	
Altered skin integrity R/T surgical wound Potential for infection at surgical site	Experience appropriate and uncomplicated wound healing Avoid fever	Use aseptic technique and teach to family and patient Enhance circulation of surgical wound site Avoid constricting bandages at surgical site Assess surgical site throughout phase II stay	Universal precautions PPE and sterile dressing supplies IV fluids Antibiotics, if ordered
Alterations in comfort—pain	Express acceptable comfort level Maintain normal cardiovascular, respiratory parameters	Administer appropriate analgesics and cold therapy Position patient for comfort Provide positive reinforcements and encourage philosophy of wellness throughout process Encourage appropriate pace for increased activities	Physician's orders for analgesics Analgesic medications Knowledge of nursing interventions, for comfort—positioning and support of body areas, breathing exercises, positive reinforcement of comfort
Alterations in comfort—nausea and vomiting	Express acceptable comfort level Avoid vomiting and retching	Encourage appropriate pace for oral intake of fluids Administer antiemetics as needed Administer IV solutions for hydration as ordered Provide positive reinforcements and encourage philosophy of wellness throughout process	Physician's orders, prescriptions for antiemetics IV fluids Literature R/T reducing gastrointestinal symptoms Appropriate food and beverages—avoidance of acid-producing juices, spicy or difficult to digest foods
Self-care deficit	Display sufficient level of alertness and self-care for safe discharge to home with RA	Provide comprehensive nursing care modified to patient's abilities Assess patient for ability to ambulate and call for assistance before discharge Ensure availability of RA before discharge	Discharge criteria

Continued

TABLE 12.2   Postsedation Patient Outcome Grids: Phase II—cont'd

Potential and Actual Problems and Nursing Diagnoses	Outcome Goals: Patient Will Be Able To:	Nursing Interventions	Resources
Actual or perceived loss of privacy or dignity	Express content at level of privacy provided Maintain dignity and sense of self-esteem	Support patient's right to privacy and dignity Promote unit philosophy that demands support of patient's right to privacy Explain and demonstrate to patient before surgery that privacy and dignity will not be invaded while patient is asleep or sedated Provide privacy—curtains, blankets, clothing that covers patient Allow patient as much decision making as is possible, and encourage RA to do same	Surroundings that are friendly, family-focused, private, and apart from view of other patients or staff Patient Bill of Rights Patient linens that provide adequate cover Cubicle curtains
Risk of hemorrhage	Maintain blood volume at normal level Maintain blood pressure at normal levels—avoid hypertension	Ensure availability of IV solutions Observe surgical site for signs of bleeding, and report to physician Administer anxiolytic and/or antihypertensive medications as ordered Instruct patient on appropriate support of surgical site	Blood bank contract and policies for rapid availability of blood products Antihypertensives Anxiolytic medications IV fluids and supplies
Anxiety R/T fear of home care without nursing support, separation from family, potential diagnosis, other issues	Express lingering fears and questions about home care or other topics Display calm demeanor Verbalize reduced anxiety Rely on RA for support in the home setting	Provide written and verbal information and ongoing explanations regarding care issues within limits of nursing Ensure home support before discharge Encourage questions from patient and RA	Verbal and written discharge instructions that include emergency contact information RA willing and able to provide home support
Potential for injury R/T faintness, weakness, fatigue, prolonged regional block, altered sensory perception	Remains free from injury Ambulates without faintness or injury	Encourage appropriate pace for progression of ambulation Monitor vital signs in relationship to ambulation Reduce obstacles to safe ambulation, such as wet floors, slippery shoes, improper fit of slings, braces, surgical shoes, and crutches Provide ongoing assessments for potential complications R/T ambulation	Safe environment Nursing attendance during ambulation attempts and while patient is in bathroom Evaluation of patient's home setting during preadmission assessment RA in home setting

ASPAN, American Society of PeriAnesthesia Nurses; *PACU,* postanesthesia care unit; *PPE,* personal protective equipment; *RA,* responsible adult; *R/T,* related to.
Adapted from Burden N. *Ambulatory Surgical Nursing.* 2nd ed. Philadelphia: WB Saunders; 2000:483–485.

safe discharge of the patient when all institutionally approved discharge criteria have been met. Use of a scoring system provides objective parameters related to the patient's postsedation recovery and readiness for discharge. Criteria-based recovery parameters provide a mechanism to assess the needs of the patient objectively. A postsedation recovery scoring mechanism was introduced into clinical practice in 1970 by Aldrete and Kroulik.[26] Through the evolution of anesthesia and surgery, variations of the Aldrete scoring system have evolved.[27,28] The original Aldrete scoring system was intended for phase I postanesthesia care use. Modifications of the Aldrete scoring system, which are more applicable for phase II patient care, are identified in Table 12.3. The modified Aldrete scoring tool assigns a predetermined

TABLE 12.3 Modified Aldrete Recovery Scoring System

Aldrete Postanesthesia Recovery Scoring System	Score
Activity	
Able to move four extremities voluntarily on command	2
Able to move two extremities voluntarily on command	1
Able to move no extremities voluntarily on command	0
Respiration	
Able to breathe deeply and cough freely	2
Dyspneic, shallow, or limited breathing	1
Apneic	0
Circulation	
Blood pressure ± 20 mm Hg of normal	2
Blood pressure ± 20–50 mm Hg of normal	1
Blood pressure ≥ 50 mm Hg of normal	0
Consciousness	
Fully awake	2
Arousable on calling	1
Not responsive	0
O_2 saturation (color)	
Able to maintain O_2 saturation > 92% on room air	2
Needs O_2 inhalation to maintain O_2 saturation > 90%	1
O_2 saturation < 90%, even with O_2 supplement	0
Dressing	
Dry	2
Wet but stationary	1
Wet but growing	0
Pain	
Pain-free	2
Mild pain handled by oral medications	1
Pain requiring parenteral medications	0
Ambulation	
Able to stand up and walk straight[a]	2
Vertigo when erect	1
Dizziness when supine	0
Fasting or Feeding	
Able to drink fluids	2
Nauseated	1
Nausea and vomiting	0
Urine Output	
Has voided	2
Unable to void but comfortable	1
Unable to void and uncomfortable	0

[a]May be substituted by Romberg's test or by picking up 12 clips in one hand.

From Aldrete JA, Kroulik D. A post anesthetic recovery score. Anesth Analg. 1970;49:924–928; data from Aldrete J, Wright A. Anesthesia News. 1992:(November): 16–17.

score to objective clinical discharge criteria that may be implemented in the postsedation setting, including the following parameters:

- Activity
- Respiration
- Circulation
- Consciousness
- Oxygen saturation
- Dressing
- Pain
- Ambulation
- Fasting and feeding
- Urine output

Application of discharge criteria includes assessment of activity level. Appropriate discharge scoring requires the patient to demonstrate controlled, coordinated movements while performing age-appropriate ambulation. Adequate discharge scoring for respiratory criteria requires the patient to retain the ability to maintain and protect his or her airway. The patient cannot display any signs of respiratory distress, including snoring, stridor, muscle retraction, decreased oxygen saturation, or elevated carbon dioxide levels. Stable vital signs for a minimum of 30 to 60 minutes generally satisfies criteria for circulatory criteria. Consciousness scoring requires the patient to be fully oriented to time, person, and place or return to baseline mentation. If dizziness is present, it cannot interfere with mobility. Oxygen saturation and color requires patients to maintain oxygen saturation of more than 95% on room air or attain preprocedure oxygen saturation values. If a therapeutic or diagnostic procedure has been performed, an evaluation of the dressing site should demonstrate that there is no bleeding and that the dressing is dry and intact. A variety of pain assessment tools may be used by the postsedation clinician. The numeric rating scale (NRS), visual analogue scale (VAS), and adjective rating scale (ARS) used to assess pain in the postsedation setting are identified in Fig. 12.2.

Patients who will be discharged to home after the procedure may generally prepare to ambulate once a postsedation score of 8 or more has been achieved (or achieve their presedation Aldrete score). Patients recovered on a gurney or recliner should be placed in a 30- to 40-degree head-up position. Dizziness or light-headedness is assessed, and the patient's activity level is advanced accordingly. If the patient tolerates the head-up position, sitting or dangling the legs for 5-minute increments precedes sitting in a chair and ambulation. The absence of diaphoresis, bradycardia, hypotension, nausea, and/or vomiting is required prior to ambulation of the patient. Assisted ambulation is recommended to assess steadiness of gait. Patients may appear alert and prepared to ambulate only to discover that they are not quite stable enough to enter the bathroom or dressing area. An assisted ambulation method may prevent

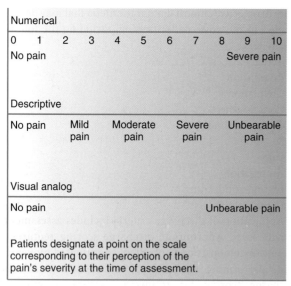

Numerical										
0	1	2	3	4	5	6	7	8	9	10
No pain										Severe pain

Descriptive				
No pain	Mild pain	Moderate pain	Severe pain	Unbearable pain

Visual analog	
No pain	Unbearable pain

Patients designate a point on the scale corresponding to their perception of the pain's severity at the time of assessment.

Fig. 12.2 Pain assessment tools. (From Potter PA, Perry AG, Stockert P, Hall A. *Essentials for Nursing Practice*. 9th ed. St. Louis: Elsevier; 2019.)

unexpected falls by patients who overextend their capabilities at any given time.

Patients who have received sedation or analgesia generally retain the ability to tolerate feedings (oral fluids) without incident. The encouragement of oral fluids is contraindicated in patients who have received oropharyngeal topical anesthetics. Prior to oral fluid intake, the presence of a gag reflex and the ability to cough must be documented. Small amounts of oral fluid may then be encouraged prior to discharge or removal of the IV catheter. Oral fluids should not be forced in the presence of nausea and vomiting. Depending on the cause of the nausea and vomiting, patients may benefit from the administration of additional IV fluids, gastrokinetic agents, multimodal analgesia, and serotonin antagonists in anticipation of discharge. The algorithm for the management of nausea and vomiting is shown in Fig. 12.3.[29] Patients with severe protracted nausea and vomiting require additional observation and should not be discharged. Additional nursing interventions that may benefit the patient in this situation include the following:

- Provide positive reinforcement to decrease anxiety.
- Avoid signs, smell, and conversations that would provoke nausea and vomiting.
- Move or ambulate the patient very slowly.
- Allow the patient to recover slowly, without aggressive stimulation.
- Advance oral intake slowly while avoiding citrus juices and coffee.

Many healthcare facilities do not require the measurement of urine output postprocedure. Patients receiving sedation or analgesia may not have urinary retention commonly experienced by postoperative surgical patients, and voiding may not be a problem. However, when opioids are used, patients may experience some urinary retention and altered bladder tone.

Patients who have not voided prior to discharge must be instructed to notify or return to the treatment facility in the event of bladder distention or the prolonged inability to void.

Once discharge criteria are met, inpatients may be transferred to their respective unit; outpatients should be discharged only in the care of a responsible adult. The responsible adult must be capable of the following[30]:

- Assisting the patient
- Ensuring patient compliance with postprocedure instruction
- Monitoring the patient's progress toward recovery

How should postsedation discharge instruction be conducted for the patient who has received moderate procedural sedation and analgesia?

Postsedation teaching should be conducted in the presence of the responsible adult who will assume care of the patient on discharge from the facility or the health care provider who is accepting care of the inpatient immediately after the procedure. Written discharge instructions (Box 12.5) should address activity level, medications, diet, and procedure-specific information. These instructions must be reviewed with each patient and responsible adult.

Postsedation discharge teaching should take place in an unhurried atmosphere, much like the presedation patient assessment process. Effective communication between the provider and patient is critically important when providing postsedation instruction. Communicating postsedation instruction should be at the sixth-grade reading level or lower. Similarly, the quantity of information may also need to be limited. A focus on repetition and reinforcement should occur with both the patient and responsible adult accompanying the patient home. Additional key education points for discharge instructions are identified in Box 12.6.

What are some mechanisms for providing postsedation patient follow-up?

A mechanism to ascertain postsedation patient status postdischarge is a required component of any risk management or quality initiative. To ascertain the postprocedure status of a patient, inpatient information may be gathered by the attending physician or health care provider who is administered sedation. Outpatient follow-up gathering is always more challenging. Data collection methods for outpatients include:

- Patient questionnaire (online or US mail delivery)
- Telephone interview
- Satisfaction survey

The purpose of postsedation assessment is to evaluate the following:

- Incidence of complications related to the administration of procedural sedation
- Delayed recovery
- Procedural complication rate
- Return to function

⚡ PATIENT SAFETY SBAR FOCUS

Postsedation Patient Care and Ensuring Patient Safety

Situation

As we were preparing to discharge one of our moderate sedation patients, our postsedation staff responded to an emergent situation that occurred in our unit. When we returned to transport the patient we discovered that he had experienced an airway obstruction. The patient is now in a long-term care facility with a diagnosis of hypoxic encephalopathy.

Background

The critical issue on the day of the event was attributed to an exceptionally busy day. During the lunch hour several of the post-sedation nurses were off the floor. The supervisor of the unit came through and requested that we expedite the discharge process for patients over the next few hours secondary to the large volume of remaining scheduled cases for the day. A root cause analysis revealed that the patient was disconnected from all monitors with the intent of moving him to the postsedation phase II area of care. During the procedure the patient received 135 micrograms of sublimaze (fentanyl) and 2 milligrams of midazolam. As the discharge process was near completion, a patient in the next recovery bay coded. All available personnel responded to the emergency leaving the patient alone for approximately 15 minutes. Returning to the patient's bedside, staff noted that the patient was not breathing and a second 'code' was called to resuscitate the patient. Unfortunately, the patient experienced significant hypoxia leading to cerebral anoxia. Documentation of the patient's respiratory pattern immediately prior to discharge revealed a respiratory rate of 10 breaths per minute.

Assessment

The pressure to 'keep patients moving through the procedural platform' must always be judiciously balanced against the interest of patient safety. Adverse events that occur in healthcare generally are the result of a single error, which when significant enough can cause patient harm. However, generally a multitude of small errors occur that align precisely at the right time and result in patient harm. Hospitals put a variety of safety mechanisms in place to prevent such occurrences. These mechanisms include in-service educational programs, safety protocols, and implementing applicable policies and procedures. The following events occurred during this particular post-sedation patient situation:

- Patient monitoring was removed from patient.
- Patient was left unmonitored by unit personnel to respond to an emergency.
- The unit was short staffed when the incident occurred (lunch hour).
- Nursing supervisor applied production pressure to "expedite the discharge process."
- Patient received 135 µg of fentanyl and 2 milligrams of midazolam.
- Patient demonstrated altered respiratory pattern (bradypnea) prior to discharge from the unit.

As demonstrated in the 'Swiss Cheese Framework Model' identified below, if one of these errors gets past one defense, another layer of defense should prevent patient harm from occurring. Adverse events occur only when all the defenses around a particular patient's situation have been circumvented by many errors. James Reason has referred to this framework for understanding adverse events as the *"Swiss Cheese Model."**

Recommendations

This cerebral anoxic event was not the result of one single error. Rather, it was the culmination of a variety of errors that led to patient harm. A number of individuals made many errors. The institution at which this adverse event occurred should consider several remedial actions to strengthen its defenses against similar incidents in the future. Policies and procedures need to reiterate that patients are never to be left unattended once monitors are removed. Regardless of unit staffing, safe patient ratios must exist during days that are considered 'high volume' and during break and lunch periods. Patients must 'score out' of the postsedation phase of care using a prescribed scoring sheet (Aldrete Score). The patient also must not be considered for discharge until an Aldrete 'respiratory criteria' has been assigned a score of 2 (breathes deeply and coughs freely). Additional take home points for the risk management department include reviewing the inadequate defenses displayed in the post-sedation setting at this facility. A review must not only analyze which adverse events occurred but also focus on methods to improve defenses. Areas of improvement should be shared with staff with appropriate education implemented to minimize future adverse events.

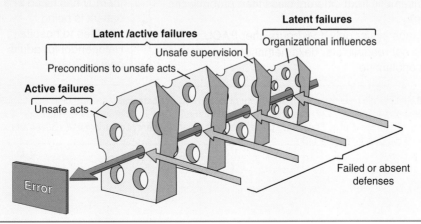

(Image from Reason J: A system approach to organizational error. *Ergonomics* 38:1708-1721, 2005.)

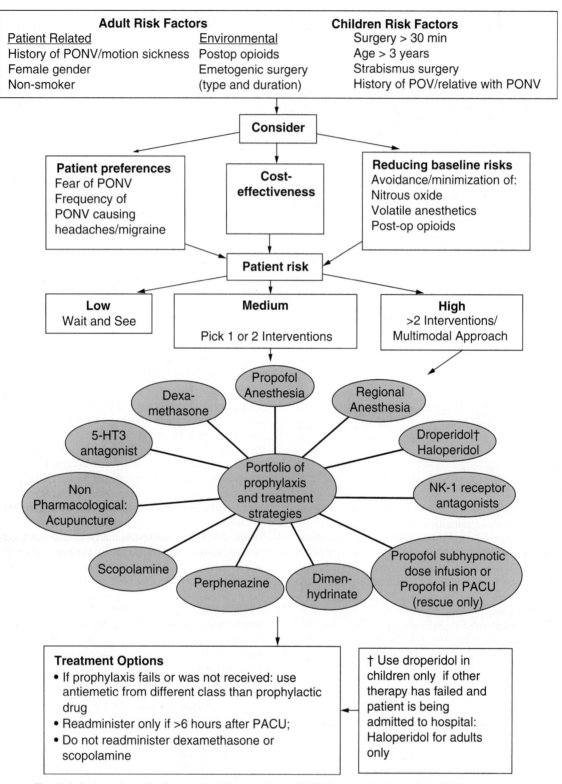

Fig. 12.3 Antiemetic medications and treatment protocol. *PACU*, Postanesthesia care unit; *PONV*, postoperative nausea and vomiting; *POV*, Postoperative vomiting. (From Gan TJ, Diemunsch P, Habib AS; Society for Ambulatory Anesthesia, et al. Consensus guidelines for the management of postoperative nausea and vomiting. Anesth Analg. 2014;118[1]:85–113.)

BOX 12.5   Postsedation Discharge Instructions

Physical Activity

- Rest today. You have received medication today that may cause drowsiness, poor balance, and instability. Do not participate in any activity that requires normal balance, strength, or coordination. If you participate in these activities, you may hurt yourself.
- Do not drive or operate machinery for 24 hours.
- Do not make important legal decisions for 24 hours.
- Avoid dangerous activities for 24 hours.
- You may (or may not) shower or bathe today. If bathing or showering is prohibited, you may shower or bathe _____ hours postprocedure.
- Notify your physician if you have not voided within 8 hours postprocedure.
- Advance your diet as tolerated.
  - You may temporarily feel nauseated or sick to your stomach, which is normal.
    - Do NOT eat too soon, because this may make you vomit—as soon as you feel like you can drink without vomiting, you should try water, juice, or low-fat soup.
    - You can progress to solid foods if the fluids do not cause nausea.
- You may return to work in _____ hours or days.

Postsedation Medications

- Unless otherwise directed by your physician, you may resume your regularly scheduled medications when you arrive home.
- Take prescribed pain medication only as directed.

Procedure Site

- There should be minimal if any blood at your procedure site.
  - If bleeding occurs, apply direct pressure to the procedure site and call your physician immediately. If you cannot reach your physician, have a responsible adult drive you to the nearest hospital emergency department.
  - There should be minimal discomfort at the procedure site. If you experience significant pain at the procedure site, contact your physician immediately.
- You may replace your dressing in ____ hours.
- Replace dressing as instructed.
- If any signs of redness, fever, exudate, swelling, or bleeding occur, contact your physician immediately.

Additional Considerations

- Contact your physician's office at (__) ____ - _____ for a follow-up appointment.
- If you are experiencing complications, contact your physician for additional directions.
  - If you are experiencing complications and cannot contact your physician, report to the nearest hospital emergency department.
  - If you report to the hospital emergency department, bring your discharge instructions with you.

BOX 12.6   Key Education Points for Discharge Instructions

Medications

- Note the name, purpose, and dosage schedule for each medication; emphasize the importance of following the directions on the label.
- The patient should resume medications taken before surgery per the physician's order.
- If pain medication is not prescribed, nonprescription, nonaspirin analgesics (e.g., acetaminophen, ibuprofen) may be effective for mild aches and pains.
- Additional pain medication may be ordered by the physician after surgery. The patient should take these medications as directed, preferably with food to prevent gastrointestinal upset.

Activity Restriction

- Advise the patient to take it easy for the remainder of the day after surgery. Dizziness or drowsiness is not unusual after surgery and anesthesia.
- For the next 24 hours, the patient should not do the following:
  - Drive a vehicle or operate machinery or power tools.
  - Consume alcohol, including beer.
  - Make important personal or business decisions or sign important documents.
- Activity level—in specific behavioral terms (e.g., do not lift objects heavier than 20 lb), describe any limitation of activities.

Diet

- Explain any dietary restrictions or instructions.
- If no dietary restriction exists, instruct the patient to progress as tolerated to a regular diet.

Surgical and Anesthesia Side Effects

- Anticipated sequelae of surgery (e.g., bleeding and pain) should be delineated.
- Common side effects associated with anesthesia include dizziness, drowsiness, myalgia, nausea and vomiting, and sore throat.

Possible Complications and Symptoms

- Instruct the patient and responsible adult about pertinent signs and symptoms that could be indicative of postoperative complications.

The patient should call the responsible physician if he or she develops the following:

- Fever > 38.3°C (101°F) orally
- Persistent, atypical pain
- Pain not relieved by medication
- Bleeding or unexpected drainage from the wound that does not stop
- Extreme redness or swelling around the incision site or drainage of pus
- Urinary retention
- Continual nausea or vomiting

Treatment and Tests

- Procedures that the patient or responsible adult is expected to perform (e.g., dressing changes, application of warm moist compresses) should be described in detail.
- A complete list of necessary supplies should be included.

Continued

BOX 12.6   Key Education Points for Discharge Instructions—cont'd

- If any postoperative tests are to be conducted, instructions as to the date, time, test location, and any previsit preparation should be listed.

Access to Postdischarge Care
- Note the telephone number of the responsible and available physician.
- Include the telephone number of the ambulatory center and hours of operation.

- Note also the name, address, and telephone number of the appropriate emergency care facility.

Follow-Up Care
- Identify the date, time, and location of the patient's scheduled return visit to the clinic or surgeon.

From Burden N. Ambulatory Surgical Nursing. 2nd ed. Philadelphia: WB Saunders; 2000:506; modified from Marley RA, Moline BM. Patient discharge from the ambulatory setting. J Post Anesth Nurs. 1996;11:39–49.

Follow-up telephone conversations provide the sedation health care provider with the ability to receive direct feedback from the patient. In addition, telephone follow-up enables the clinician to collect quality assurance outcome data.[31] Consistent postsedation assessment is an accurate method to identify complications and ensure the delivery of quality sedation services.

SUMMARY

Use of specific discharge criteria in the postsedation phase of patient care provides the health care provider with the ability to assess, diagnose, and treat complications associated with the administration of procedural sedation. They also provide the clinician with the ability to verify the patient's return to presedation physiologic status. Postsedation teaching and providing discharge instructions properly prepare the patient for return to the inpatient setting or home.

REFERENCES

1. The Joint Commission. *The Joint Commission Standards and Elements of Performance Standards for Sedation and Anesthesia Care. Provision of Care, Treatment, and Services PC.03.01.01. Comprehensive Accreditation Manual.* Oakbrook Terrace, IL: Joint Commission Resources; 2018.
2. American Society of Anesthesiologists Task Force on Moderate Procedural Sedation and Analgesia. Practice guidelines for moderate procedural sedation and analgesia 2018. *Anesthesiology.* 2018; 128:437–479.
3. Association of Perioperative Registered Nurses. Guideline for care of the patient receiving moderate sedation/analgesia. In: *Guidelines for Perioperative Practice.* Denver, CO: AORN; 2016.
4. Scott AM, Li J, Oyewole-Eletu S, et al. Understanding facilitators and barriers to care transitions: Insights from Project ACHIEVE site visits. *The Joint Commission Journal on Quality and Patient Safety.* 2017; 43:433–447. https://doi.org/10.1016/j.jcjq.2017.02.012.
5. CRICO Strategies. *Malpractice risks in communication failures: 2015 annual benchmarking report.* Boston, MA: The Risk Management Foundation of the Harvard Medical Institutions, Inc.; 2016, February.
6. The Joint Commission Center for Transforming Health Care. *Improving transitions of care: Hand-off communications.* Oakbrook Terrace, IL: The Joint Commission; 2014, December 22:2014.
7. Institute for Health Care Improvement. SBAR technique or communication: a situational briefing model. http://www.ihi.org/knowledge/Pages/Tools/SBARTechniquefor CommunicationASituationalBriefing Model.aspx.
8. Jackson PD, Biggins MS, Cowan L, et al. Evidence summary and recommendations for improved communication during care transitions. *Rehabilitation Nursing.* 2016; 41:135–148. https://doi.org/10.1002/rnj.230.
9. The Joint Commission Center for Transforming Health Care. *Targeted Solutions Tool for Hand-Off Communications.* Oakbrook Terrace, IL: The Joint Commission; 2017.
10. Natafgi N, Zhu X, Baloh J, et al. Critical access hospital use of TeamSTEPPS to implement shift-change handoff communication. *Journal of Nursing Care Quality.* 2018; 32:77–86.
11. Patton LJ, Tidwell JD, Falder-Saeed KL, et al. Ensuring safe transfer of pediatric patients: A quality improvement project to standardize handoff communication. *Journal of Pediatric Nursing.* 2017; 34:44–52.
12. Zou XJ, Zhang YP. Rates of nursing errors and handoffs-related errors in a medical unit following implementation of a standardized nursing handoff form. *Journal of Nursing Care Quality.* 2016; 31:61–67.
13. Agency for Healthcare Research and Quality. TeamSTEPPS Team strategies & tools to enhance performance & patient safety. http://teamstepps.ahrq.gov.
14. Agency for Healthcare Research and Quality. *TeamSTEPPS 2.0 Pocket Guide: Team strategies & tools to enhance performance and patient safety.* https://www.ahrq.gov/sites/default/files/publications/files/pocketguide.pdf; 2013.
15. Moon TS, Gonzales MX, Woods AP. A mnemonic to facilitate the handover from the operating room to intensive care unit: "I PUT PATIENTS FIRST." *Journal of Anesthesia and Clinical Research.* 2015; 6:545.
16. Heinrichs WL, Bauman EB, Dev P. SBAR 'flattens the hierarchy' among caregivers. *Studies in Health Technology and Informatics.* 2012; 173:175–182.
17. Cudjoe KG. Add identity to SBAR. *Nursing Made Incredibly Easy.* 2016; 14:6–7.
18. Labson M. *SBAR—a powerful tool to help improve communication!* www.jointcommission.org/At_home_with_the_joint_commission/sbar%E2%80%93_a_powerful_tool_to_help_improve_communication/; 2013.
19. Bonacum D. Profiles in improvement: *Institute for health care improvement.* http://www.ihi.org/knowledge/Pages/AudioandVideo/ProfilesinImprovementDougBonacu; 2008.

20. The Joint Commission. *Sentinel event alert 58: Inadequate hand-off communication.* https://www.jointcommission.org/sentinel_event_alert_58_inadequate_handoff_communications; 2017.

21. Chard R, Makary M. 8 checklist mistakes to avoid. *AORN Periop Insider.* 2013; 329–342.

22. Mentis HM, Chellali A, Manser K, et al. A systematic review of the effect of distraction on surgeon performance: Directions for operating room policy and surgical training. *Surgical Endoscopy.* 2016; 30:1713–1724. https://doi.org/10.1007/s00464-015-4443-z.

23. Thomas EJ, Helmreich RL. Will airline safety models work in health care? In: Rosenthal MM, Sutcliffe KM, eds. *Medical error: What do we know? What do we do?* San Francisco, CA: Jossey Bass; 2002:217–234.

24. Gordon S, Mendenhall P, O'Connor BB. *Beyond the checklist: What else health care can learn from aviation teamwork and safety.* Ithaca, NY: Cornell University Press; 1981.

25. Federal Aviation Administration. *Sec. 121.542 Flight crewmember duties. Doc. No. 20661, 46 FR 5502.* Washington, DC: Government Printing Office; 1981.

26. Aldrete JA, Kroulik D. A postanesthetic recovery score. *Anesthesia and Analgesia.* 1970; 49:924.

27. Trevisani L, Cifalà V, Gilli G, et al. Post-anaesthetic discharge scoring system to assess patient recovery and discharge after colonoscopy. *World Journal of Gastrointestinal Endoscopy.* 2013; 5:502–507. https://doi.org/10.4253/wjge.v5.i10.502.

28. Aldrete JA. Postanesthesia recovery score revisited. *Journal of Clinical Anesthesia.* 1995; 7:89–91.

29. Gan T, Diemunsch P, Habib AS, et al. Consensus guidelines for the management of postoperative nausea and vomiting. *Anesthesia and Analgesia.* 2014; 118:85–113.

30. Marley RA, Moline BM. Patient discharge from the ambulatory care setting. *Journal of Post Anesthesia Nursing.* 1996; 11:39–49.

31. Kleinpell RM. Improving telephone follow-up after ambulatory surgery. *Journal of Perianesthesia Nursing.* 1997; 12:336–340.

CHAPTER 12: REVIEW QUESTIONS

1. The primary purpose of postsedation monitoring is to _____.
   A. Ensure the return of physiologic function
   B. Administer additional postsedation medications
   C. Prepare the patient to resume presedation nutrition
   D. Allow time to ambulate the patient immediately postsedation

2. Characteristics unique to phase II perianesthesia nursing practice include which of the following?
   A. Patient preparation (physical and emotional)
   B. Implementation of nursing care to provide a safe transition from the fully anesthetized state to a physiologic state requiring less acute care
   C. Implementation of nursing care to prepare the patient for self-care or to be cared for by another caretaker
   D. Data collection, assessment, and planning

3. Postsedation recovery should be which of the following?
   A. Minimum of 30 minutes
   B. Minimum of 60 minutes
   C. Minimum of 90 minutes
   D. Immediate initiation at the end of the procedure

4. An assessment tool that incorporates predetermined parameters to assess clinical criteria associated with patient recovery objectively is identified as which of the following?
   A. Sedation flowsheet
   B. Postsedation scoring mechanism
   C. Mallampati classification system
   D. Subjective scoring mechanism

5. The Aldrete scoring system assigns a predetermined score to basic objective criteria, including which of the following?
   A. Activity level, respiration, circulation, level of consciousness, and oxygenation
   B. Activity level, eye movement, circulation, and level of consciousness

   C. Activity level, respirations, swallowing reflex, and circulation
   D. Respiration, swallowing reflex, circulation, and patient temperature

6. The Aldrete scoring system's circulatory criteria applies a minimum numeric score of ___ for maintenance of the patient's heart rate and blood pressure at ± 20% to 50% of presedation values.
   A. 0
   B. 1
   C. 2
   D. 3

7. Which of the following statements related to postsedation teaching and instruction is false?
   A. Instructions should be given in an unhurried atmosphere.
   B. Instructions must address medications, diet, activity, and procedure-specific information.
   C. Instructions must be given to the patient only, immediately postsedation.
   D. Instructions should be reviewed in the presence of a responsible adult.

8. A method to reduce interruptions during handoff or sign out procedures is identified as which of the following?:
   A. No discussion protocol
   B. Dialogue-free patient handoff
   C. No-interruption zone communication(s)
   D. Sterile cockpit rule

9. Which of the following mnemonics is not an evidence-based handoff protocol?
   A. SBAR
   B. I PASS (THE) BATON
   C. I PUT PATIENTS FIRST
   D. BAR READBACK

10. Which of the following statements represents sound clinical judgment with respect to postsedation patient care?
    A. All patients may be discharged 2 hours postsedation.
    B. Postsedation patient care must be individualized; patients may be discharged after all institutionally approved discharge criteria are met.
    C. Patients who receive oral or intramuscular sedation do not require postsedation recovery or observation.
    D. Postsedation recovery is only required for intravenously administered sedative and analgesic agents.

11. Which of the following organizations requires a standardized handoff process?
    A. The Joint Commission
    B. Respective State Board of Nursing
    C. American Nurses Association
    D. Agency for Healthcare and Quality

12. Postsedation discharge instructions should be provided to the patient at a maximum _____-grade reading level.
    A. sixth
    B. eighth
    C. tenth
    D. twelfth

Answers can be found in Appendix A.

Sedation Simulation: Design and Risk Management Strategies

John O'Donnell

At the completion of this chapter, the learner shall:
- Define what is meant by simulation in the context of patient sedation.
- Identify best simulation practices and standards that can be integrated into sedation simulation exercises.
- Review types of simulation, including task training, standardized patients, augmented and virtual reality, and team training.
- Review evidence with respect to the impact of sedation simulation training on provider readiness.

- Review evidence with respect to the impact of sedation simulation training on patient care practices.
- Identify opportunities to improve patient safety through sedation simulation.
- Describe approaches to the management of risk through simulation educational methods.
- Develop a working knowledge of the foundational terms in simulation educational methods.

COMPETENCY STATEMENT

The health care provider will identify opportunities to improve patient safety through sedation simulation.

Why do educators discuss the adoption of simulation educational methods as a revolution in health care education?

Health care simulation has been defined as "a technique, not a technology, to replace or amplify real experiences with guided experiences that evoke or replicate substantial aspects of the real world in a fully interactive manner."[1] Professional health care educators around the world have now adopted simulation educational approaches for multiple reasons, including to reinforce concepts of basic science, such as pharmacology, help students prepare for entry into clinical practice, evaluate new devices, enhance professionalism skills, and develop psychomotor skill in the area of competency demonstration, interprofessional education (IPE), and the development of teamwork skills.[2-18] The simulation approach also offers an opportunity to prepare students for aspects of clinical care that include crisis events such as fires, anaphylaxis, and hemorrhage, as well as in high-risk procedure training such as central venous catheter (CVC) insertion, management of rare but life-threatening events, such as malignant hyperthermia, and development of teamwork skills.[19-29] Simulation can be used as a primary educational method but is most often used as one component of an integrated training curriculum that supplements both classroom teaching and actual clinical experience. Simulation literature is available in journals throughout the health professions, with numerous meta-analyses and systematic reviews published that describe simulation education practices, optimal conditions for teaching and learning, and a wide variety of outcomes in the simulation laboratory (e.g., changes in knowledge, skill, and confidence), in the clinical setting (e.g., provider change in care practices), patient outcomes, and even in financial benefit (e.g., return on investment of simulation education dollars).[30-48]

More recent focus in simulation education has been on introducing the use of simulation into actual patient care areas—sometimes called *in situ simulation*—to prepare for health care epidemics such as an Ebola outbreak, evaluate patient safety threats, and evaluate patient care processes.[5,49-57] Improvements in simulator technology, widespread adoption across the industry, focus on how simulation improvements in the laboratory translate to clinical care (simulation translational science), and development of international accreditation processes (for simulation centers) and certification examinations (for individuals) represent some of the most important innovations in health care education that have occurred over the last 25 years.[58-66]

What is the typical design of a simulation course?

The design of a health care simulation course depends on available resources, the needs of the students, and the preparation of faculty. Many health care simulation activities include a spectrum of tools and devices, and it is important to try to match the capabilities of the simulator being used to the requirements of the simulation activity being attempted. For example, in sedation simulation training, if it is important that the participant have an extended conversation (e.g., conduct a preoperative evaluation) and a physical examination, a human actor or standardized patient (SP) is likely to be the best choice.[67] If it is critical that the sedation nurse develop

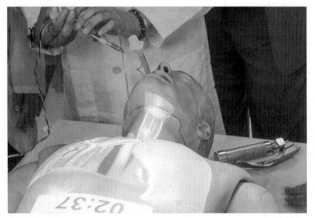

Fig. 13.1 These computerized high-fidelity simulators can be used to present a spectrum of human-like physiology and responses for use during sedation simulation. (Courtesy Winter Institute for Simulation Education and Research, University of Pittsburgh, Pittsburgh, PA.)

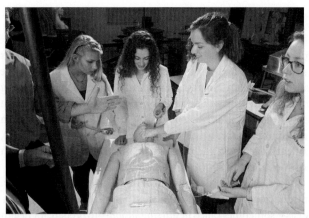

Fig. 13.2 Undergraduate nursing students performing an assessment of a pediatric patient experiencing a desaturation episode. (Courtesy Winter Institute for Simulation Education and Research, University of Pittsburgh, Pittsburgh, PA.)

psychomotor skills in the insertion of an intravenous (IV) catheter, then a partial task trainer, such as the computerized Laerdal Virtual IV system (Laerdal Medical, Wappingers Falls, NY), or a low-technology IV insertion arm might be chosen, depending on resources available. These IV devices, identified as part or partial task trainers, are intended to facilitate the development of a specific skill set. Full-body simulators that incorporate vital sign monitoring (Fig. 13.1) afford the learner a higher fidelity learning opportunity (Fig. 13.2). Furthermore, if the sedation nurse is also going to be performing airway management interventions, the computerized simulator must include an airway with enough realism to allow for the placement of appropriate devices and also respond physiologically to correct (and incorrect) airway interventions. Examples of computerized mannequins include the Gaumard HAL Advanced Multipurpose Adult Simulator (Gaumard Scientific, Miami), the Laerdal Sim Man 3-G, and the CAE Human Patient Simulator (HPS; CAE Healthcare, Sarasota, FL).[68-70]

Importantly, one of the fastest growing areas in simulation education is in the use of virtual reality and augmented reality systems. Virtual reality systems allow providers to put on headsets and other feedback devices (e.g., sensory gloves) that allow them to interact virtually with a computer-generated environment. Augmented reality systems are a combination of physical devices and computer-generated images. Both augmented and virtual reality simulations can serve as supplements or even alternatives to traditional mannequin-based learning activities.[71-74] An example of an exciting new simulation device being developed at the University of Pittsburgh is the BodyExplorer. The BodyExplorer augmented reality simulation system, identified in Fig. 13.3, offers users a form of x-ray vision as they practice skills such as medication administration, airway management, and anatomy. Students can interact with projected anatomy and physiology to see the internal consequences of external actions. A demonstration video can be viewed using this link: https://www.youtube.com/watch?v=AUa3q_jvAJo&t=18s. An automated tutoring system is built into the system to afford students 24/7 practice opportunities and also to reduce faculty and other personnel costs.[74]

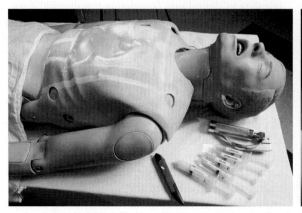
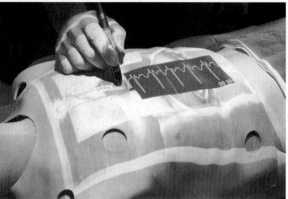

Fig. 13.3 BodyExplorer. This is an augmented reality simulation system being developed at the University of Pittsburgh. (Courtesy Winter Institute for Simulation Education and Research, University of Pittsburgh, Pittsburgh, PA.)

How can I rapidly master this new educational simulation language?

Several attempts have been made to develop a standard language or nomenclature for simulation educators and participants in simulation to use in describing their work and educational experience. Two recent and parallel projects have been developed by the International Nursing Association of Clinical Simulation and Learning (INACSL) and the Society for Simulation in Healthcare (SSiH). The INACSL work was first published in 2011 and revised in 2013 and 2016 as the "Standards of Best Practice: Simulation." The standards include a subsection titled "Simulation Glossary," which provides key terms and definitions.[69] The SSiH work resulted in publication of the *Healthcare Simulation Dictionary* in 2016. This initiative was supported by 18 simulation societies across four continents, including INACSL.[75] The following terms and definitions are some of the most important for individuals teaching with simulation or serving as participants.

Clinical scenario. This is "A deliberately designed simulation experience (also known as a case), that provides participants with an opportunity to meet identified objectives. The scenario provides a context for the simulation and can vary in length and complexity, depending on the objectives."[69]

Debriefing. "Debriefing is a facilitator-led participant discussion of events, reflection, and assimilation of activities into the participants' cognition to produce long-lasting learning."[76] The purpose of a debriefing is to create a meaningful dialogue that helps the participants of the simulation gain a better understanding of their performance during the session. Key features include obtaining feedback from facilitators, verbalizing their own impressions, reviewing actions, and sharing perceptions of the experience. Debriefing is often noted as one of the more important opportunities for deep learning during health care simulation and is acknowledged as a best practice. How much participants learn and later incorporate into their practice depends in part on the effectiveness of the debriefing. Structuring the debriefing conversation is now recognized as a key element of debriefings. Sawyer et al. have published a meta-analysis of all current debriefing methods and noted that a commonality among all approaches is structure. They noted in their review that no debriefing method has been demonstrated to be clearly superior but that structure appears to benefit both facilitators and students.[77]

O'Donnell et al. have worked in conjunction with the American Heart Association to develop a structured and supported debriefing (SSD) model as an online interactive software system for faculty development.[78] This method is sometimes referred to as the *gather, analyze, and summarize (GAS) approach* and was developed with speed of debriefing skill acquisition and ease of use as primary goals (Table 13.1). Other authors have published derivations of this model or have adapted their debriefing methods to ensure that structure is a core element.[79,80] Structuring the debriefing in a way that maintains continuous focus on the specific learning objectives and also addresses other behaviors or actions has great value. Use of policies,

standards of care, algorithms, and event logs (created by computerized mannequins or documented by observers) are important supportive elements for the structured conversation. Furthermore, asking participants to compare simulation experiences to events from their actual clinical lives is called *normalizing* and helps participants integrate the new information and recognize the value of the activity toward improving their care of patients.

Also important is a conclusion to the debriefing. During this phase, the facilitator guides a review of effective and ineffective actions and also guides a summary of the most important take-home points. This clears up any confusion about the overall objectives and helps create a culture of personal quality improvement, which is critical to ongoing professional development.

Evaluation. This is "A broad term for appraising data or placing a value on data gathered through one or more measurements. It involves rendering a judgment, including strengths and weaknesses. Evaluation measures quality and productivity against a standard of performance."[69]

Facilitation. This is "A method and strategy that occurs throughout (before, during, and after) simulation-based encounters (SBEs) in which a person (facilitator) helps to bring about an outcome(s) by providing guidance."[69]

Feedback. This is "An activity where information is relayed back to a learner; feedback should be constructive, address specific aspects of the learner's performance, and be focused on the learning objectives."[75] Feedback has been identified by numerous authors as a best practice and is essential for helping participants understand the most important points of the exercise and their performance.[81,82] Additionally, many authors now have incorporated the feedback lessons into their clinical teaching and practice.[83]

In situ simulation. "Simulation taking place in the actual patient care setting/environment is an effort to achieve a high level of fidelity and realism; this training is particularly suitable for difficult work environments, due to space constraints or noise. This training is valuable to assess, troubleshoot, or develop new system processes."[75]

Interprofessional education. This is "An educational environment where students from two or more professions learn about, from, and with each other to enable effective collaboration and improve health outcomes."[84]

Normalize. This is "A facilitator-led process in which the simulation event is connected to 'norms' or standards for clinical care. For example, participants are asked to reflect upon (thoroughly think about) the simulation event, identify a similar clinical event, compare the two events, and then describe a correct management approach. Establishing the connection between the simulation and 'real life' events is thought to support transfer of learning."[85]

Objectives. These are "Statements of specific measurable results that participants are expected to achieve during a SBE. Statements may encompass cognitive (knowledge), affective (attitude), or psychomotor (skills) domains of learning that match the learners' level of knowledge and experience."[69]

TABLE 13.1   Modified GAS Debriefing Tool[a]

Phase	Goal	Actions	Sample Questions	Time
Gather	Question participant(s) to gauge emotional readiness and gain understanding of what they believe occurred	• Request narrative from sedation provider • Request clarifying or supplemental information from other team members	• All: Do you feel prepared to debrief the sedation simulation? • Team leader: Can you tell us what happened? • Team members: Can you add to the account?	25%

Analyze	Facilitate participants' reflection on and analysis of their actions	• Review accurate record of simulation events
		• Report observations (correct and incorrect actions)
		• Ask a series of questions to reveal participants' thinking processes
		• Assist participants to reflect on performances
		• Direct and redirect participants to ensure continuous focus on session objectives
			• Directive statements
			  • I noticed...
			  • Tell me more about...
			  • How did you feel about...
			  • What were you thinking when...
			  • Help me to understand....
			• Redirect: I see; however, can you tell me about "X" aspect of the scenario...
			• Rephrase and summarize: OK, so in other words, you are saying "X" occurred?
			• Conflict resolution: Let's refocus: What's important is not who is right but what is right for the patient...
				50%

Summarize	Facilitate identification and review of lessons learned	• Participants identify positive aspects of team or individual behaviors and behaviors that require change
		• Summary of comments or statements
			• Wrap-up
			  • List two actions or events that you thought were effective or well done.
			  • Describe two areas that you think you or the team need to work on...
				25%

GAS, Gather, analyze, and summarize.
[a]This tool is a component of the structured and supported debriefing model.
Courtesy Winter Institute for Simulation Education and Research, University of Pittsburgh, Pittsburgh, PA.

Outcomes. These are "Measurable results of the participants' progress toward meeting a set of objectives. Expected outcomes are the change in knowledge, skills, or attitudes as a result of the simulation experience."[69]

Reflective learning. This is "A facilitator-guided process where the participant is encouraged to review, explore, and internally examine an issue of concern triggered by the simulation experience. This review helps to create and clarify the meaning of the experience for the participant, with opportunity for change in perspective and future behavior."[86-88]

Simulation fidelity. This is "The degree to which the simulation replicates the real event and/or workplace; this includes physical, psychological, and environmental elements."[75] Computerized mannequins are usually the focal point of simulation training and education. One outcome that has resulted from this focus on high-technology devices is the widespread use of the term *fidelity* to describe how closely simulators can mimic human responses or physiology. There are also other aspects of fidelity, which include environmental (how close the setting is to the real thing) and psychological (how close the situation is to a real situation). Fidelity is often described along a continuum (low, medium, high), with high-technology simulators often being touted as superior training devices, although the evidence for their superiority has not been clearly established.[89-92]

Prebriefing. This is "An information or orientation session held prior to the start of a simulation activity in which instructions or preparatory information is given to the participants. The purpose of the prebriefing is to set the stage for a scenario and assist participants in achieving scenario objectives."[69]

Psychological safety. This is "A feeling (explicit or implicit) within a simulation-based activity that participants are comfortable participating, speaking up, sharing thoughts, and asking for help as needed without concern for retribution or embarrassment."[75]

Safe learning environment. This is "A learning environment where it is clarified that learners feel physically and psychologically safe to make decisions, take actions, and interact in the simulation."[75]

Scenario. This is "A deliberately designed simulation experience (also known as a case), that provides participants with an opportunity to meet identified objectives. The scenario provides a context for the simulation and can vary in length and complexity, depending on the objectives."[69]

Standardized or simulated patient. This involves "Human 'role players' who are trained to interact with learners in a wide range of contexts including education and research. These individuals are described by such terms as *standardized* or *simulated patients* or *simulated participants* (SP[s])."[67]

Standardized patients have emerged as an important supplemental application in nursing education for several reasons. First, they provide the opportunity for every student to gain an authentic experience with a patient interview or interaction. Second, if the SP individuals have received special training, they can be used for objective, structured clinical examinations (OSCEs), which allow objective and detailed evaluation of student performances from the instructor's perspective and also from the SP's perspective.[93,94] Third, SPs can be prepared to present a variety of medical conditions or patient care situations (e.g., upset family) in a standardized manner. Examples of SP use in simulation sedation education could include preoperative evaluation, head to toe physical assessment, demonstration of professionalism behaviors, and demonstration of effective patient communication.[95,96] Nursing educational efforts in the use of SPs have lagged behind medical education because OSCE training is a core required component of the US Medical Licensure Examination (USMLE) in the United States and in medical training across the world.[67,97]

Task trainer or partial task trainer. This is "A device designed to train in just the key elements of the procedure or skill being learned, such as lumbar puncture, chest tube insertion, central line insertion, or part of a total system."[75]

Are there best practices in simulation education that can be included in our sedation simulation course?

A number of reviews and meta-analyses have identified best practices in simulation education, as well as comparing simulation to standard educational approaches.[38,45,98-100] Perhaps most well-known are the series of reviews conducted by Issenberg et al. and McGaghie et al., which critically reviewed the available simulation literature to extract common themes within simulation educational design and published practices.[45,100] As outlined in Box 13.1, these best practices remain relevant today, despite the intervening years.

Cook et al. have conducted a series of systematic reviews focused on simulation education versus standard education, the translational impact of simulation, and the importance of feedback (debriefing), as well as other key variables important to this educational approach.[38,44,101] In a 2012 publication in the *Journal of the American Medical Association* (JAMA), Cook et al. reported that technology-enhanced education was consistently associated with large outcomes for knowledge, skill, and behavior and moderate effects for patient-related outcomes when compared against no

intervention.[39] Furthermore, in stratifying the impact of specific educational design features, Cook et al. identified features (Box 13.2) with significant impact on learning outcomes.[38] Note that although not a duplicate of the previous list, there are many overlaps and commonalities.

The INACSL used these resources, among others, to develop standards for simulation educators in 2010. These were most recently revised in 2016 and 2017. Each of these INACSL standards is defined and includes criteria for performance, as well as specific required elements. The list of INACSL standards identified in Box 13.3 includes nine areas; each area includes criteria for performance, as well as specific required elements.

BOX 13.1 Best Practices in Simulation

Feedback
Deliberate practice
Curriculum integration
Outcome measurement
Simulation fidelity
Skill acquisition and maintenance
Mastery learning
Transfer to practice
Team training
High-stakes testing
Instructor training
Educational and professional context

BOX 13.2 Design Features with Significant Impact on Learning Outcomes

Range of difficulty
Repetitive practice (at one time)
Distributed practice (across time)
Cognitive interactivity
Multiple learning strategies
Individualized learning
Mastery learning (to a particular standard)
Feedback
Longer training time

BOX 13.3 Standards of Best Practice: Simulation

Simulation design
Outcomes and objectives
Facilitation
Debriefing
Participant evaluation
Professional integrity
Simulation-enhanced interprofessional education
Simulation glossary
Operations

INACSL, International Nursing Association of Clinical Simulation and Learning.
Adapted from references 14, 69, 70, 102-107.

Some sedation colleagues go to simulation centers and practice as teams, and other centers have simulators and instructors brought into their clinical practice setting. How does point of care simulation education work?

There are many examples of point of care or in situ simulation approaches, with numerous advantages to this approach. First, completing the simulation training in the actual sedation practice environment allows practitioners to use the equipment and environment of care with which they are familiar. Furthermore, this approach allows an evaluation of environment and process issues of the facility in combination with the training of the practitioners.

Kobayashi et al. used an in situ approach in a pilot study to evaluate procedural sedation in an emergency department (ED) environment.[108] Attending ED physicians and residents went through two sedation simulation scenarios. The focus of the study was on the use of protocols for preparing for the sedation, the level of vigilance during sedations, adverse event management, and evaluation of the patients after the sedation. The authors concluded that the course was effective for the development of safety skills in emergency room procedural sedation.

In a follow-up study, Siegel et al. conducted a randomized controlled trial of the ED sedation simulations with 24 emergency room residents.[109] Both groups received simulation with the experimental group, also using an experimental informatics reminder system to remind them of needed actions. The authors concluded that the simulations could be used to evaluate safety behavior skills of the residents.

Hadfield et al. have described an in situ simulation designed for dental simulation.[110] Dentists and dental nurses who administered sedation were included in the study. After completing the simulations, semistructured interviews were conducted. Participants reported that the sessions were "worthwhile, realistic, challenging and emotionally positive." These practitioners also reported that they thought their knowledge and ability to implement "human factors skills" (e.g., improved communication) were improved. Other benefits reported were that the simulations revealed process and supply flaws in the actual clinical environment.

Is simulation education or actual clinical practice more effective?

The substitution simulation training for clinical practice training has been a subject of national and international interest. Numerous examples exist in the surgical and medical training literature demonstrating improvement in specific procedural skills, knowledge, teamwork, and decision making, with substantial progress reported in validating the approach.[111-113]

The best-known example demonstrating the effective replacement of actual clinical training with simulation is in the nursing profession. In 2014, Hayden et al. conducted a longitudinal study looking at the replacement of undergraduate clinical education with simulation.[62] The study was supported by the National Council of State Boards of Nursing (NCSBN) in partnership with the National League for Nursing (NLN). This study used the INACSL standards to help design scenarios and teaching activities. A total of six schools of nursing participated, including both Bachelor's and Associate Degree nursing schools. The study required replacement of actual clinical training hours with structured simulation activities. The control group replaced 10% of clinical training, and the experimental groups replaced 25% and 50% of all clinical training with simulation activities. The assessment methods were rigorous and followed the students postgraduation. No differences were found in board pass rates, clinical competence, knowledge, or attitudes, including prior to graduation and into actual professional practice. Based on this study, US boards of nursing began allowing replacement of clinical training with simulation. Furthermore, Alexander et al. published NCSBN guidelines for simulation use in undergraduate nursing educational programs.[60] These NCSBN guidelines are based on the INACSL standards and other best practice recommendations.

Is there evidence to demonstrate that simulation training for sedation can improve sedation care processes as well as patient care?

A large body of publications target the area of sedation simulation but little definitive evidence exists regarding what design works best for sedation simulation education. The following are selected examples of papers describing outcomes, providing a review of the current state of sedation simulation, discussing the value of the approach in provider preparation, and highlighting important design features that remain best practices today.

Sedation simulation has been a focus of academic inquiry since at least 2000.[120] evaluated the use of simulation for teaching sedation skills to 20 nurses.[114] Precourse preparation consisted of a review of the American Society of Anesthesiologists (ASA) practice guidelines for sedation and analgesia by nonanesthesiologists.[115] All nurses received a knowledge pretest. Following four practice sessions, in which each nurse gained experience providing sedation to a computerized anesthesia simulator, the nurses had a practical simulation examination followed by a knowledge posttest. Improvements were reported in the areas of knowledge and skill, with the course highly rated (3.75/4.0, with 1 = poor and 4 = excellent).

Caparelli-White and Urman have also described the development of hospital policies for sedation administration.[116] They suggested that these efforts should involve multiple disciplines and include clinicians, administrators, and risk managers. Noting that local, regional, and national policies and standards must be considered, they discussed the process of clinician preparation, including simulation training as one essential element for improving quality of care and patient safety.

Pisansky et al. published a review paper noting the massive increase in the numbers and types of procedures, including sedation being done outside of operating rooms and without the involvement of anesthesia providers.[117] These authors are anesthesiologists and, in this review, discussed evidence regarding how to improve patient safety for nonanesthesia providers involved in administering deep sedation. The authors identified the ASA recommendations, which are now consensus recommendations of numerous professional organizations, as an important guide for improving the safety of sedation practice and, more specifically, for cases when deep sedation is a target. The authors acknowledged that there is little evidence to support that these guidelines are actually adhered to in most sedation practices. They also suggested that a component critical to patient safety is some sort of formalized educational program, including simulation experiences that can be used to develop and evaluate key competencies, including "preprocedural evaluation, understanding sedation levels, airway management, documentation, emergency life support skills, teamwork and quality improvement." They discussed the high variability in provider training in the sedation domain and suggested that one of the more comprehensive programs in preparation for deep sedation is the ASA Safe Sedation Training—Deep, available at https://www.asahq.org/education.[117]

Sauter et al. have developed, implemented, and evaluated a mandatory interprofessional simulation-based sedation training program for practicing doctors (26) and nurses (24) in a Swedish emergency department setting.[118] They designed a curriculum that consisted of a precourse learning module, separate airway training course, three practice simulations, and a final testing simulation. The investigators used a precourse/postcourse design; the curriculum consisted of an individual self-learning module, an airway skill training course, three simulation-based team training cases, and a final practical learning course in the operating room. Before and after each training session, self-efficacy, awareness of emergency procedures, knowledge of sedation medication, and crisis resource management were assessed with a questionnaire. Changes in these measures were compared; it was found that there was a large increase in self-efficacy and knowledge that was independent of profession and experience level. They conducted clinical evaluation after implementation and found no major complications among the sedations performed. They concluded that interprofessional and interdisciplinary simulation-based sedation training was both an efficient and effective way to implement conscious sedation training for ED personnel.

What type of competencies should be developed during a sedation simulation session?

There are many decisions to be made when designing a successful simulation encounter. It is important that there be a structure to the design process to ensure that all key elements are included. When designing a simulation activity, it is useful to use a checklist to ensure that nothing important is missed. The Scenario Development and Testing Process Checklist identified in Box 13.4 can be used for general organization, as well as to make sure that the simulation works effectively and to verify that faculty are prepared and in agreement with how the simulation should run. As highlighted in Fig. 13.4, it is important to understand the "anatomy" of simulation scenario

---

> **BOX 13.4 Scenario Development and Testing Process Checklist**
>
> 1. Identify topic.
> 2. Determine learner level.
> 3. Create specific learning objectives.
> 4. Develop the story.
> 5. Develop flow of the scenario.
> 6. Compile comprehensive equipment lists.
> 7. Establish feedback/debriefing plan.
> 8. Determine assessment strategy.
> 9. Complete facilitation instructions.
> 10. Perform scenario testing (α, β).
>
> Courtesy Winter Institute for Simulation Education and Research, University of Pittsburgh, Pittsburgh, PA; and from Henrichs T, Thompson J: A Resource for Nurse Anesthesia Educators. 2nd ed. Park Ridge, IL: American Association of Nurse Anesthetists; 2017.

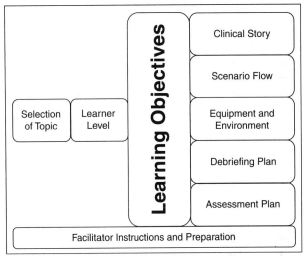

Fig. 13.4 The anatomy of a scenario dissected into its component parts. (From Henrichs T, Thompson J. A Resource for Nurse Anesthesia Educators. 2nd ed. Park Ridge, IL: American Association of Nurse Anesthetists; 2017.)

design.[119] Following are examples of scenarios that follow this development pattern, with the exception of a detailed assessment plan. Such a plan will require development of facility-specific assessment rubrics based on institutional policy.

Gastrointestinal Endoscopy Laboratory Scenario: Example 1. This involves adult sedation simulation, pharmacology, and monitoring.

Overall topic. This refers to titration of sedation medications to specific procedural goals of amnesia, anxiolysis, and analgesia for an adult patient undergoing screening colonoscopy.

Learner level. This is aimed at practicing sedation providers (individual or team simulation).

Objectives

Participants will do the following:
- Identify the sedation goals for the procedure.
- Demonstrate the ability to safely prepare the patient for sedation.
- Demonstrate the ability to titrate medications safely.

- Use monitoring data and patient assessment information to inform medication titration.

Patient stem or story. Mr. Smith is a 50-year-old patient who is presenting for a screening colonoscopy. He has a past medical history significant for hypertension, smoking, and heavy alcohol use. He is 72 inches tall and weighs 280 pounds (body mass index [BMI], 38).

Scenario story flow. Mr. Smith is very nervous and will require substantial doses of sedation medication because of his anxiety, alcohol use disorder, and weight. He will demonstrate substantial tolerance to the effects of the sedation medications. The specific doses that will provide adequate sedation will need to be agreed on by the team ahead of time. Without adequate sedation, Mr. Smith will complain of pain and discomfort and will move during the colonoscopy. The proceduralist will complain that conditions are not adequate to complete the examination.

List of supplies and materials

- Simulator and monitor with ability to display vital signs, including electrocardiogram (ECG), blood pressure (BP), heart rate (HR), and SaO_2
- Sedation scale—use the scale that is implemented at the clinical facility; otherwise, select a recognized sedation scale. (**Note:** Remember that some aspects of sedation assessment scales cannot easily be evaluated using a simulator; therefore, the in-room facilitator will need to provide feedback regarding patient response.)
- Monitoring devices
- IV setup with a drainage bag so that medications can be given
- Syringes, medications, and labels
- IV infusion pump (for sedation medications or IV line)
- Alcohol wipes
- Suction
- Oxygen delivery system
- Emergency supplies
- Airway equipment (airways, endotracheal tubes, syringes, laryngoscopes, suction devices, oxygen delivery devices)

Key debriefing points to be discussed

- How are the goals of a sedation agreed on?
- How rapidly should specific medications be titrated?
- What is the pharmacology of the sedation medications selected?
- What are the monitoring requirements for this procedure, and how can they be used to guide the administration of sedation medications?
- What factors would predict that Mr. Smith would be a challenge to sedate?
- What are the postprocedure implications of giving large doses of sedation medications?

It is often useful to repurpose a simulation scenario to have participants demonstrate other aspects important to competence in sedation practice. As noted earlier in the chapter, this could include teamwork skills (e.g., communication, situational awareness), preoperative evaluation (using a standardized patient for the history sand physical components), or management of complications. For Example 2, we will consider modifying Example 1 to address several of these alternative goals.

Gastrointestinal Endoscopy Laboratory Scenario: Example 2. This involves adult sedation simulation and management of a complication, hypertension.

Overall topic. This refers to hypertensive complications during the titration of sedation medications for a colonoscopy.

Learner level. This is aimed at practicing sedation providers (individual or team simulation).

Objectives

- Titrate sedation medications for a screening colonoscopy.
- Identify hemodynamic instability (significant hypertension) during the procedure.
- Demonstrate the ability to work effectively with other team members to treat the hypertension.
- Provide an effective report to the proceduralist regarding the situation.
- Prepare and administer antihypertensive and additional sedation medication (as ordered).

Patient stem or story. Mr. Smith is a 50-year-old patient who is presenting for a screening colonoscopy. He has a past medical history significant for hypertension, smoking, and heavy alcohol use. He is 72 inches tall and weighs 280 pounds (BMI, 38).

Scenario story flow. Mr. Smith is very nervous and will require substantial doses of sedation medication because of his anxiety, alcohol use disorder, and weight. He will demonstrate substantial tolerance to the effects of the sedation medications. Despite appearing to be adequately sedated, Mr. Smith will demonstrate substantial hypertension (mean arterial pressure [MAP] increases more than 20% from baseline) during the colonoscopy. It does not resolve with additional sedation and, if the sedation provider does not administer an antihypertensive agent, the patient will begin to complain of chest discomfort. Obtaining an order for the antihypertensive will require providing a concise report (e.g., situation-background-assessment-recommendation [SBAR] or other structured report) to the proceduralist and then preparing and administering the medication and evaluating the response.

List of supplies and materials. The only substantial changes to the supply list from Example 1 would be ensuring that appropriate antihypertensive medications are available.

Key debriefing points

- What is the magnitude of BP change that should trigger treatment during procedural sedation?
- What are the potential consequences of not treating the hypertensive episode?
- What are the elements of an effective report of a clinical problem?
- What is the pharmacology of commonly used antihypertensive agents available in the sedation setting?
- How should this patient be evaluated and managed in the postprocedure area?

Again, it is often useful to repurpose simulation scenarios (clinical stories) to have the participants demonstrate other aspects important to their competence in sedation practice.

It is also useful to continue to evolve a particular scenario during a training session as the participants will become familiar with the "patient" and will be able to absorb additional details cognitively. For Example 3, we will consider modifying the situation in Examples 1 and 2 to the point of the patient suffering a cardiac arrest because of his hypertensive response to the procedure. This scenario could be implemented in a simulation facility or as in situ simulation in an actual procedural area. The advantage of the in situ simulation is in the evaluation of more team members and facility processes for addressing emergency situations.

Several key decisions will need to be made ahead of time for this next scenario. First, will the procedural sedation team be aware that a cardiac arrest or other major complication is a possibility? Second, if a code is called, will the facility be aware ahead of time, or will this be done with no warning? If the facility is notified, the focus would be shifted to performance of key tasks and skills. If the facility is not notified, the focus could be shifted to response time and other measures of rapid response team (RRT) function and the process of care handoff, as well as preparing the patient for transfer.

Gastrointestinal Endoscopy Laboratory Scenario: Example 3. This involves an in situ simulation to determine emergency response readiness of the sedation provider, other staff, and the facility.

Overall topic. This refers to cardiac arrest during the sedation of a severely hypertensive patient during screening colonoscopy.

Learner level(s). This could include practicing sedation providers, proceduralist, support personnel, rapid response team members, and administrators.

Objectives
- Titrate sedation medications during screening colonoscopy.
- Monitor for and identify hemodynamic instability.
- Identify cardiac arrest (e.g., ventricular tachycardia).
- Activate the RRT.
- Implement initial Advanced Cardiac Life Support (ACLS) interventions (e.g., cardiopulmonary resuscitation [CPR], automated external defibrillator [AED] placement, airway management) prior to the arrival of the RRT.
- Plan for patient transfer on return of spontaneous circulation (ROSC).

Patient stem or story. Mr. Smith is a 50-year-old patient who is presenting for a screening colonoscopy. He has a past medical history significant for hypertension, smoking, and heavy alcohol use. He is 72 inches tall and weighs 280 pounds (BMI, 38).

Scenario story flow. Mr. Smith is very nervous and requires substantial doses of sedation medication because of his anxiety, alcohol use disorder, and weight. During the sedation, Mr. Smith will complain of pain and discomfort and become increasingly hypertensive. He will demonstrate ST segment elevation and then experience cardiac arrest. The ECG will show ventricular tachycardia. After ROSC, prepare to send Mr. Smith to the intensive care unit (ICU) or to the cardiac catheterization laboratory, depending on facility policy.

List of supplies and materials. The only substantial changes to the supply list from Examples 1 and 2 would be ensuring that a code cart is available, including medications and defibrillator.

Key debriefing points
- When should a sedation case be cancelled or diverted to an operating room setting?
- What activities should occur while awaiting the arrival of the RRT?
- How should report be given to RRT members?
- Review ACLS protocols for cardiac arrest, including CPR, defibrillation, medications, and airway management.
- On ROSC, where should Mr. Smith be sent?

I have attended a meeting with the hospital's risk management officer to discuss a patient outcome from last week. During the event, it was noted that respiratory depression was not assessed properly by the sedation provider during a gastrointestinal (GI) procedure. After review, she recommended sedation simulation as a way to reduce future patient safety risks. Can simulation be used as a risk management strategy?

There are numerous publications that have addressed the use of simulation and its impact on patient risk. Simulation team performance, as well as code team response efficiency and other patient safety hazards, can be directly measured with several simulation strategies. One approach is in the pre- and postimplementation analyses of actual events after a simulation training has been conducted (e.g., a cardiac arrest event during a simulation). Another could be achieved in the careful application of the failure, mode, effects, and analysis (FMEA) model applied to areas of latent threats identified through in situ simulation efforts, with a prospective calculation of cost savings resulting from avoidance of actual patient harm. An early and rigorous example of this FMEA method was reported by Blike et al.[120] This team described the evaluation of latent patient safety threats during pediatric simulation. This was an in situ study and focused on more than 300 personnel comprising the sedation and critical event response teams in the areas of radiology and ED. All providers in these areas were notified that patient safety drills using simulation were going to be conducted.

Pediatric respiratory events (including respiratory arrest) were the most common serious event and remain a key concern in pediatric patient sedation management today. A 4-year-old child was represented by a pediatric simulator, which was programmed to experience respiratory arrest with consequent bradycardia (in response to hypoxia) and hypotension leading to eventual arrest, without proper intervention. An exemplar exercise incorporating experienced anesthesia personnel for the management of the simulated sedation emergencies was used to establish a gold standard comparator. Construct validity was established comparing medical student versus second-year anesthesia resident performance. All sessions were videotaped for analysis. Numerous latent system and human factor failures were noted, including timely identification of the problem, communication of an emergency, and initiation of correct treatment. The exemplar patient experienced no hypoxia or hypotension due to prompt rescue and treatment; the radiology team cases experienced hypoxia and hypotension that lasted on average 4.5 minutes and the ED teams an average of 5.5 minutes, respectively. This study is a powerful example of the value of simulation in a demonstration of how latent system safety threats can be probed and analyzed using simulation methods.

At the macro level, the risk environment of an entire hospital and its staff can be assessed. Adler et al. have described the use of a simulation program to test systems and prepare their staff for the move to a new hospital.[121] They described the development of a comprehensive series of simulations, which resulted in 258 hours of simulation activities for 514 hospital workers of all types. They focused on the identification of latent patient safety threats and the establishment of safe workflows. More than 600 issues were identified, and postsimulation surveys demonstrated that the simulations were positively received by most respondents.

SUMMARY

Simulation educational methods are now being used worldwide as a way to supplement, support, and even replace clinical experiences. It is estimated that over the past 20 years, more than 15,000 papers have been published in the health care literature in the area of simulation educational methods. As a result, educational best practices and standards have been identified and are being advocated. Simulation for sedation practice has been used for more than 2 decades, and inquiry is now focusing on how to design and implement simulation into cutting edge sedation training. The use of simulation for sedation competence assessment, team skills, and risk assessment at the individual and facility levels has been reported. It is clear that given the absence of risk to actual patients, and the potential for substantial gains in knowledge and skill, simulation will continue to be used for the preparation of sedation professionals.

REFERENCES

1. Gaba D. The future vision of simulation in health care. *Qual Saf Health Care.* 2004;13(Suppl 1):i2–i10.
2. Nguyen N, Watson WD, Dominguez E. An event-based approach to design a teamwork training scenario and assessment tool in surgery. *J Surg Educ.* 2016;73 (2):197–207.
3. Mahramus TL, Penoyer DA, Waterval EM, et al. Two hours of teamwork training improves teamwork in simulated cardiopulmonary arrest events. *Clin Nurse Spec.* 2016; 30(5):284–291.
4. Salas E, Rosen MA. Building high reliability teams: progress and some reflections on teamwork training. *BMJ Quality & Safety.* 2013;22(5):369–373.
5. Patterson MD, Geis GL, Falcone RA, et al. In situ simulation: detection of safety threats and teamwork training in a high risk emergency department. *BMJ Quality & Safety.* 2013; 22(6):468–477.
6. Capella J, Smith S, Philp A, et al. Teamwork training improves the clinical care of trauma patients. *J Surg Educ.* 2010; 67(6):439–443.
7. Lind MM, Corridore M, Sheehan C, et al. A multidisciplinary approach to a pediatric difficult airway simulation course. *Otolaryngol Head Neck Surg.* 2018;159(1):127–135.
8. Ajdari A, Boyle LN, Kannan N, et al. Simulation of the emergency department care process for pediatric traumatic brain injury. *J Healthc Qual.* 2018;40(2):110–118.
9. Schornack LA, Baysinger CL, Pian-Smith MCM. Recent advances of simulation in obstetric anesthesia. *Curr Opin Anaesthesiol.* 2017;30(6):723–729.
10. Chang E. The role of simulation training in obstetrics: a health care training strategy dedicated to performance improvement. *Curr Opin Obstet Gynecol.* 2013;25(6):482–486.
11. King J, Beanlands S, Fiset V, et al. Using interprofessional simulation to improve collaborative competences for nursing, physiotherapy, and respiratory therapy students. *J Interprof Care.* 2016;1–7.
12. Sigalet EL, Donnon TL, Grant V. Insight into team competence in medical, nursing and respiratory therapy students. *J Interprof Care.* 2015;29(1):62–67.
13. Stockert B, Ohtake PJ. A national survey on the use of immersive simulation for interprofessional education in physical therapist education programs. *Simul Healthc.* 2017;12 (5):298–303.
14. International Association for Clinical Simulation & Learning. Standards of best practice: simulation: simulation-enhanced interprofessional education (Sim-IPE). *Clinical Simulation In Nursing.* 2016;12:S34–S38.
15. Meyer BA, Seefeldt TM, Ngorsuraches S, et al. Interprofessional education in pharmacology using high-fidelity simulation. *Curr Pharm Teach Learn.* 2017;9(6):1055–1062.
16. Thompson TL, Bonnel WB. Integration of high-fidelity patient simulation in an undergraduate pharmacology course. *J Nurs Educ.* 2008;47(11):518–521.
17. Seropian M, Dillman D, Lasater K, Gavilanes J. Mannequin-based simulation to reinforce pharmacology concepts. *Simul Healthc.* 2007;2(4):218–223.
18. Wali E, Pinto JM, Cappaert M, et al. Teaching professionalism in graduate medical education: What is the role of simulation? *Surgery.* 2016;160(3):552–564.
19. Barsuk JH, Cohen ER, Nguyen D, et al. Attending physician adherence to a 29-component central venous catheter bundle checklist during simulated procedures. *Crit Care Med.* 2016; 44(10):1871–1881.
20. Mok M, Ker J. Developing clinical skills bundles. *Clin Teach.* 2015;12(5):403–407.
21. Craft C, Feldon DF, Brown EA. Instructional design affects the efficacy of simulation-based training in central venous catheterization. *American Journal of Surgery.* 2014;207(5): 782–789.
22. Barsuk JH, Cohen ER, Potts S, et al. Dissemination of a simulation-based mastery learning intervention reduces central line-associated bloodstream infections. *BMJ Quality & Safety.* 2014;23(9):749–756.
23. Cain CL, Riess ML, Gettrust L, Novalija J. Malignant hyperthermia crisis: optimizing patient outcomes through simulation and interdisciplinary collaboration. *AORN Journal.* 2014;99(2):301–308. quiz 309–311.
24. Hotchkiss MA, Mendoza SN. Update for nurse anesthetists. Part 6. Full-body patient simulation technology: gaining

experience using a malignant hyperthermia model. *AANA J.* 2001;69(1):59–65.

25. Schwid HA, O'Donnell D. Educational computer simulation of malignant hyperthermia. *J Clin Monit.* 1992;8(3): 201–208.

26. Coppens I, Verhaeghe S, Van Hecke A, Beeckman D. The effectiveness of crisis resource management and team debriefing in resuscitation education of nursing students: a randomised controlled trial. *J Clin Nurs.* 2018;27 (1-2):77–85.

27. Weinger MB, Banerjee A, Burden AR, et al. Simulation-based assessment of the management of critical events by board-certified anesthesiologists. *Anesthesiology.* 2017;127(3): 475–489.

28. Yee B, Naik VN, Joo HS, et al. Nontechnical skills in anesthesia crisis management with repeated exposure to simulation-based education. *Anesthesiology.* 2005;103(2):241–248.

29. O'Donnell J, Fletcher J, Dixon B, Palmer L. Planning and implementing an anesthesia crisis resource management course for student nurse anesthetists. *CRNA.* 1998;9(2):50–58.

30. Shin S, Park JH, Kim JH. Effectiveness of patient simulation in nursing education: meta-analysis. *Nurse Educ Today.* 2015;35(1):176–182.

31. Oh PJ, Jeon KD, Koh MS. The effects of simulation-based learning using standardized patients in nursing students: A meta-analysis. *Nurse Educ Today.* 2015;35(5):e6–e15.

32. Lee J, Oh PJ. Effects of the use of high-fidelity human simulation in nursing education: a meta-analysis. *J Nurs Educ.* 2015;54(9):501–507.

33. Cheng A, Lockey A, Bhanji F, et al. The use of high-fidelity manikins for advanced life support training-a systematic review and meta-analysis. *Resuscitation.* 2015;93:142–149.

34. Brydges R, Manzone J, Shanks D, et al. Self-regulated learning in simulation-based training: a systematic review and meta-analysis. *Med Educ.* 2015;49(4):368–378.

35. Cook DA. How much evidence does it take? A cumulative meta-analysis of outcomes of simulation-based education. *Med Educ.* 2014;48(8):750–760.

36. Cheng A, Lang TR, Starr SR, et al. Technology-enhanced simulation and pediatric education: a meta-analysis. *Pediatrics.* 2014;133(5). e1313.1323.

37. Lorello GR, Cook DA, Johnson RL, Brydges R. Simulation-based training in anaesthesiology: a systematic review and meta-analysis. *British Journal of Anaesthesia.* 2014; 112(2):231–245.

38. Cook DA, Hamstra SJ, Brydges R, et al. Comparative effectiveness of instructional design features in simulation-based education: systematic review and meta-analysis. *Medical Teacher.* 2013;35(1):e867–e898.

39. Cook DA, Hatala R, Brydges R, et al. Technology-enhanced simulation for health professions education: a systematic review and meta-analysis. *JAMA.* 2011;306(9):978–988.

40. Salas E, DiazGranados D, Klein C, et al. Does team training improve team performance? A meta-analysis. *Human Factors.* 2008;50(6):903–933.

41. Hegland PA, Aarlie H, Stromme H, Jamtvedt G. Simulation-based training for nurses: Systematic review and meta-analysis. *Nurse Educ Today.* 2017;54:6–20.

42. O'Leary JA, Nash R, Lewis PA. High-fidelity patient simulation as an educational tool in paediatric intensive care: A systematic review. *Nurse Educ Today.* 2015;35(10):e8–e12.

43. Kirkman MA, Ahmed M, Albert AF, et al. The use of simulation in neurosurgical education and training. A systematic review. *J Neurosurg.* 2014;121(2):228–246.

44. Cook DA, Brydges R, Hamstra SJ, et al. Comparative effectiveness of technology-enhanced simulation versus other instructional methods: a systematic review and meta-analysis. *Simul Healthc.* 2013;7(5):308–320.

45. Issenberg SB, McGaghie WC, Petrusa ER, et al. Features and uses of high-fidelity medical simulations that lead to effective learning: a BEME systematic review. *Med Teach.* 2005;27(1):10–28.

46. McGaghie WC, Issenberg SB, Barsuk JH, Wayne DB. A critical review of simulation-based mastery learning with translational outcomes. *Med Educ.* 2014;48(4):375–385.

47. Barsuk JH, Cohen ER, Feinglass J, et al. Cost savings of performing paracentesis procedures at the bedside after simulation-based education. *Simul Healthc.* 2014; 9(5):312–318.

48. Cohen ER, Feinglass J, Barsuk JH, et al. Cost savings from reduced catheter-related bloodstream infection after simulation-based education for residents in a medical intensive care unit. *Simul Healthc.* 2010;5(2):98–102.

49. Knight P, MacGloin H, Lane M, et al. Mitigating latent threats identified through an embedded in situ simulation program and their comparison to patient safety incidents: a retrospective review. *Front Pediatr.* 2017;5:281.

50. Lopez C. National risk manager leading simulation education. *J Nurses Prof Dev.* 2015;31(2):124–125.

51. Walsh K. Simulation is the way to bring risk management and patient safety together. *Acad Med.* 2011;86(10):1193–1194.

52. Hunt EA, Nelson KL, Shilkofski NA. Simulation in medicine: addressing patient safety and improving the interface between health care providers and medical technology. *Biomed Instrum Technol.* 2006;40(5):399–404.

53. Petrosoniak A, Auerbach M, Wong AH, Hicks CM. In situ simulation in emergency medicine: moving beyond the simulation lab. *Emerg Med Australas.* 2017;29(1):83–88.

54. Yajamanyam PK, Sohi D. In situ simulation as a quality improvement initiative. *Arch Dis Child Educ Pract Ed.* 2015.

55. Ventre KM, Barry JS, Davis D, et al. Using in situ simulation to evaluate operational readiness of a children's hospital-based obstetrics unit. *Simul Healthc.* 2014;9(2):102–111.

56. Phrampus PE, O'Donnell JM, Farkas D, et al. Rapid development and deployment of Ebola readiness training across an academic health system: the critical role of simulation education, consulting, and systems integration. *Simul Healthc.* 2016;11(2):82–88.

57. Gaba DM. Simulation as a critical resource in the response to Ebola virus disease. *Simul Healthc.* 2014;9(6):337–338.

58. Rogers DA, Peterson DT, Ponce BA, et al. Simulation and faculty development. *Surg Clin North Am.* 2015;95(4):729–737.

59. Decker SIL. *Simulation as an educational strategy in the development of critical and reflective thinking: a qualitative exploration. PhD thesis.* Denton, TX: Texas Woman's University; 2007.

60. Alexander M, Durham CF, Hooper JI, et al. NCSBN simulation guidelines for prelicensure nursing programs. *Journal of Nursing Regulation.* 2015;6(3):39–42.

61. O'Donnell JM, Decker S, Howard V, et al. NLN/Jeffries simulation framework state of the science project: simulation learning outcomes. *Clinical Simulation In Nursing.* 2014;10(7):373–382.

62. Hayden JK, Smiley RA, Alexander M, et al. The NCSBN National Simulation Study: A longitudinal, randomized, controlled study replacing clinical hours with simulation in prelicensure nursing education. *Journal of Nursing Regulation.* 2014;5(2 Suppl):S1–S41.

63. Schwab B, Hungness E, Barsness KA, McGaghie WC. The role of simulation in surgical education. *J Laparoendosc Adv Surg Tech A.* 2017;27(5):450–454.

64. McGaghie WC, Issenberg SB, Cohen ER, et al. Translational educational research: a necessity for effective health-care improvement. *Chest.* 2012;142(5):1097–1103.

65. Society for Simulation in Healthcare. SSH certification programs. http://www.ssih.org/Certification.

66. Society for Simulation in Healthcare. Full accreditation. http://www.ssih.org/Accreditation/Full-Accreditation.

67. Lewis KL, Bohnert CA, Gammon WL, et al. The Association of Standardized Patient Educators (ASPE) standards of best practice (SOBP). *Adv Simul (Lond).* 2017;2:10.

68. Cooper JB, Taqueti VR. A brief history of the development of mannequin simulators for clinical education and training. *Qual Saf Health Care.* 2004;13(Suppl 1):i11–i18.

69. International Association for Clinical Simulation and Learning. Standards of best practice: simulation glossary. *Clinical Simulation In Nursing.* 2016;12:S39–S47.

70. International Association for Clinical Simulation and Learning. Standards of best practice: simulation design. *Clinical Simulation In Nursing.* 2016;12:S5–S12.

71. McGrath JL, Taekman JM, Dev P, et al. Using virtual reality simulation environments to assess competence for emergency medicine learners. *Acad Emerg Med.* 2018;25(2):186–195.

72. Elessawy M, Wewer A, Guenther V, et al. Validation of psychomotor tasks by Simbionix LAP Mentor simulator and identifying the target group. *Minim Invasive Ther Allied Technol.* 2017;26(5):262–268.

73. Zaveri PP, Davis AB, O'Connell KJ, et al. Virtual reality for pediatric sedation: a randomized controlled trial using simulation. *Cureus.* 2016;8(2):e486.

74. Foronda CL, Alfes CM, Dev P, et al. Virtually nursing: emerging technologies in nursing education. *Nurse Educ.* 2016.

75. Lopreiato JOE, Downing D, Gammon W, et al. *Health care simulation dictionary.* http://www.ssih.org/dictionary; 2016. Accessed July 25, 2016.

76. Fanning RM, Gaba DM. The role of debriefing in simulation-based learning. *Simul.* 2007;2(2):115–125.

77. Sawyer T, Eppich W, Brett-Fleegler M, et al. More than one way to debrief: a critical review of health care simulation debriefing methods. *Simul Healthc.* 2016;11(3):209–217.

78. O'Donnell JM, Rodgers D, Lee W, et al. *Structured and supported debriefing [interactive multimedia program].* Dallas: American Heart Association (AHA); 2009.

79. Cheng A, Grant V, Robinson T, et al. Promoting Excellence and Reflective Learning in Simulation (PEARLS) approach to health care debriefing: a faculty development guide. *Clinical Simulation in Nursing.* 2016;12(10):419–428.

80. Palaganas JC, Fey M, Simon R. Structured debriefing in simulation-based education. *AACN Adv Crit Care.* 2016;27(1):78–85.

81. Burns CL. Using debriefing and feedback in simulation to improve participant performance: an educator's perspective. *Int J Med Educ.* 2015;6:118–120.

82. Ramani S. Reflections on feedback: closing the loop. *Med Teach.* 2016;38(2):206–207.

83. Hunter LA. Debriefing and feedback in the current health care environment. *J Perinat Neonatal Nurs.* 2016;30(3):174–178.

84. World Health Organization. World Health Organization (WHO) framework for action on interprofessional education and collaborative practice. In: *Paper presented at the Interprofessional Education Collaborative.* Switzerland: Geneva; 2010.

85. Merriam-Webster. *Merriam-Webster Unabridged Online Dictionary.* Springfield: MA; 2008.

86. Boyd EM, Fales AW. Reflective learning: key to learning from experience. *Journal of Humanistic Psychology.* 1983;23(2):99–117.

87. Rudolph JW, Simon R, Dufresne RL, Raemer DB. There's no such thing as "nonjudgmental" debriefing: a theory and method for debriefing with good judgment. *Simul Healthc.* 2006;1(1):49–55.

88. Rudolph JW, Simon R, Rivard P, et al. Debriefing with good judgment: combining rigorous feedback with genuine inquiry. *Anesthesiol Clin.* 2007;25(2):361–376.

89. Lee J, Cheng A, Angelski C, Allain D, Ali S. High-fidelity simulation in pediatric emergency medicine: a national survey of facilitator comfort and practice. *Pediatr Emerg Care.* 2015;31(4):260–265.

90. Ignacio J, Dolmans D, Scherpbier A, et al. Comparison of standardized patients with high-fidelity simulators for managing stress and improving performance in clinical deterioration: A mixed methods study. *Nurse Educ Today.* 2015;35(12):1161–1168.

91. Schulz CM, Skrzypczak M, Raith S, et al. High-fidelity human patient simulators compared with human actors in an unannounced mass-casualty exercise. *Prehosp Disaster Med.* 2014;29(2):176–182.

92. Paige JT, Garbee DD, Kozmenko V, et al. Getting a head start: high-fidelity, simulation-based operating room team training of interprofessional students. *Journal of the American College of Surgeons.* 2014;218(1):140–149.

93. Kelly MA, Mitchell ML, Henderson A, et al. OSCE best practice guidelines-applicability for nursing simulations. *Adv Simul (Lond).* 2016;1:10.

94. Rushforth HE. Objective structured clinical examination (OSCE): review of literature and implications for nursing education. *Nurse Education Today.* 2007;27(5):481–490.

95. Turner TR, Scerbo MW, Gliva-McConvey GA, Wallace AM. Standardized patient encounters: periodic versus postencounter evaluation of nontechnical clinical performance. *Simul Healthc.* 2016;11(3):164–172.

96. Plaksin J, Nicholson J, Kundrod S, et al. The benefits and risks of being a standardized patient: a narrative review of the literature. *Patient.* 2016;9(1):15–25.

97. Peitzman SJ, Cuddy MM. Performance in physical examination on the USMLE Step 2 Clinical Skills examination. *Acad Med.* 2015;90(2):209–213.

98. Salas E, Klein C, King H, et al. Debriefing medical teams: 12 evidence-based best practices and tips. *Jt Comm J Qual Patient Saf.* 2008;34(9):518–527.

99. Bremner MN, Aduddell K, Bennett DN, Van Geest JB. The use of human patient simulators: best practices with novice nursing students. *Nurse Educ.* 2006;31(4):170–174.

100. McGaghie WC, Issenberg SB, Petrusa ER, Scalese RJ. A critical review of simulation-based medical education research: 2003-2009. *Med Educ.* 2010;44(1):50–63.

101. Cook DA, Brydges R, Zendejas B, et al. Technology-enhanced simulation to assess health professionals: a systematic review of validity evidence, research methods, and reporting quality. *Academic Medicine*. 2013;88(6):872–883.

102. International Association for Clinical Simulation and Learning. Standards of best practice: simulation: outcomes and objectives. *Clinical Simulation In Nursing*. 2016;12:S13–S15.

103. International Association for Clinical Simulation and Learning. Standards of best practice: simulation: professional integrity. *Clinical Simulation In Nursing*. 2016;12:S30–S33.

104. International Association for Clinical Simulation and Learning. Standards of best practice: simulation: facilitation. *Clinical Simulation In Nursing*. 2016;12:S16–S20.

105. International Association for Clinical Simulation and Learning. Standards of best practice: simulation: participant evaluation. *Clinical Simulation In Nursing*. 2016;12:S26–S29.

106. International Association for Clinical Simulation and Learning. Standards of best practice: simulation: debriefing. *Clinical Simulation in Nursing*. 2016;12:S21–S25.

107. International Association for Clinical Simulation and Learning. Standards of best practice: simulation: operations. *Clinical Simulation In Nursing*. 2017;13:681–687.

108. Kobayashi L, Dunbar-Viveiros JA, Devine J, et al. Pilot-phase findings from high-fidelity in situ medical simulation investigation of emergency department procedural sedation. *Simul Healthc*. 2012;7(2):81–94.

109. Siegel NA, Kobayashi L, Dunbar-Viveiros JA, et al. In situ medical simulation investigation of emergency department procedural sedation with randomized trial of experimental bedside clinical process guidance intervention. *Simul Healthc*. 2015;10(3):146–153.

110. Hadfield A, Thompson S, Hall J, Diaz-Navarro C. Perception of simulation training in emergencies for dental sedation practitioners. *Clin Teach*. 2018;15(1):52–56.

111. Johnston MJ, Paige JT, Aggarwal R, et al. An overview of research priorities in surgical simulation: what the literature shows has been achieved during the 21st century and what remains. *Am J Surg*. 2016;211(1):214–225.

112. Van Nortwick SS, Lendvay TS, Jensen AR, et al. Methodologies for establishing validity in surgical simulation studies. *Surgery*. 2010;147(5):622–630.

113. Aucar JA, Groch NR, Troxel SA, Eubanks SW. A review of surgical simulation with attention to validation methodology. *Surgical Laparoscopy, Endoscopy & Percutaneous Techniques*. 2005;15(2):82–89.

114. Farnsworth ST, Egan TD, Johnson SE, Westenskow D. Teaching sedation and analgesia with simulation. *J Clin Monit Comput*. 2000;16(4):273–285.

115. A report by the American Society of Anesthesiologists Task Force on Sedation and Analgesia by Non-Anesthesiologists. *Anesthesiology*. 1996;84(2):459–471.

116. Caperelli-White L, Urman RD. Developing a moderate sedation policy: essential elements and evidence-based considerations. *AORN J*. 2014;99(3):416–430.

117. Pisansky AJ, Beutler SS, Urman RD. Education and training for nonanesthesia providers performing deep sedation. *Curr Opin Anaesthesiol*. 2016;29(4):499–505.

118. Sauter TC, Hautz WE, Hostettler S, et al. Interprofessional and interdisciplinary simulation-based training leads to safe sedation procedures in the emergency department. *Scand J Trauma Resusc Emerg Med*. 2016;24:97.

119. O'Donnell JM, Phrampus P. Simulation in Nurse Anesthesia Education and Practice. In: Henrichs BT, JA, ed. *A Resource for Nurse Anesthesia Educators*. 2nd ed. Elsevier; 2017:261–294.

120. Blike GT, Christoffersen K, Cravero JP, Andeweg SK, Jensen J. A method for measuring system safety and latent errors associated with pediatric procedural sedation. Anesthesia & Analgesia. 2005;101(1):48–58.

121. Adler MD, Mobley BL, Eppich WJ, et al. Use of simulation to test systems and prepare staff for a new hospital transition. *J Patient Saf*. 2015.

CHAPTER 13: REVIEW QUESTIONS

1. Health care simulation education is _____.
   - A. An attempt to duplicate the clinical world exactly
   - B. A technology involving computerized mannequins
   - C. A training technique used to augment clinical experience
   - D. Untested, with no evidence of effectiveness

2. Simulation educational methods are being used _____.
   - A. Mainly in nursing education in developing countries
   - B. Only in nursing and medical education in developed nations
   - C. For 100% of clinical experiences in some professions
   - D. In nearly every country and health care profession

3. In using simulation to train for a full presedation evaluation (history and physical), the best approach would be to have students _____.
   - A. Interview each other
   - B. Engage in an extended conversation with a computerized mannequin
   - C. Interact with well-trained standardized patients
   - D. Work through an interview using a screen-based simulation program

4. Debriefing is important in simulation education because it _____.
   - A. Allows instructors to tell students about the errors in their performance
   - B. Clearly establishes the hierarchy between participants and instructors
   - C. Is where all the learning takes place during simulation
   - D. Promotes a clear understanding of individual and team performance

5. The GAS debriefing tool mnemonic stands for gather, analyze, and _____
   - A. Safety
   - B. Summarize
   - C. Specify
   - D. Status

6. Facilitation during a simulation activity typically involves which of the following?
   A. The instructor providing guidance to the participants
   B. The computerized mannequin demonstrating changes in vital signs (e.g., ECG, heart rate)
   C. Stopping the simulation to point out errors and then continuing
   D. Placing the simulator in an actual patient care setting

7. In situ simulation _____.
   A. Can be used to evaluate key safety processes in the actual care setting
   B. Is conducted in the simulation laboratory
   C. Must always include a computerized mannequin
   D. Has no demonstrated value and should not be used as a method

8. The term fidelity in relation to simulation is defined as _____.
   A. Loyalty to one type of simulator (e.g., Laerdal SimMan)
   B. The amount of learning that occurs during a particular simulation event
   C. How close the simulation is to a real clinical event
   D. The connection of the simulation event to simulation best practices

9. The use of an upper torso, head. and airway to practice ventilation and airway management skills in a simulation laboratory would typically be considered as which of the following?
   A. Partial task training
   B. High-fidelity simulation
   C. High-stakes testing
   D. In situ simulation

10. Which of the following statements is most accurate?
    A. The impact of simulation methods in sedation education is well established
    B. All aspects of a sedation simulation course should involve computerized mannequins (high fidelity)
    C. There are only a few studies that have looked at simulation for the verification of sedation skills.
    D. Sedation simulation can fully replace orientation of personnel in a procedural sedation setting

11. Design characteristics unique to an augmented reality simulation include which of the following?
    A. Use of projected displays of anatomy and physiology controlled by software in combination with physical devices
    B. Engagement in a fully immersive online simulation program in which the participant chooses an avatar (online character) to act out clinical interventions
    C. Prebriefing and debriefing of the simulation events, with stimulation of active reflection
    D. Linking of participant actions with simulated patient (mannequin or standardized patient) responses, including verbal responses and physiologic data streams (e.g., ECG, BP, HR)

12. Which of the following is (are) simulation best practices?
    A. Feedback
    B. Deliberate practice
    C. Transfer to practice
    D. All of the above

Answers can be found in Appendix A.

Care of the Moderate Procedural Sedation and Analgesia Patient: Unfolding Clinical Case Study

LEARNING OUTCOMES

At the completion of this chapter, the learner shall:
- Identify select components of preprocedural, procedural, and postprocedural patient care associated with moderate procedural sedation and analgesia.
- State competency requirements for the professional administering or monitoring the patient receiving moderate sedation and analgesia.

- Identify the indications, side effects, and clinical pharmacology associated with sedative, hypnotic, and analgesic medications administered in the moderate procedural sedation and analgesia settings.

Nurse educators may use this unfolding case scenario to assess staff members' clinical development.

Staff members: Please complete the first section of the chapter by answering all questions.

Nurse educators: Review the unfolding clinical case scenario after your staff member completes it by comparing his or her answers to the provided rationales featured at the end of this chapter.

STAFF MEMBERS: COMPLETE THE UNFOLDING CLINICAL CASE STUDY BELOW

Molly, a registered nurse, recently accepted a transfer from the emergency department to the moderate procedural sedation and analgesia patient care team. The human resources department requires the following competencies:
- Advanced Cardiac Life Support (ACLS) course completion
  - Online course content completion
  - Skills station competency verification
- Pediatric Advanced Life Support (PALS) course completion
  - Online course content completion
  - Skills station competency verification
- Venipuncture
  - Online learning module course completion
- Pharmacology competencies
  - Sedation unit orientation week
- Procedural patient care competencies
  - Sedation unit orientation week
- Postprocedure patient care competencies
  - Sedation unit orientation week

Exercise 1 (Short Essay)

Identify any concerns associated with the facility's onboarding process for Molly.

1. _____
2. _____
3. _____

Molly arrived at the hospital early for her first day as a sedation nurse. She was told to report to the interventional platform. The nursing supervisor informed her that there were two call-outs for the day. Molly was instructed "to go and orient in the GI suite." Although Molly was new to the unit, she noted that most of the day's GI patients could not be easily aroused. They did not respond purposefully to repeated or painful stimulation and could not maintain a patent airway independently. Ventilatory function was impaired. However, cardiovascular function was maintained.

Exercise 2 (Select the Appropriate Response)

At the end of the day, Molly met with the unit's nurse educator. After a lengthy discussion regarding the levels of sedation, Molly recognized that her attending physician had been maintaining patients in a state of _____ for their GI procedures.
☐ Minimal sedation
☐ Moderate sedation
☐ Deep sedation
☐ General anesthesia

As orientation to the sedation unit progressed, the nurse manager informed Molly that all sedation unit policies and procedures were created using the American Society of

Anesthesiologists (ASA) Practice Guidelines for Moderate Procedural Sedation and Analgesia 2018.[1]

Exercise 3 (Select the Appropriate Response)

Molly's appropriate response to the nurse manager should have included the following information:

☐ Inform the nurse manager that the current policies and procedures are based on current information and guidelines.

☐ Request that the nurse manager appoint a committee to update hospital sedation policies and procedures based on the 2018 practice guidelines for moderate procedural sedation and analgesia.[1]

☐ Defer all decisions to the attending physician of choice regarding levels of sedation and appropriate monitoring strategies.

☐ Defer decision-making authority related to sedation policy and procedure development to the Hospital Chair, Department of Anesthesia.

After a lengthy conversation, the nurse manager and Molly discussed deferring to the state board of nursing regarding the administration of procedural sedation by nurses within their state for additional guidance. After reviewing the Nurse Practice Act together, they recognize that it permits registered nurses within their state to provide the following level of procedural sedation:

• A drug-induced depression of consciousness during which patients respond purposefully to verbal commands, either alone or accompanied by light tactile stimulation. No interventions are required to maintain a patent airway, and spontaneous ventilation is adequate. Cardiovascular function is usually maintained.

Exercise 4 (Fill in the Blank)

The definition outlined above is identified as _____.

After 3 weeks of employment, Molly noticed that many of the patients receiving moderate procedural sedation drift between levels of sedation. Meeting criteria of various levels of sedation occurs secondary to each patient's response to sedative and analgesic medications based on the medication administered, dosage, technique of administration, and presence of concomitant disease states.

Exercise 5 (Select the Appropriate Response)

The rationale for alternating between the various levels of sedation (minimal, moderate, deep) is defined as the _____.

☐ Variety of sedative states
☐ Criteria for sedation
☐ Lability of sedation
☐ Continuum of sedation

The goals of moderate procedural sedation and analgesia may vary based on procedural requirements, prescribing physician preference, and sedation technique selected. One of our emergency department (ED) physicians recently provided an in-service to our staff and mentioned that the goal of moderate sedation in the ED is to produce an unconscious patient. One of the nurses questioned this practice and was told that EDs may provide deep sedation and general anesthesia for diagnostic or therapeutic procedures.

Exercise 6 (Select All That Apply)

Based on the definitions of moderate procedural sedation and analgesia, the above statement is false; the actual goals include the following:

☐ Maintaining ventilator rate at < 10 breaths/min
☐ Maintaining patient safety and welfare
☐ Minimizing physical pain and discomfort
☐ Providing a state of anxiolysis
☐ Guaranteeing an amnestic state for the duration of the procedure
☐ Controlling behavior and movement to allow safe performance of procedures

Emmie is the nurse assigned to a 49-year-old male patient named Will who presents to the ED. Physician evaluation and radiologic imaging confirm that the patient has a shoulder disclocation requiring reduction. Procedural sedation and analgesia is ordered to assist with the reduction process. Emmie is a relatively new nurse to the ED and has not completed the procedural sedation and analgesia education competency verification required per hospital policy and procedure. Bringing this to the charge nurse's attention, she is informed that the department is short-staffed. Tyler, the ED nurse manager, reiterates "just get in there, give the meds and let them pop the shoulder back; it's no big deal."

Exercise 7 (Short Essay)

Based on knowledge of hospital sedation policy and procedure and state board of nursing requirements, Emmie's appropriate response to Tyler's directive includes the following:

1. _____
2. _____
3. _____

Emmie refused to administer or monitor the patient receiving procedural sedation for the shoulder reduction. However, her initial nursing assessment revealed another potential risk factor for the patient scheduled for shoulder reduction.

Exercise 8 (Select the Appropriate Response)

The patient's body mass index (BMI) on admission is 31, classifying him as _____.

☐ Underweight
☐ Normal weight
☐ Overweight
☐ Obese

An experienced sedation provider would recognize that obesity predisposes the patient to increased morbidity during the administration of moderate procedural sedation and analgesia.

Exercise 9 (Select All That Apply)

The multisystemic effects of obesity include the following:
☐ Increased carbon dioxide production
☐ Decreased oxygen consumption
☐ Decreased work of breathing
☐ Increased intraabdominal pressure
☐ Increased risk of aspiration
☐ Decreased stroke volume
☐ Decreased pulmonary compliance

Another nurse was assigned to complete the presedation patient assessment and prepare the patient for shoulder reduction. Vital signs on initial assessment included the following:

$$Heart\ rate = 92$$

$$Blood\ pressure = 146/92\ \ mm\ Hg$$

$$Oxygen\ saturation = 94\%$$

Exercise 10 (Select the Appropriate Response)

Proper classification of the patient's blood pressure is

_____.

☐ Normal
☐ Elevated
☐ Stage I, high blood pressure
☐ Stage II, high blood pressure

Exercise 11 (Short Essay)

Presedation concerns associated with the hypertensive patient presenting with a long-standing history of hypertension include the following:

1. _____
2. _____
3. _____
4. _____

During further review of systems, the patient revealed that he currently sees an endocrinologist, who is attempting to "regulate my thyroid gland." The patient confirmed that he continued to have intolerance to cold and bradycardia. A chest x-ray revealed slight cardiomegaly. These symptoms confirmed the ongoing presence of hypothyroidism.

Exercise 12 (True or False)

It is important to inform the physician prescribing moderate procedural sedation and analgesia medications about these particular findings because hypothyroid patients frequently demonstrate a decreased sensitivity to anxiolytic, sedative, and analgesic medications.
☐ True
☐ False

Completing the presedation assessment, the attending physician, Dr. Ella inquired about the patient's social history.

The patient stated that he "currently did not use any illicit substances." However, "I do smoke cigarettes … three packs a day, and I have been smoking for about 21 years."

Exercise 13 (Select the Appropriate Response)

Summarizing the presedation assessment, the patient's pack-year smoking history was recorded as _____ pack-years.
☐ 21
☐ 42
☐ 63
☐ 85

Exercise 14 (Short Essay)

A comprehensive metabolic profile revealed that the patient's albumin and plasma proteins are significantly decreased. Upon reviewing the plan of sedation care with the attending physician, the nurse discussed the pharmacologic ramifications associated with administering procedural sedation and analgesia to a patient with decreased protein levels. These pharmacologic and patient care considerations include:

1. _____
2. _____
3. _____
4. _____

Prior to administering sedation for the procedure, the physician engaged the nurse in a pharmacodynamics discussion and asked, "What are all the medications that work on the GABA site?"

Exercise 15 (Select All That Apply)

A knowledgeable sedation provider would identify the following medications that exert their pharmacologic effect on the gamma-amino butyric acid (GABA) receptor complex:
☐ Benzodiazepines
☐ Opioids
☐ Alkylphenols
☐ Dissociatives
☐ Local anesthetics

As the procedure commenced, the patient became bradycardic (heart rate = 54 beats/min) and was complaining of pain. The physician ordering the procedural sedation stated, "Please administer a narcotic that does not cause bradycardia."

Exercise 16 (Select All That Apply)

Which of the following opioids cause bradycardia?
☐ Fentanyl
☐ Sufentanil
☐ Alfentanil
☐ Morphine
☐ Demerol

After additional opioid was administered, the patient's respiratory rate decreased to three breaths/min. The opioid antagonist naloxone (Narcan) was ordered by the proceduralist.

Exercise 17 (Select the Appropriate Response)

The appropriate dose of intravenous naloxone to reverse respiratory depression associated with opioid administration is _____.

☐ 0.2 mg
☐ 0.4 mg
☐ 1 to 4 micrograms per kilogram
☐ 4 to 8 micrograms per kilogram

Exercise 18 (Select All That Apply)

In the event that naloxone does not "chemically reverse" the respiratory depressant effects associated with opioid administration, which of the following respiratory events may occur?

☐ Respiratory insufficiency
☐ Upper airway obstruction
☐ Respiratory arrest
☐ Pulmonary aspiration

The patient responded to the administration of naloxone. Vital signs following naloxone administration include the following:

$$\text{Heart rate} = 68 \text{ beats/min}$$

$$\text{Blood pressure} = 134/85 \text{ mm Hg}$$

$$\text{Oxygen saturation} = 96\%$$

Exercise 19 (Fill in the Blank)

Will, the sedation provider noted at the conclusion of the procedure that the patient had some preexisting physical signs that could predispose him to difficult airway management. In the event that naloxone did not reverse the respiratory depressant effects and the patient obstructed, identify three characteristics on physical examination that may predispose the patient to difficult airway management.

1. _____
2. _____
3. _____

Anesthesia was called to evaluate the patient after further radiologic evaluation revealed that surgery was required to reduce a forearm fracture. Prior to leaving, the anesthesia provider stated that the patient had a Mallampati class IV airway.

Exercise 20 (True or False)

A Mallampati class IV airway indicates that the patient would be an easy intubation, generally requiring minimal effort.

☐ True
☐ False

A last minute decision was made to postpone the surgery until the next morning. Prior to sending the patient to the medical surgical floor, the following level of care is required:

• Focused postsedation patient care to prepare the patient for additional inpatient care, discharge to self-care, or care to be provided by another caregiver

Exercise 21 (Select the Appropriate Response)

The level of postsedation care outlined above is defined as

_____.

☐ Phase I
☐ Phase II
☐ Phase III
☐ Phase IV

Exercise 22 (Short Essay)

The patient satisfactorily scored out of the postsedation phase of care. Preparation was being made to hand off the patient to the medical surgical nursing unit. Delineate the specific benefits associated with incorporating handoff mnemonics in clinical practice.

1. _____
2. _____
3. _____

NURSE EDUCATORS: UNFOLDING CLINICAL CASE STUDY RATIONALES

Note: Answers and rationales are shown in **bold**.

Molly, a registered nurse, recently accepted a transfer from the ED to the moderate procedural sedation and analgesia patient care team. The Human Resource Department requires the following competencies:

- ACLS course completion
  - Online course content completion
  - Skills station competency verification
- PALS course completion
  - Online course content completion
  - Skills station competency verification
- Venipuncture
  - Online learning module course completion
- Pharmacology competencies
  - Sedation unit orientation week
- Procedural patient care competencies
  - Sedation unit orientation week
- Postprocedure patient care competencies
  - Sedation unit orientation week

Exercise 1 (Short Essay)

Identify any concerns associated with the facility's onboarding process for Molly.

Part of the onboarding process for Molly must also include familiarizing herself with individual state board of nursing requirements related to moderate procedural sedation and analgesia patient care. Laws by state related to the administration of moderate procedural sedation and analgesia for registered nurses may be reviewed at the following websites: https://sedationcertification.com/resources/position-statements/position-statements-by-state/clickable-map and http://www.sedationconsulting.com/laws-by-state.

Clinical practice standards, guidelines, and position statements also need to be reviewed by Molly because they form the basis for hospital sedation policy. Hospital policy and procedure related to moderate procedural sedation patient care must be understood prior to providing direct patient care. The pursuit of best sedation practice in the interest of patient safety should be reflected in Molly's human resource department expanded credentialing process to ensure that she receives the required education and meets the requisite moderate procedural sedation and analgesia qualifications for her new position.

Molly arrived at the hospital early for her first day as a sedation nurse. She was told to report to the interventional platform. The nursing supervisor informed her that there were two call-outs for the day. Molly was instructed "to go and orient in the GI suite." Although Molly was new to the unit, she noted that most of the day's GI patients could not be easily aroused. They did not respond purposefully to repeated or painful stimulation and could not maintain a patent airway independently. Ventilatory function was impaired. However, cardiovascular function was maintained.

Exercise 2 (Select the Appropriate Response)

At the end of the day, Molly met with the unit's nurse educator. After a lengthy discussion regarding the levels of sedation, Molly recognized that her attending physician had been maintaining patients in a state of _____ for their GI procedures.

- ☐ Minimal sedation
- ☐ Moderate sedation
- ☐ Deep sedation
- ☐ General anesthesia

The goals of moderate procedural sedation and analgesia may vary based on procedural requirements, prescribing physician preference, and sedation technique selected. Regardless of the variables outlined above, the primary goal of moderate procedural sedation and analgesia include administering the lowest dose of medication to do the following:

- **Maintain patient safety and welfare.**
- **Minimize physical pain and discomfort.**
- **Control anxiety, minimize psychological trauma, and maximize amnesia.**
- **Control behavior and movement to allow safe performance of procedures.**

The term *moderate procedural sedation and analgesia* **is defined as a drug-induced depression of consciousness during which patients respond purposefully to verbal commands, either alone or accompanied by light tactile stimulation. No interventions are required to maintain a patent airway, and spontaneous ventilation is adequate. Cardiovascular function is usually maintained. The goal of the attending physician should be focused on maintaining a state of moderate sedation. Deep sedation or general anesthesia may predispose the patient to an increased incidence of respiratory depression, decreased response to the hypoxic drive, and the potential for cardiovascular depression. It is critically important to recognize that deep levels of sedation are not the objectives of moderate procedural sedation and analgesia.**

As orientation to the sedation unit progressed, the nurse manager informed Molly that all sedation unit policies and procedures were created using the (ASA) Practice Guidelines for Moderate Procedural Sedation and Analgesia 2018.[1]

Exercise 3 (Select the Appropriate Response)

Molly's appropriate response to the nurse manager should have included the following information:

- ☐ Inform the nurse manager that the current policies and procedures are based on current information and guidelines.
- ☐ **Request that the nurse manager appoint a committee to update hospital sedation policies and procedures based on the 2018 practice guidelines for moderate procedural sedation and analgesia.[2]**
- ☐ Defer all decisions to the attending physician of choice regarding levels of sedation and appropriate monitoring strategies.
- ☐ Defer decision-making authority related to sedation policy and procedure development to the Hospital Chair, Department of Anesthesia.

In October 2014, the ASA Committee on Standards and Practice Parameters recommended that updated practice guidelines addressing moderate procedural sedation and analgesia be developed; these were published in March 2018. These updated guidelines replaced the 2002 practice guidelines for sedation and analgesia by nonanesthesiologists.[1] The 2018 sedation guidelines were developed by a multidisciplinary task force of physicians from several medical and dental specialty organizations and specifically addressed moderate procedural sedation provided by any medical specialty in any location. These updated guidelines include new recommendations that addressed the following:

- Patient evaluation and preparation
- Continual monitoring of ventilatory function with capnography to supplement standard monitoring by observation and pulse oximetry
- The presence of an individual in the procedure room with the knowledge and skills to recognize and treat airway complications
- Sedatives and analgesics not intended for general anesthesia (e.g., benzodiazepines, dexmedetomidine)
- Sedatives and analgesics intended for general anesthesia (e.g., propofol, ketamine, etomidate)
- Recovery care
- Creation and implementation of quality improvement processes

After a lengthy conversation, the nurse manager and Molly discussed deferring to the state board of nursing regarding the administration of procedural sedation by nurses in their state for additional guidance. After reviewing the Nurse Practice Act together, they recognized that it permits registered nurses in their state to provide the following level of procedural sedation:

- A drug-induced depression of consciousness during which patients respond purposefully to verbal commands, either alone or accompanied by light tactile stimulation. No interventions are required to maintain a patent airway, and spontaneous ventilation is adequate. Cardiovascular function is usually maintained.

Exercise 4 (Fill in the Blank)

The definition outlined above is identified as **moderate sedation and analgesia or procedural sedation and analgesia.**

After 3 weeks of employment, Molly noticed that many of the patients receiving moderate procedural sedation drift between levels of sedation. Meeting criteria of various levels of sedation occurs secondary to each patient's response to sedative and analgesic medications based on the medication administered, dosage, technique of administration, and presence of concomitant disease states.

Exercise 5 (Select the Appropriate Response)

The rationale for alternating between the various levels of sedation (minimal, moderate, deep) is defined as the

☐ Variety of sedative states
☐ Criteria for sedation
☐ Lability of sedation
☐ **Continuum of sedation**

Because sedation is a continuum, it is not always possible to predict how an individual patient will respond. Hence, practitioners intending to produce a given level of sedation should be able to rescue patients whose level of sedation becomes deeper than initially intended. Rescue of a patient from a deeper level of sedation than intended is an intervention by a practitioner who is proficient in airway management and advanced life support. The qualified practitioner corrects adverse physiologic consequences of the deeper than intended level of sedation (e.g., hypoventilation, hypoxia, hypotension) and returns the patient to the originally intended level of sedation. It is not appropriate to continue the procedure at an unintended level of sedation.

The goals of moderate procedural sedation and analgesia may vary based on procedural requirements, prescribing physician preference, and sedation technique selected. One of our ED physicians, Dr. Tyler recently provided an in-service to our staff and mentioned that the goal of moderate sedation in the ED is to produce an unconscious patient. One of the nurses questioned this practice and was told that EDs may provide deep sedation and general anesthesia for diagnostic or therapeutic procedures.

Exercise 6 (Select All That Apply)

Based on the definitions of moderate procedural sedation and analgesia, the above statement is false; the actual goals include the following:

☐ Maintaining ventilator rate at < 10 breaths/min
☐ **Maintaining patient safety and welfare**
☐ **Minimizing physical pain and discomfort**
☐ **Providing a state of anxiolysis**
☐ Guaranteeing an amnestic state for the duration of the procedure
☐ Controlling behavior and movement to allow safe performance of procedures

Emmie is the nurse assigned to a 49-year-old male patient named Will who presents to the ED. Physician evaluation and radiologic imaging confirm that the patient has a shoulder dislocation requiring reduction. Procedural sedation and analgesia is ordered to assist with the reduction process. Emmie is a relatively new nurse to the ED and has not completed the procedural sedation and analgesia education competency verification required per hospital policy and procedure. Bringing this to the charge nurse's attention, she is informed that the department is short-staffed. Tyler, the ED nurse manager reiterates "just get in there, give the meds and let them pop the shoulder back; it's no big deal."

Exercise 7 (Short Essay)

Based on knowledge of hospital sedation policy and procedure and respective state board of nursing, Emmie's appropriate response to Tyler's directive includes the following:

The best course of action for the clinical scenario outlined includes Emmie reiterating to her nurse manager that she has not completed the required educational components as outlined by the hospital sedation and analgesia policy and procedure.

An offer to switch patient assignments may be an effective solution to de-escalate the situation outlined.

Emmie refused to administer or monitor the patient receiving procedural sedation for the shoulder reduction. However, her initial nursing assessment revealed another potential risk factor for the patient scheduled for shoulder reduction.

Exercise 8 (Select the Appropriate Response)

The patient's body mass index (BMI) on admission is 31, classifying him as _____.
- ☐ Underweight
- ☐ Normal weight
- ☐ Overweight
- ☐ **Obese**

BMI is calculated as follows:

$$BMI = weight(lb)/[height(inches)]^2 \times 703$$

Calculate BMI by dividing weight in pounds (lb) by height in inches squared and multiplying by a conversion factor of 703.

Example:

$$Weight = 150 \ lb$$
$$Height = 5'5''(65'')$$

Calculation: $(150 \div [65])^2) \times 703 = 24.96$

Body mass index weight status includes the following metrics:

Below 18.5—Underweight
18.5–24.9—Normal or healthy weight
25.0–29.9—Overweight
30.0 and above—Obese

An experienced sedation provider would recognize that obesity predisposes the patient to increased morbidity during the administration of moderate procedural sedation and analgesia.

Exercise 9 (Select All That Apply)

The multisystemic effects of obesity include the following:
- ☐ **Increased carbon dioxide production**
- ☐ **Decreased oxygen consumption**
- ☐ Decreased work of breathing
- ☐ **Increased intraabdominal pressure**
- ☐ Increased risk of aspiration
- ☐ Decreased stroke volume
- ☐ **Decreased pulmonary compliance**

Another nurse was assigned to complete the presedation patient assessment and prepare the patient for shoulder reduction. Vital signs on initial assessment included the following:

$$Heart \ rate = 92 \ beats/min$$
$$Blood \ pressure = 146/92 \ mm \ Hg$$
$$Oxygen \ saturation = 94\%$$

Exercise 10 (Select the Appropriate Response)

Proper classification of the patient's blood pressure is _____.
- ☐ Normal
- ☐ Elevated
- ☐ Stage I, high blood pressure
- ☐ **Stage II, high blood pressure**

High blood pressure used to be defined as 140/90 mm Hg. The new blood pressure guidelines, published in November 2017 by the American College of Cardiology, were designed to help people take steps to control their blood pressure earlier in the disease process.[3] High blood pressure is a major risk factor for heart disease and stroke, the two leading causes of death in the world. The guideline change now recognizes 46% of the US adult population as having high blood pressure, compared with 32% under the previous definition. Classification of systemic blood pressure for adults is shown in Table 14.1.

TABLE 14.1	Systemic Blood Pressure (BP) for Adults		
Category	Systolic (mm Hg)	Diastolic (mm Hg)	Recommendations
Normal	<120	Less than 80	Healthy lifestyle choices and yearly checks
Elevated blood pressure	120–129 or	Less than 80	Healthy lifestyle changes, reassessed in 3–6 months
High blood pressure, stage 1	130–139 or	80–89	10-year heart disease and stroke risk assessment; if <10% risk, lifestyle changes, reassessed in 3–6 months; if higher, lifestyle changes and medication, with monthly follow-ups until BP is controlled
High blood pressure, stage 2	≥140 or	≥90	Lifestyle changes and two different classes of medicine, with monthly follow-ups until BP is controlled

Exercise 11 (Short Essay)

Presedation concerns associated with the hypertensive patient presenting with a long-standing history of hypertension include the following:

1. **Duration of hypertension**
2. **Effectiveness of prescribed treatment plan**
3. **Identification of medication and dosage used to treat hypertension**
4. **Identification of the patient's presedation anxiety level**

During further review of systems, the patient revealed that he currently sees an endocrinologist, who is attempting to "regulate my thyroid gland." The patient confirmed that he continued to have intolerance to cold and bradycardia. The chest x-ray revealed slight cardiomegaly. These symptoms confirmed the ongoing presence of hypothyroidism.

Exercise 12 (True or False)

It is important to inform the physician prescribing moderate procedural sedation and analgesia medications about these particular findings because hypothyroid patients frequently demonstrate a decreased sensitivity to anxiolytic, sedative, and analgesic medications.

☐ True
☐ False

Hypothyroid patients generally have a marked or increased sensitivity to intravenous sedatives, analgesics, and hypnotics. Hypothyroidism also reduces the ventilatory response to $Paco_2$ and Pao_2. This marked sensitivity requires a reduction in the dose of sedative and analgesic medications administered to the patient. Careful titration of sedatives, analgesics, and hypnotics is required because even markedly reduced doses have resulted in profound central nervous system (CNS) and respiratory depression.

Completing the presedation assessment, the nurse inquired about the patient's social history. The patient stated that he "currently did not use any illicit substances." However, "I do smoke cigarettes … three packs a day, and I have been smoking for about 21 years."

Exercise 13 (Select the Appropriate Response)

Summarizing the presedation assessment, the patient's pack-year smoking history was recorded as _____ pack-years.

☐ 21
☐ 42
☐ **63**
☐ 85

A tobacco use history is best quantified in pack-years and documented on the presedation assessment form:

> Pack-years = number of packs smoked per day
> multiplied by the number of years smoked

Patients with a smoking history present a multitude of physiologic changes for the sedation provider to consider. The inhaled components of smoke are associated with the development of coronary artery disease, peripheral vascular disease, cerebrovascular disease, stroke, chronic obstructive pulmonary disease (COPD), peptic ulcer disease, esophageal reflux, and lung cancer. Nicotine produces an increase in heart rate, blood pressure, myocardial contraction, myocardial oxygen consumption, and myocardial excitement. These sympathetic nervous system changes are undesirable in a patient presenting for moderate procedural sedation who may already be apprehensive and anxious. Whenever possible, patients should be counseled to consider cessation of smoking 12 to 48 hours prior to the procedure. Even short-term smoking cessation (12 hours) prior to the planned procedure has been shown to reduce the deleterious effects of nicotine and carbon monoxide on cardiopulmonary function, resulting in a reduced heart rate, blood pressure, and circulating catecholamine levels. Additionally, the moderate procedural sedation practitioner caring for the pediatric patient subjected to second-hand smoke must be prepared to handle complications associated with children who are exposed to passive smoke. These complications include increased reactive airway disease, abnormal pulmonary function tests, increased respiratory tract infection, laryngospasm, and postsedation oxygen desaturation.

Exercise 14 (Short Essay)

A comprehensive metabolic profile revealed that the patient's albumin and plasma protein levels are significantly decreased. On reviewing the plan of sedation care with the attending physician, the nurse discussed the pharmacologic ramifications associated with administering procedural sedation and analgesia to a patient with decreased protein levels. These pharmacologic and patient care considerations include the following:

1. **Patients with nutritional disorders, carcinoma, recent weight loss, renal disease, or decreased plasma protein levels may demonstrate enhanced or exaggerated effects from pharmacologic adjuncts used to achieve a state of sedation or analgesia.**
2. **Patients with decreased plasma proteins or physical conditions associated with altered plasma proteins require careful titration of all CNS depressant medications.**
3. **Small incremental doses, administered slowly over several minutes, allow the clinician the ability to assess the pharmacologic effects of the medication fully.**

Prior to administering sedation for the procedure, the physician engaged the nurse in a pharmacodynamics discussion and asked, "What are all the medications that work on the GABA site?"

Exercise 15 (Select All That Apply)

A knowledgeable sedation provider would identify the following medications that exert their pharmacologic effect on the GABA receptor complex.

Benzodiazepines. Benzodiazepines bind to specific receptor sites in the CNS within the GABA receptor complex. This binding does not result in opening of the chloride ion channel, but potentiates opening in response to GABA. GABA therefore triggers a burst of channel openings, and these bursts increase in number if additional receptor sites are concurrently activated by benzodiazepines.

Opioids. Opioids do not work on the GABA receptor complex. The administration of opioids results in binding to specific opiate receptors located within the central nervous system. Opioids occupy mu, delta, and kappa receptor subtypes and produce analgesia, drowsiness, and mood alteration. The pharmacologic effects of opioids depend on the specific receptor subtypes stimulated. Opioids suppress pain by their action in the brain, spinal cord, and peripheral nervous system through their pharmacologic effect on the mu, delta, and kappa receptor subtypes,

Alkylphenols. Propofol exerts its pharmacologic effect at the GABA receptor complex. Through an interaction at this GABA receptor complex, opening of the chloride ion channel results in hyperpolarization of cell membranes. Neuroinhibition in the central nervous system is produced, resulting in sedation, hypnosis, and unconsciousness. Additional pharmacodynamic research on propofol has revealed that it produces widespread inhibition of the *N*-methyl-D-aspartate (NMDA) subtype of glutamate receptor through modulation of sodium channel gating, an action that also may contribute to the drug's CNS effects. Additional pharmacodynamic effects associated with propofol use include the following:

- Direct depressant effect on neurons of the spinal cord
- Increase in dopamine concentrations in the nucleus accumbens
- Decreased serotonin levels in the area postrema, resulting in an antiemetic effect

Dissociatives. Dissociative anesthetic agents do not work at the GABA receptor complex. Ketamine (Ketalar, Ketaject) is a derivative of phencyclidine that produces a dissociative state. In subanesthetic doses, ketamine provides profound analgesia. Ketamine yields dissociative anesthetic effects secondary to antagonistic actions at the phencyclidine site of the NMDA receptor (NMDAR). NMDAR is a glutamate receptor and ion channel protein found in nerve cells. Characteristic appearance of the dissociative state includes the following:

- Intense analgesia
- Cataleptic state
- Nystagmus
- Open-eyed gaze
- Noncommunicative patient
- Skeletal muscle movement

Local Anesthetics. Local anesthetics do not work at the GABA receptor complex. Local anesthetics prevent the development of the action potential required for depolarization of nerve cells by blocking sodium channels. For transmission of impulses to occur, movement of sodium and potassium ions via these channels is required. Depolarization occurs when sodium ions move from extracellular fluid to the intracellular space. Repolarization occurs when potassium ions move from the intracellular to the extracellular space.

As the procedure commenced, the patient became bradycardic (heart rate = 54 beats/min) and was complaining of pain. The physician ordering the procedural sedation stated, "Please administer a narcotic that does not cause bradycardia."

Exercise 16 (Select All That Apply)

Which of the following opioids cause bradycardia?
- ☐ **Fentanyl**
- ☐ **Sufentanil**
- ☐ **Alfentanil**
- ☐ Morphine
- ☐ Demerol

Opioids alter the cardiovascular system through a variety of physiologic mechanisms. With the exception of meperidine and the fentanyl derivatives, opioids are devoid of major cardiovascular effects. Meperidine produces tachycardia because of its vagolytic effect. In comparison, fentanyl derivatives (fentanyl, sufentanil, alfentanil) produce a vagally mediated bradycardia. Blood pressure may decrease secondary to bradycardia, decreased systemic vascular resistance, and alterations in the sympathetic nervous system. Meperidine and morphine sulfate release histamine, which may significantly decrease systemic vascular resistance and produce bronchoconstriction.

After additional opioid was administered, the patient's respiratory rate decreased to 3 breaths/min. The opioid antagonist naloxone (Narcan) was ordered by the proceduralist.

Exercise 17 (Select the Appropriate Response)

The appropriate dose of intravenous naloxone to reverse respiratory depression associated with opioid administration is _____.
- ☐ 0.2 mg
- ☐ 0.4 mg
- ☐ **1 to 4 micrograms per kilogram**
- ☐ 4 to 8 micrograms per kilogram

The CNS and respiratory depressant effects of opioids can be reversed with the administration of naloxone (Narcan). As identified in Fig. 4.4 (see Chapter 4), naloxone is a pure opioid antagonist that competitively binds at the opiate receptor site. One to 4 mcg, titrated in 0.1-mg increments, promptly reverses opioid-induced analgesia and depression of ventilation.

Exercise 18 (Select All That Apply)

In the event that naloxone does not chemically reverse the respiratory depressant effects associated with opioid administration, which of the following respiratory events may occur?
- ☐ **Respiratory insufficiency**
- ☐ Upper airway obstruction
- ☐ Respiratory arrest
- ☐ Pulmonary aspiration

Binding to the mu receptor results in respiratory depression. The ventilatory response associated with the administration of procedural opioids may lead to increased arterial carbon dioxide levels, decreased response to carbon

dioxide, decreased respiratory rate, and increased minute ventilation (dose dependent).

The patient responded to the administration of naloxone. Vital signs following naloxone administration include the following:

$$Heart\ rate = 68\ beats/min$$

$$Blood\ pressure = 134/85\ mm\ Hg$$

$$Oxygen\ saturation = 96\%$$

Exercise 19 (Fill in the Blank)

At the conclusion of the procedure, the nurse noted that the patient had some preexisting physical signs that could predispose him to difficult airway management. In the event that naloxone did not reverse the respiratory depressant effects, and the patient obstructed, identify three characteristics on physical examination that may predispose the patient to difficult airway management.

There are a variety of characteristics that may assist in identifying a difficult airway management patient. In the assessment of the temporomandibular joint (TMJ, interincisor distance) is conducted with the patient's mouth opened as wide as possible. In the adult, the distance between the upper and lower central incisors is normally 4 to 6 cm (2.54 cm = 1 inch). An adult should be able to open the mouth at least 40 cm (two large fingerbreadths) between the upper and lower incisors. An interincisor gap of less than two fingerbreadths may be associated with difficult endotracheal intubation. The presence of a clicking sound, pain associated with opening of the mouth, or a reduced ability to open the mouth indicates reduced TMJ mobility. Patients with preexisting TMJ disease may have limited airway mobility if mechanical conduits (e.g., oropharyngeal airway, endotracheal tube, laryngeal mask airway) are required to treat respiratory distress during procedural sedation care.

Another airway assessment technique measures thyromental distance. Thyromental distance is the distance between the prominence of the thyroid cartilage and the bony point of the lower mandibular border; it should be more than 7 cm (three fingerbreadths). A distance of less than 7 cm may indicate that the patient may be difficult to intubate if needed during an airway emergency secondary to the inability to align the oral, pharyngeal, and laryngeal access, which is required for direct visualization and intubation of the larynx.

Additionally, side to side movement, neck extension, and neck flexion must be assessed prior to the procedure. Alignment of the three axes required for successful endotracheal intubation (oral, pharyngeal, laryngeal) requires a combination of flexion and extension with a goal of attainment of the so-called sniffing position. Limitations in the ability to achieve this position can impair laryngoscopy and endotracheal intubation during emergency airway maneuvers. Additional physical characteristics that may indicate the potential for difficult airway management include the following:

1. Hyponathic (recessed) jaw
2. Hypernathic (protruding) jaw
3. Deviated trachea
4. Large tongue
5. Short, thick neck
6. Protruding teeth
7. High arched palate

Anesthesia was called to evaluate the patient after further radiologic evaluation revealed that surgery was required to reduce a forearm fracture. Prior to leaving, the anesthesia provider stated that the patient had a Mallampati class IV airway.

Exercise 20 (True or False)

A Mallampati airway class IV indicates that the patient would be an easy intubation, generally requiring minimal effort.

☐ True

☐ **False**

The modified Mallampati airway classification system, described in 1983, attempts to grade the degree of difficulty of endotracheal intubation from grade I to IV. The examination is conducted with the patient in a sitting position. The patient's head is maintained in a neutral position and the mouth is opened as wide as possible (50–60 mm). Classification of the patient's airway is based on a description of the anatomic area visualized; see Table 14.3.

Decreased visualization of anatomic landmarks correlates with the anticipated difficulty of airway management or endotracheal intubation.[3] After physical examination of the patient's airway, a Mallampati score of 4 led the anesthesia provider to the assumption that the patient is a potentially "difficult airway."

A last minute decision was made to postpone the surgery until the next morning. Prior to sending the patient to the medical surgical floor, the following level of care is required:

- Focused postsedation patient care to prepare the patient for additional inpatient care, discharge to self-care, or care to be provided by another caregiver

TABLE 14.3	Classification of the Patient's Airway
Mallampati Classification	**Visualization**
Class I	Soft palate, fauces, anterior pillar and posterior pillar
Class II	Soft palate, fauces, and entire uvula
Class III	Soft palate and base of uvula
Class IV	Hard palate only; soft palate not visible

Exercise 21 (Select the Appropriate Response):

The level of postsedation care outlined above is defined as _____.

☐ Phase I

☐ **Phase II**

☐ Phase III

☐ Phase IV

There are two phases of postsedation or postanesthesia care. These include the following.

Phase I. The patient is required to be closely monitored and continuously assessed as he or she returns to presedation physiologic status. Phase I postsedation patients should never be left unattended. Nursing care remains focused on ensuring that the patient maintains a patent airway, demonstrates hemodynamic stability, recovers with manageable pain levels, and successfully returns to a presedation cognitive level.

Phase II. Phase II postsedation care focuses on preparing the patient for additional inpatient care, discharge to self-care, or care to be provided by another caregiver.

Exercise 22 (Short Essay)

The patient satisfactorily scored out of the postsedation phase of care. Preparation was being made to hand off the patient to the medical surgical nursing unit. Delineate the specific benefits associated with incorporating handoff mnemonics in clinical practice.

Improved handoffs, which incorporate a variety of evidence-based mnemonics, tools, forms, and checklists, are available for use in the sedation setting. A number of mnemonics are available in clinical practice, such as the following:

- **I PASS THE BATON**
- **I PUT PATIENTS FIRST**
- **PATIENT**
- **SBAR**
- **ISBAR**

An effective mnemonic example is **I PUT PATIENTS FIRST**, which serves as a guideline to improve the effectiveness of the handover process from the operating room to the intensive care unit. **I PUT PATIENTS FIRST** can standardize the handoff process and serve as an educational tool for all health care providers.

REFERENCES

1. Practice Guidelines for Moderate Procedural Sedation and Analgesia 2018: A Report by the American Society of Anesthesiologists Task Force on Moderate Procedural Sedation and Analgesia, the American Association of Oral and Maxillofacial Surgeons, American College of Radiology, American Dental Association, American Society of Dentist Anesthesiologists, and Society of Interventional Radiology. *Anesthesiology*. 2018;128(3):437–479.

2. Whelton PK, Carey RM, Aronow WS, et al; 2017 ACC/AHA/ AAPA/ABC/ ACPM/AGS/APhA/ASH/ASPC/NMA/PCNA Guideline for the Prevention, Detection, Evaluation, and Management of High Blood Pressure in Adults: A Report of the American College of Cardiology/American Heart Association Task Force on Clinical Practice Guidelines. *J Am Coll Cardiol*. 2018;71:e127–e248.

3. Safavi M, Honarmand A, Amoushahi M. Prediction of difficult laryngoscopy: Extended mallampati score versus the MMT, ULBT and RHTMD. *Adv Biomed Res*. 2014;3:133.

Answer Key for Chapter Review Questions

CHAPTER 1

1. D
2. B
3. B
4. C
5. A
6. A
7. C
8. A
9. A & C
10. D
11. C
12. B

CHAPTER 2

1. B
2. B
3. B
4. D
5. C
6. A
7. C
8. A
9. D
10. B
11. D
12. C
13. B
14. A
15. B

CHAPTER 3

1. D
2. B
3. A
4. A
5. B
6. D
7. A
8. C
9. D

10. B
11. D
12. C

CHAPTER 4

1. B
2. D
3. A
4. B
5. C
6. D
7. B
8. B
9. D
10. C
11. D
12. B

CHAPTER 5

1. A
2. B
3. A
4. D
5. D
6. A
7. C
8. D
9. D
10. B
11. A
12. C

CHAPTER 6

1. A
2. A
3. C
4. C
5. A
6. D
7. A
8. C

9. B
10. B
11. D
12. B

CHAPTER 7

1. D
2. D
3. C
4. C
5. B
6. B
7. C
8. C
9. D
10. D
11. B
12. B

CHAPTER 8

1. B
2. D
3. D
4. C
5. B
6. B
7. C
8. A
9. A
10. D
11. B
12. B

CHAPTER 9

1. C
2. D
3. A
4. B
5. C
6. C
7. A
8. B
9. C
10. B
11. D
12. D

CHAPTER 10

1. D
2. D
3. A

4. B
5. A
6. A
7. B
8. B
9. B
10. D
11. C
12. C

CHAPTER 11

1. D
2. C
3. A
4. A
5. C
6. B
7. A
8. B
9. C
10. D
11. D
12. D

CHAPTER 12

1. A
2. C
3. D
4. B
5. A
6. B
7. C
8. D
9. D
10. B
11. A
12. A

CHAPTER 13

1. C
2. D
3. C
4. D
5. B
6. A
7. A
8. C
9. A
10. C
11. A
12. D

ASA Practice Guidelines for Moderate Procedural Sedation and Analgesia 2018[a]

UPDATE HIGHLIGHTS

In October 2014, the American Society of Anesthesiologists Committee on Standards and Practice Parameters recommended that new practice guidelines addressing moderate procedural sedation and analgesia be developed. These new guidelines:

- Replace the "Practice Guidelines for Sedation and Analgesia by Non-Anesthesiologists: An Updated Report by the American Society of Anesthesiologists Task Force on Sedation and Analgesia by Non-Anesthesiologists," published in 2002.[b]
- Specifically address moderate sedation. They do not address mild or deep sedation and do not address the educational, training, or certification requirements for providers of moderate procedural sedation. (Separate Practice Guidelines are under development that will address deep procedural sedation.)
- Differ from previous guidelines in that they were developed by a multidisciplinary task force of physicians from several medical and dental specialty organizations with the intent of specifically addressing moderate procedural sedation provided by any medical specialty in any location.

New recommendations include:

- Patient evaluation and preparation
- Continual monitoring of ventilatory function with capnography to supplement standard monitoring by observation and pulse oximetry
- The presence of an individual in the procedure room with the knowledge and skills to recognize and treat airway complications
- Sedatives and analgesics not intended for general anesthesia (e.g., benzodiazepines and dexmedetomidine)
- Sedatives and analgesics intended for general anesthesia (e.g., propofol, ketamine and etomidate)
- Recovery care
- Creation and implementation of quality improvement processes.

SUMMARY OF RECOMMENDATIONS

Patient Evaluation

- Review previous medical records and interview the patient or family to identify:
  - Abnormalities of the major organ systems (e.g., cardiac, renal, pulmonary, neurologic, sleep apnea, metabolic, endocrine)
  - Adverse experience with sedation/analgesia, as well as regional and general anesthesia
  - History of a difficult airway
  - Current medications, potential drug interactions, drug allergies, and nutraceuticals
  - History of tobacco, alcohol or substance use or abuse
  - Frequent or repeated exposure to sedation/analgesic agents
- Conduct a focused physical examination of the patient (e.g., vital signs, auscultation of the heart and lungs, evaluation of the airway, and when appropriate to sedation, other organ systems in which major abnormalities have been identified.)
- Review available laboratory test results.
  - Order additional laboratory tests guided by a patient's medical condition, physical examination, and the likelihood that the results will affect the management of moderate sedation/analgesia.
  - Evaluate results of these tests before sedation is initiated.
- If possible, perform the preprocedure evaluation well enough in advance (e.g., several days to weeks) to allow for optimal patient preparation.[a]
- Reevaluate the patient immediately before the procedure.

Preprocedure Patient Preparation

- Consult with a medical specialist (e.g., physician anesthesiologist, cardiologist, endocrinologist, pulmonologist, nephrologist, pediatrician, obstetrician, or otolaryngologist),

---

[a]Practice Guidelines for Moderate Procedural Sedation and Analgesia 2018: A Report by the American Society of Anesthesiologists Task Force on Moderate Procedural Sedation and Analgesia, the American Association of Oral and Maxillofacial Surgeons, American College of Radiology, American Dental Association, American Society of Dentist Anesthesiologists, and Society of Interventional Radiology. Anesthesiology 2018;128(3):437–479.

[b]American Society of Anesthesiologists: Practice guidelines for sedation and analgesia by non-anesthesiologists: An updated report. Anesthesiology. 2002; 96:1004–1017.

[a]This may not be feasible for urgent or emergency procedures, interventional radiology or other radiology settings.

when appropriate before the administration of moderate procedural sedation to patients with significant underlying conditions.

- If a specialist is needed, select a specialist based on the nature of the underlying condition and the urgency of the situation.
- For severely compromised or medically unstable patients (e.g., ASA status IV, anticipated difficult airway, severe obstructive pulmonary disease, coronary artery disease, or congestive heart failure) or if it is likely that sedation to the point of unresponsiveness will be necessary to obtain adequate conditions, consult with a physician anesthesiologist.

- Before the procedure, inform patients or legal guardians of the benefits, risks, and limitations of moderate sedation/analgesia and possible alternatives, and elicit their preferences.[a]
- Inform patients or legal guardians before the day of the procedure that they should not drink fluids or eat solid foods for a sufficient period of time to allow for gastric emptying before the procedure.[b]
- On the day of the procedure, assess the time and nature of last oral intake
  - Evaluate the risk of pulmonary aspiration of gastric contents when determining (1) the target level of sedation and (2) whether the procedure should be delayed.
- In urgent or emergent situations where complete gastric emptying is not possible, do not delay moderate procedural sedation based on fasting time alone.

Patient Monitoring

Monitoring Patient Level of Consciousness

- Periodically (e.g., at 5-min intervals) monitor a patient's response to verbal commands during moderate sedation, except in patients who are unable to respond appropriately (e.g., patients where age or development may impair bidirectional communication) or during procedures where movement could be detrimental.
- During procedures where a verbal response is not possible (e.g., oral surgery, restorative dentistry, upper endoscopy), check the patient's ability to give a "thumbs up" or other indication of consciousness in response to verbal or tactile (light tap) stimulation; this suggests that the patient will be able to control his airway and take deep breaths if necessary.[c]

Monitoring Patient Ventilation and Oxygenation

- Continually[a] monitor ventilatory function by observation of qualitative clinical signs.
- Continually monitor ventilatory function with capnography unless precluded or invalidated by the nature of the patient, procedure, or equipment.
  - For uncooperative patients, institute capnography after moderate sedation has been achieved.
- Continuously monitor all patients by pulse oximetry with appropriate alarms.

Monitoring Hemodynamics

- Determine blood pressure before sedation/analgesia is initiated unless precluded by lack of patient cooperation.
- Once moderate sedation/analgesia is established, continually monitor blood pressure (e.g., at 5-min intervals) and heart rate during the procedure unless such monitoring interferes with the procedure (e.g., magnetic resonance imaging where stimulation from the blood pressure cuff could arouse an appropriately sedated patient).
- Use electrocardiographic monitoring during moderate sedation in patients with clinically significant cardiovascular disease or those who are undergoing procedures where dysrhythmias are anticipated.

Contemporaneous Recording of Monitored Parameters

- Record patients' level of consciousness, ventilatory and oxygenation status, and hemodynamic variables at a frequency that depends on the type and amount of medication administered, the length of the procedure, and the general condition of the patient.
  - At a minimum, this should occur: (1) before the administration of sedative/analgesic agents[b], (2) after administration of sedative/analgesic agents, (3) at regular intervals during the procedure, (4) during initial recovery, and (5) just before discharge.
- Set device alarms to alert care team to critical changes in patient status.

Availability of An Individual Responsible for Patient Monitoring

- Ensure that a designated individual other than the practitioner performing the procedure is present to monitor the patient throughout the procedure.

---

[a]This may not be feasible for urgent or emergency procedures.

[b]See American Society of Anesthesiologists: Practice guidelines for preoperative fasting and the use of pharmacologic agents to reduce the risk of pulmonary aspiration: Application to healthy patients undergoing elective procedures: An updated report. Anesthesiology. 2017; 126:376–393.

[c]A response limited to reflex withdrawal from a painful stimulus is not considered a purposeful response and thus represents a state of general anesthesia.

---

[a]The term "continual" is defined as "repeated regularly and frequently in steady rapid succession" whereas "continuous" means "prolonged without any interruption at any time" (see Standards for Basic Anesthetic Monitoring, American Society of Anesthesiologists. Approved by the ASA House of Delegates October 21, 1986, and last amended October 28, 2015. http://www.asahq.org/quality-and-practice-management/standards-andguidelines/search?)q=basic anesthesia monitoring.

[b]For rare uncooperative patients (e.g., children with autism spectrum disorder or attention-deficit disorder) recording oxygenation status or blood pressure may not be possible until after sedation.

○ The individual responsible for monitoring the patient should be trained in the recognition of apnea and airway obstruction and be authorized to seek additional help.

○ The designated individual may assist with minor, interruptible tasks once the patient's level of sedation/analgesia and vital signs have stabilized, provided that adequate monitoring for the patient's level of sedation is maintained.

Supplemental Oxygen

- Use supplemental oxygen during moderate procedural sedation/analgesia unless specifically contraindicated for a particular patient or procedure.

Emergency Support

- Assure that pharmacologic antagonists for benzodiazepines and opioids are immediately available in the procedure suite or procedure room.[a]
- Assure that an individual is present in the room who understands the pharmacology of the sedatives/analgesics administered (e.g., opioids and benzodiazepines) and potential interactions with other medications and nutraceuticals the patient may be taking.
- appropriately sized equipment for establishing a patent airway is available.
- at least one individual capable of establishing a patent airway and providing positive pressure ventilation is present in the procedure room.
- suction, advanced airway equipment, a positive-pressure ventilation device, and supplemental oxygen are immediately available in the procedure room and are in good working order.
  ○ a member of the procedural team is trained in the recognition and treatment of airway complications (e.g., apnea, laryngospasm, airway obstruction), opening the airway, suctioning secretions, and performing bag-valve-mask ventilation.
- a member of the procedural team has the skills to establish intravascular access.
- a member of the procedural team has the skills to provide chest compressions.
- a functional defibrillator or automatic external defibrillator is immediately available in the procedure area.
- an individual or service (e.g., code blue team, paramedic-staffed ambulance service) with advanced life support skills (e.g., tracheal intubation, defibrillation, resuscitation medications) is immediately available.
- members of the procedural team are able to recognize the need for additional support and know how to access emergency services from the procedure room (e.g., telephone, call button).

Sedative or Analgesic Medications Not Intended for General Anesthesia

- Combinations of sedative and analgesic agents may be administered as appropriate for the procedure and the condition of the patient.[a]
  ○ Administer each component individually to achieve the desired effect (e.g., additional analgesic medication to relieve pain; additional sedative medication to decrease awareness or anxiety.)
- Dexmedetomidine may be administered as an alternative to benzodiazepine sedatives on a case-by-case basis.
- In a patient receiving intravenous medications for sedation/analgesia, maintain vascular access throughout the procedure and until the patient is no longer at risk for cardiorespiratory depression.
- In patients who have received sedation/analgesia by non-intravenous routes or whose intravenous line has become dislodged or blocked, determine the advisability of reestablishing intravenous access on a case-by-case basis.
- Administer intravenous sedative/analgesic drugs in small, incremental doses, or by infusion, titrating to the desired endpoints.
  ○ Allow sufficient time to elapse between doses so the peak effect of each dose can be assessed before subsequent drug administration.
- When drugs are administered by nonintravenous routes (e.g., oral, rectal, intramuscular, transmucosal), allow sufficient time for absorption and peak effect of the previous dose to occur before supplementation is considered.

Sedative/Analgesic Medications Intended for General Anesthesia

- When moderate procedural sedation with sedative/analgesic medications for general anesthesia by any route is intended, provide care consistent with that required for general anesthesia.
- Assure that practitioners administering sedative/analgesic medications intended for general anesthesia are able to reliably identify and rescue patients from unintended deep sedation or general anesthesia.
- For patients receiving intravenous sedatives/analgesics intended for general anesthesia, maintain vascular access throughout the procedure and until the patient is no longer at risk for cardiorespiratory depression.
- In patients who have received sedative/analgesic medications intended for general anesthesia by nonintravenous routes or whose intravenous line has become dislodged

---

[a]"Immediately available in the procedure room" refers to accessible shelving, unlocked cabinetry, and other measures to ensure that there is no delay in accessing medications and equipment during the procedure.

[a]The propensity for combinations of sedative and analgesic agents to cause respiratory depression and airway obstruction emphasizes the need to appropriately reduce the dose of each component as well as the need to (continually) monitor respiratory function. Knowledge of each drug's time of onset, peak response, and duration of action is important. Titration of drug to effect is an important concept; one must know whether the previous dose has taken to full effect before administering additional drug.

or blocked, determine the advisability of reestablishing intravenous access on a case-by-case basis.

- Administer intravenous sedative/analgesic medications intended for general anesthesia in small, incremental doses, or by infusion, titrating to the desired endpoints.
  - Allow sufficient time to elapse between doses so the peak effect of each dose can be assessed before subsequent drug administration.
- When drugs intended for general anesthesia are administered by nonintravenous routes (e.g., oral, rectal, intramuscular, transmucosal), allow sufficient time for absorption and peak effect of the previous dose to occur before supplementation is considered.

Reversal Agents

- Assure that specific antagonists are immediately available in the procedure room whenever opioid analgesics or benzodiazepines are administered for moderate procedural sedation/analgesia, regardless of route of administration.
- If patients develop hypoxemia, significant hypoventilation or apnea during sedation/analgesia: (1) encourage or physically stimulate patients to breathe deeply, (2) administer supplemental oxygen, and (3) provide positive-pressure ventilation if spontaneous ventilation is inadequate.
- Use reversal agents in cases where airway control, spontaneous ventilation, or positive-pressure ventilation is inadequate.
  - Administer naloxone to reverse opioid-induced sedation and respiratory depression.[a]
  - Administer flumazenil to reverse benzodiazepine-induced sedation and respiratory depression.
- After pharmacologic reversal, observe and monitor patients for a sufficient time to ensure that sedation and cardiorespiratory depression does not recur once the effect of the antagonist dissipates.
- Do not use sedation regimens that are intended to include routine reversal of sedative or analgesic agents.

Recovery Care

- After sedation/analgesia, observe and monitor patients in an appropriately staffed and equipped area until they are near their baseline level of consciousness and are no longer at increased risk for cardiorespiratory depression.
- Monitor oxygenation continuously until patients are no longer at risk for hypoxemia.
- Monitor ventilation and circulation at regular intervals (e.g., every 5 to 15 min) until patients are suitable for discharge.
- Design discharge criteria to minimize the risk of central nervous system or cardiorespiratory depression after discharge from observation by trained personnel.

Creation and Implementation of Patient Safety Processes

- Create and implement a quality improvement process based upon established national, regional, or institutional reporting protocols (e.g., adverse events, unsatisfactory sedation).
  - Periodically update the quality improvement process to keep up with new technology, equipment, or other advances in moderate procedural sedation/analgesia.
- Strengthen patient safety culture through collaborative practices (e.g., team training, simulation drills, development and implementation of checklists).
- Create an emergency response plan (e.g., activating "code blue" team or activating the emergency medical response system: 911 or equivalent).

Adapted from Practice Guidelines for Moderate Procedural Sedation and Analgesia 2018: A Report by the American Society of Anesthesiologists Task Force on Moderate Procedural Sedation and Analgesia, the American Association of Oral and Maxillofacial Surgeons, American College of Radiology, American Dental Association, American Society of Dentist Anesthesiologists, and Society of Interventional Radiology. Anesthesiology. 2018;128(3):437–479.

---

[a]Practitioners are cautioned that acute reversal of opioid-induced analgesia may result in pain, hypertension, tachycardia, or pulmonary edema.

AORN Competency Verification Tool—Moderate Sedation and Analgesia, Care of the Patient Receiving—RN

[Sample Facility Name]

Name: _____   Date: _____

Competency Statement: The perioperative RN has completed facility or health care organization–required education and competency verification activities related to care of the patient receiving moderate sedation and analgesia.[a]

Outcome Statement:
- The patient receives correctly administered medication(s).[b]
- The patient's respiratory status is maintained or improved from baseline levels.[c]
- The patient's cardiac status is maintained or improved from baseline levels.[d]
- The patient demonstrates or reports adequate pain control.[e]

Competency Statements and Performance Criteria	Verification Method [Select applicable code from legend at bottom of page.]						Not Met (explain why)
	DEM/ DO/DA	KAT	S/SBT/ CS	V	RWM/ P&P	O	
Patient Assessment							
1. Recognizes that the patient's suitability for moderate sedation and analgesia is determined based on selection criteria established by an interdisciplinary team.							
2. Performs a nursing assessment before administering moderate sedation that includes a review of the patient's:							
a. Consent explaining the risks, benefits, and alternatives to sedation							
b. Medical history							
c. Age, height, weight, and BMI (body mass index)							
d. Pregnancy test results, when applicable							
e. Current medications (prescribed, over-the-counter, alternative or complementary therapies, supplements), dosage, last dose, and frequency							
f. Drug use (e.g., marijuana, street drugs, nonprescribed prescription drugs)							
g. Tobacco and alcohol use							
h. Laboratory test results							
i. Diagnostic test results							
j. Baseline cardiac status (e.g., heart rate, blood pressure)							
k. Baseline respiratory status (e.g., rate, rhythm, blood oxygen level [SpO$_2$])							

DEM/DO/DA = Demonstration/Documentation/Documentation Audit
S/SBT/CS = Skills Laboratory/Scenario-based Training/Controlled Simulation
RWM/P&P = Review of Written or Visual Materials/Policy/Procedure Review (Specify P&P #s _____)

KAT = Knowledge Assessment Test
V = Verbalization
O = Other: _____

[a] Guideline for care of the patient receiving moderate sedation. In: Association of periOperative Registered Nurses (AORN). Guidelines for Perioperative Practice. Denver: AORN; 2016:617–648.
[b] Petersen C, ed. Medication administration. In: Perioperative Nursing Data Set. 3rd ed. Denver: AORN;2011:203–210.
[c] Petersen C, ed. Respiratory status. In: Perioperative Nursing Data Set. 3rd ed. Denver: AORN;2011:294–300.
[d] Petersen C, ed. Cardiac status. In: Perioperative Nursing Data Set. 3rd ed. Denver: AORN; 2011:301–307.
[e] Petersen C, ed. Pain control. In: Perioperative Nursing Data Set. 3rd ed. Denver: AORN; 2011:308–311.

Competency Statements and Performance Criteria	Verification Method [Select applicable code from legend at bottom of page.]						Not Met (explain why)
	DEM/ DO/DA	KAT	S/SBT/ CS	V	RWM/ P&P	O	
l. Allergies and sensitivities (e.g., medications, latex, chemical agents, foods, adhesives, tapes)							
m. NPO status							
n. Ability to tolerate and maintain the required position for the duration of the planned procedure							
o. Need for IV access							
p. Previous adverse experiences with moderate sedation including: • Delayed emergence from anesthesia or sedation • Postprocedure nausea and vomiting • Adverse effects from anesthetic or sedative medications • Airway or breathing problems							
q. Sensory impairment (e.g., visual, auditory)							
r. Level of anxiety							
s. Level of pain							
t. Arrangement for a responsible adult caregiver to escort patient home							
3. Uses the American Society of Anesthesiologists (ASA) Physical Status Classification to determine patient acuity							
4. Identifies patients who are classified as ASA I, ASA II, and medically stable ASA III as appropriate for RN-administered moderate sedation and analgesia							
5. Assesses the patient for characteristics that may indicate difficulty with mask ventilation, including the following:							
a. Age > 55 years							
b. BMI $\geq$ 30 kg/m^2							
c. Missing teeth							
d. Presence of a beard							
e. Short neck							
f. Limited neck extension							
g. Small mouth opening							
h. Jaw abnormalities							
i. Large tongue							
j. Nonvisible uvula							

DEM/DO/DA = Demonstration/Documentation/Documentation Audit
S/SBT/CS   = Skills Laboratory/Scenario-based Training/Controlled Simulation
RWM/P&P = Review of Written or Visual Materials/Policy/Procedure Review (Specify P&P #s _____)

KAT = Knowledge Assessment Test
V   = Verbalization
O   = Other: _____

Competency Statements and Performance Criteria	Verification Method [Select applicable code from legend at bottom of page.]						Not Met (explain why)
	DEM/ DO/DA	KAT	S/SBT/ CS	V	RWM/ P&P	O	
k. History of snoring, stridor, or sleep apnea							
l. History of problems with anesthesia or sedation							
m. Advanced rheumatoid arthritis							
n. Chromosomal abnormality (e.g., trisomy 21)							
o. Tonsillar hypertrophy							
6. Assesses the patient for obstructive sleep apnea using a sleep apnea assessment screening tool							
7. Screens pediatric patients for obstructive sleep apnea; recognizes that screening criteria may include: a. Weight > 95th percentile for age and gender							
b. Intermittent vocalization during sleep							
c. Parental report of restless sleep, difficulty breathing, struggling respiratory effort during sleep							
d. Night terrors							
e. Unusual sleep positions							
f. New onset of enuresis							
g. Somnolence (e.g., appears sleepy during the day, is difficult to arouse at usual awakening time)							
h. Easily distracted							
i. Overly aggressive							
j. Irritability							
k. Difficulty concentrating							
8. Consults with an anesthesia professional if the patient presents with a history of obstructive sleep apnea							
9. Implements additional precautions (e.g., noninvasive positive pressure ventilation with continuous positive airway pressure [CPAP] or bilevel positive airway pressure, careful titration of opioids, nonopioid analgesia techniques, multimodal pain management) for a patient with sleep apnea who will undergo moderate sedation							
10. Consults with an anesthesia professional and develops a perioperative plan of care if the patient presents with any of the following: a. Known history of respiratory or hemodynamic instability							

DEM/DO/DA = Demonstration/Documentation/Documentation Audit
S/SBT/CS = Skills Laboratory/Scenario-based Training/Controlled Simulation
RWM/P&P = Review of Written or Visual Materials/Policy/Procedure Review (Specify P&P #s _____)

KAT = Knowledge Assessment Test
V   = Verbalization
O   = Other: _____

Competency Statements and Performance Criteria	Verification Method [Select applicable code from legend at bottom of page.]						Not Met (explain why)
	DEM/ DO/DA	KAT	S/SBT/ CS	V	RWM/ P&P	O	
b. History of coagulation abnormality							
c. History of neurologic or cardiac disease that may be affected by medications administered for moderate sedation and analgesia							
d. Previous difficulties with anesthesia or sedation							
e. Severe sleep apnea or other airway-related issues							
f. One or more significant comorbidities							
g. Pregnancy							
h. Inability to communicate (e.g., aphasic)							
i. Inability to cooperate							
j. Multiple drug allergies							
k. Multiple medications with potential for drug interaction with sedative analgesics							
l. Current substance use (e.g., street drugs, herbal supplements, nonprescribed prescription drugs)							
m. ASA physical classification of unstable ASA III, or							
n. ASA physical classification of ASA IV or above							
Patient Monitoring							
11. Collaborates with licensed independent practitioner (e.g., physician, podiatrist, dentist) in developing and documenting the sedation and analgesia plan of care that includes the following: a. Medications and route of administration							
b. Predetermined depth of sedation to complete the procedure							
c. Length of the procedure and sedation							
d. Recovery time							
12. Recognizes that the perioperative RN monitors the patient and administers medications under the direct supervision of a licensed independent practitioner							
13. Recognizes that the supervising licensed independent practitioner is to be physically present and immediately available in the procedure suite for diagnosis, treatment, and management of complications while the patient is sedated							

DEM/DO/DA = Demonstration/Documentation/Documentation Audit
S/SBT/CS = Skills Laboratory/Scenario-based Training/Controlled Simulation
RWM/P&P = Review of Written or Visual Materials/Policy/Procedure Review (Specify P&P #s _____)

KAT = Knowledge Assessment Test
V = Verbalization
O = Other: _____

Competency Statements and Performance Criteria	Verification Method [Select applicable code from legend at bottom of page.]						Not Met (explain why)
	DEM/ DO/DA	KAT	S/SBT/ CS	V	RWM/ P&P	O	
14. Verbalizes the location of emergency resuscitation equipment and supplies and recognizes that emergency resuscitation equipment and supplies are to be immediately available in every location in which moderate sedation is administered							
15. Verbalizes the location of oxygen sources and recognizes that supplemental oxygen is to be immediately available for the patient receiving moderate sedation and analgesia							
16. Identifies opioid antagonists (i.e., naloxone) and benzodiazepine antagonists (i.e., flumazenil) and recognizes they are to be readily available whenever opioids and benzodiazepines are administered							
17. Verifies that emergency equipment and supplies are age- and size-appropriate							
18. Administers moderate sedation and analgesia within the scope of nursing practice							
19. Verbalizes the recommended dose, recommended dilution, onset, duration, effects, potential adverse reactions, drug compatibility, and contraindications for each medication used during moderate sedation							
20. Recognizes that two perioperative RNs will be assigned to care for the patient receiving moderate sedation and analgesia. One RN will administer the sedation medication and monitor the patient and the other RN will perform the circulating role							
21. Recognizes that the perioperative RN monitoring the patient is to have no competing responsibilities that would compromise continuous monitoring assessment of the patient during the administration of moderate sedation							
22. Recognizes that the perioperative RN providing moderate sedation and analgesia is to be in constant attendance with unrestricted immediate visual and physical access to the patient							
23. Recognizes that the perioperative RN caring for the patient receiving moderate sedation and analgesia may perform short interruptible tasks (e.g., opening additional sutures, tying a gown) to assist the perioperative team while remaining in the operating or procedure room							
24. Recognizes that the perioperative RN providing moderate sedation and analgesia will not perform short interruptible tasks when propofol is used and that the RN is to monitor the patient without interruption							

DEM/DO/DA = Demonstration/Documentation/Documentation Audit
S/SBT/CS = Skills Laboratory/Scenario-based Training/Controlled Simulation
RWM/P&P = Review of Written or Visual Materials/Policy/Procedure Review (Specify P&P #s _____)

KAT = Knowledge Assessment Test
V = Verbalization
O = Other: _____

Competency Statements and Performance Criteria	Verification Method [Select applicable code from legend at bottom of page.]						Not Met (explain why)
	DEM/ DO/DA	KAT	S/SBT/ CS	V	RWM/ P&P	O	
25. Monitors and documents the patient's physiologic and psychological responses, identifies nursing diagnoses based on assessment of the data, and implements the plan of care							
26. Obtains and documents baseline patient monitoring of the following:							
a. Pulse							
b. Blood pressure							
c. Respiratory rate							
d. SpO_2 by pulse oximetry							
e. End-tidal carbon dioxide by capnography							
f. Pain level							
g. Anxiety level							
h. Level of consciousness							
27. Obtains and documents intraoperative patient monitoring of the following:							
a. Cardiac rate and rhythm							
b. Blood pressure							
c. Respiratory rate							
d. SpO_2 by pulse oximetry							
e. End-tidal carbon dioxide by capnography							
f. Depth of sedation assessment							
g. Pain level							
h. Anxiety level							
i. Level of consciousness							
28. Obtains and documents postoperative patient monitoring of the following:							
a. Cardiac rate and rhythm							
b. Blood pressure							
c. Respiratory rate							
d. SpO_2 by pulse oximetry							
e. Pain level							
f. Sedation level							
g. Level of consciousness							

DEM/DO/DA = Demonstration/Documentation/Documentation Audit
S/SBT/CS   = Skills Laboratory/Scenario-based Training/Controlled Simulation
RWM/P&P   = Review of Written or Visual Materials/Policy/Procedure Review (Specify P&P #s _____)

KAT = Knowledge Assessment Test
V   = Verbalization
O   = Other: _____

Competency Statements and Performance Criteria	Verification Method [Select applicable code from legend at bottom of page.]						Not Met (explain why)
	DEM/ DO/DA	KAT	S/SBT/ CS	V	RWM/ P&P	O	
h. Intravenous line (e.g., patency, site, type of fluid)							
i. Condition of dressing and wound							
j. Type and patency of drainage tubes							
29. Verifies that monitoring equipment, oxygen source, masks and cannulas, suction source, tubing and tips, and oral and nasal airways are working correctly and are immediately available in the room where the procedure will be performed							
30. Verifies that clinical alarms are audible and set to alert for critical changes in the patient's status							
31. Verifies that the emergency resuscitation cart is immediately available in the location where moderate sedation will be administered							
32. Verifies that opioid antagonists (i.e., naloxone) and benzodiazepine antagonists (i.e., flumazenil) are readily available when administering opioids and benzodiazepines							
33. Before administering medications: a. Verifies the licensed independent practitioner's order							
b. Verifies the correct dosing parameters							
c. Identifies the patient-specific maximum dose by consulting the medication formulary, pharmacist, physician, or product information sheet or other published reference material							
34. Administers intravenous medications one at a time, in incremental doses, and titrated to desired effect (i.e., moderate sedation that enables the patient to maintain his or her protective reflexes, airway patency, and spontaneous ventilation)							
35. Adjusts doses of sedatives and analgesics when caring for an older adult, as directed by the licensed independent practitioner							
36. Allows sufficient time for drug absorption and onset before considering additional medications when administering medications by a nonintravenous route (e.g., oral, rectal, intramuscular, intranasal, transmucosal)							
37. Assesses the patient's level of consciousness by evaluating the patient's ability to respond purposefully to verbal commands, either alone or with light tactile stimulation							
38. Assesses and documents the depth of sedation using the [facility-specific objective scale]							

DEM/DO/DA = Demonstration/Documentation/Documentation Audit
S/SBT/CS   = Skills Laboratory/Scenario-based Training/Controlled Simulation
RWM/P&P = Review of Written or Visual Materials/Policy/Procedure Review (Specify P&P #s _____)

KAT = Knowledge Assessment Test
V   = Verbalization
O   = Other: _____

Competency Statements and Performance Criteria	Verification Method [Select applicable code from legend at bottom of page.]						Not Met (explain why)
	DEM/ DO/DA	KAT	S/SBT/ CS	V	RWM/ P&P	O	
39. Determines the necessity, method, and flow rate of oxygen administration under the direction of the supervising licensed independent practitioner based on the patient's optimal level of oxygen saturation as measured with pulse oximetry							
40. Documents the moderate sedation and analgesia medications administered, including the following:							
a. Medication							
b. Strength							
c. Total amount administered							
d. Route							
e. Time							
f. Patient response							
g. Adverse reactions							
Patient Discharge							
41. Recognizes that medical supervision of patient recovery and discharge after moderate sedation and analgesia is the responsibility of the operating practitioner or licensed independent practitioner							
42. Recognizes that a qualified provider defined by **[facility-specific policy]** will be available in the facility to discharge the patient in accordance with established discharge criteria							
43. Recognizes that discharge criteria are established by a multidisciplinary team							
44. Evaluates the patient for discharge readiness based on established discharge criteria that includes the following:							
a. Return to baseline mental status (e.g., alert and oriented)							
b. Stable vital signs							
c. Sufficient time interval (e.g., 2 hours) since the last administration of an antagonist (e.g., naloxone, flumazenil)							
d. Use of an objective patient assessment discharge scoring system (e.g., Aldrete Recovery Score, Post-Anesthetic Discharge Scoring System)							
e. Absence of protracted nausea							
f. Intact protective reflexes							
g. Adequate pain control							
h. Return of motor and sensory control							
i. Ability to remain awake for at least 20 minutes							

DEM/DO/DA = Demonstration/Documentation/Documentation Audit
S/SBT/CS   = Skills Laboratory/Scenario-based Training/Controlled Simulation
RWM/P&P   = Review of Written or Visual Materials/Policy/Procedure Review (Specify P&P #s _____)

KAT = Knowledge Assessment Test
V   = Verbalization
O   = Other: _____

Verification Method
[Select applicable code from legend at bottom of page.]

Competency Statements and Performance Criteria	DEM/DO/DA	KAT	S/SBT/CS	V	RWM/P&P	O	Not Met (explain why)
j. Arrangement for safe transport from the facility							
45. Evaluates the need for delaying discharge when the patient:							
a. Has obstructive sleep apnea							
b. Receives morphine							
c. Receives dexmedetomidine							
d. Receives an antagonist or							
e. Experiences postoperative nausea and vomiting							
46. Evaluates the need for prolonged pediatric patient discharge when:							
a. The child receives a medication with a long half-life (e.g., chloral hydrate) and							
b. Only one responsible adult is accompanying a child recovering from moderate sedation and analgesia							
47. Provides additional discharge instruction for the adult responsible for care of an infant or toddler riding home in a car seat, including the need for the following:							
a. Careful observation of the child's position to avoid airway obstruction							
b. Care by two responsible adults (i.e., driver and observer)							
48. Verifies that the patient or a responsible adult is able to verbalize an understanding of the discharge instructions							
49. Gives the patient and his or her caregiver verbal and written discharge instructions							
50. Places a copy of the written discharge instructions in the patient's medical record							
51. Documents care of the patient receiving moderate sedation and analgesia accurately, completely, and legibly according to facility or health care organization policies and procedures throughout the continuum of care							
52. Verbalizes a review of facility or health care organization policies and procedures related to care of the patient receiving moderate sedation and analgesia							
53. Participates in assigned quality improvement activities related to care of the patient receiving moderate sedation and analgesia							

Concurrent competency verification of the following is recommended

- [Additional competencies related to care of the patient receiving moderate sedation and analgesia as determined by the facility or health care organization]

DEM/DO/DA = Demonstration/Documentation/Documentation Audit
S/SBT/CS   = Skills Laboratory/Scenario-based Training/Controlled Simulation
RWM/P&P = Review of Written or Visual Materials/Policy/Procedure Review (Specify P&P #s _____)

KAT = Knowledge Assessment Test
V   = Verbalization
O   = Other: _____

AANA Latex Allergy Management Guidelines[a]

OVERVIEW

Definition of Latex Allergy

In recent years, natural rubber latex (NRL or latex) allergy has been recognized as a significant problem for both patients and healthcare employees.[1] Latex allergy is an IgE-mediated (immunologic) reaction to the proteins present in NRL that come from the milky fluid of the Brazilian rubber tree, *Hevea Brasiliensis*.[2] Many medical or dental supplies and devices, such as latex gloves, syringes, and catheters, are manufactured from NRL, and can trigger allergies in some individuals. Such allergic reactions typically manifest in the form of redness or itching and can progress to more severe symptoms, such as asthma and anaphylaxis.[2,3] Although there is no cure for latex allergy, prompt diagnosis and management can significantly minimize the risk of this serious reaction.[2]

Groups at Risk for Latex Allergy

While the general population has a low incidence of latex allergy, ranging from 1.0% to 6.7%, certain groups remain at high risk. These groups include **healthcare workers** who frequently wear latex gloves (8-16%) and **children with spina bifida, spinal cord trauma, and urogenital malformations** who may have had repeated exposure to latex products because of multiple surgeries (24-64%).[4] Other groups at risk for latex allergy include:

- Workers with occupational exposure to latex (e.g., hairdressers, latex glove manufacturers or housekeeping personnel).[5]
- Patients with a history of asthma, dermatitis or eczema.[5]
- Patients exposed to repeated bladder catheterization as a result of spinal cord trauma or neurogenic bladder.
- Patients with food allergy, especially to bananas, avocados, kiwi, or chestnuts.[1,6]
- Patients with a history of anaphylaxis of uncertain etiology, especially during past surgeries, hospitalization or dental visits.[1,7]

---

[a]Developed in 1993 by the Infection and Environmental Control Task Force.
Revised by the Occupational Safety and Hazard Committee and approved by AANA Board of Directors in 1998.
Revised as *Latex Allergy Management, Guidelines* by AANA Board of Directors in July 2014.
Reaffirmed by the AANA Board of Directors in September 2018.

- Patients with a history of multiple surgeries or medical procedures during childhood.[6]
- Female patients facing greater exposure to latex-containing products due to obstetric procedures, gynecological examinations, and contact with contraceptives.[8]

Routes of Exposure and Reactions to Latex

Latex allergy usually occurs when latex-containing products (especially **powdered gloves**) come in direct contact with the skin, mucous membranes (eyes, mouth, vagina, and rectum), or the bloodstream. The powder in gloves can absorb latex proteins and then become an airborne carrier. Individuals may develop allergic reactions through merely inhaling latex-containing dust.[1,9] Latex allergy symptoms can range from mild (e.g., redness) to severe (e.g., anaphylaxis) and are typically classified into three major types:[1,10]

- **Immediate hypersensitivity (type I)** - This is an IgE-mediated (immune) response that typically has an immediate reaction (within 5-30 minutes of initial contact). Symptoms can include urticarial, asthma, rhinitis, conjunctivitis, orbit edema, angioedema, lip edema, and anaphylaxis.
- **Delayed hypersensitivity (type IV)** - This is an immune reaction that takes place several hours after initial contact (within 6-48 hours). Common symptoms include erythema, swelling, cracking, itching, weeping, and dryness of the skin.
- **Irritant contact dermatitis** - This is a non-allergic reaction, typically occurring in frequent glove users. The reaction may appear within minutes to hours of glove contact. Symptoms may include redness, chapping, chafing, drying, and scaling and cracking. This condition may not be necessarily attributable to contact with latex, as other products (e.g., household cleaning supplies) may also be responsible for this type of skin reaction.

MANAGEMENT

Latex Allergy Management Initiative

Management of latex allergy requires identifying the problem and taking appropriate actions to protect both patients and healthcare workers. Healthcare settings should consider forming a multidisciplinary committee consisting of representatives from the medical staff, clinical staff, and ancillary departments. The committee should be responsible for developing **policies**, **procedures** and **consultation services** related to managing latex allergies. The focus of the initiative should be concentrated in four main areas:[4]

- Identifying and protecting patients at risk;
- Determining whether certain employees are at higher risk;
- Accommodating employees with allergies; and
- Educating and raising awareness among patients and employees.

All gloves used by staff in the facility need to be evaluated for effectiveness (i.e., appropriate barrier protection). Given that latex gloves are the main source of allergies, high-quality non-powdered, low protein gloves should be used as standard across all healthcare settings.[9,11-13]

Latex-Safe Environment

A latex-safe environment should be provided and appropriately managed in all healthcare facilities. Many facilities in the United States are now latex-safe. However, maintaining a latex-safe environment is not always easy as it involves considerable resources in terms of time and money. Leadership, organizational readiness for change, and continued education are equally important in creating and maintaining a latex-safe environment.[12]

Areas designated as latex-safe need to be closely supervised to ensure availability of latex-safe carts with non-latex medical products in all patient care areas.[13]

The facility should develop, maintain, and regularly update a database system that contains all latex products, their substitutes and documents cases with latex-related reactions.[13] Updated lists of non-latex products are available on the following websites: the Spina Bifida Association of America (www.sbaa.org) and American Latex Allergy Association (http://latexallergyresources.org/medical-products).

Healthcare professionals working or volunteering in developing countries need to be aware that facilities may not be latex-safe.

MANAGING HIGH RISK PATIENTS

Successful management of high risk patients (immediate hypersensitivity, type I) involves early diagnosis and emergency treatment.

1. *Pre-operative Assessment*
   All patients should be assessed for latex allergy before anesthesia. Detailed patient history is obtained to identify patients at risk, including:[1,14]
   - Patient history of latex allergy.
   - Occupation/employment history.
   - The presence of symptoms, such as itchy, swollen eyes, runny nose, and sneezing. Some people may develop asthma (symptoms may include chest tightness, wheezing, coughing and shortness of breath) after contact with latex-containing products (e.g., allergic reaction after blowing a balloon).
   - Any history of fruit allergy.
   - Spina bifida and multiple surgical procedures during childhood.

If any of the above symptoms are present, patients should be treated as if they are allergic to latex.

2. *Pre-operative Diagnostic Testing*
   A health care provider should advise his/her patient with suspected latex allergy to undergo further testing. It is especially important to rule out IgE-mediated sensitivity. In the United States, there are three different FDA-approved serum tests to detect and quantify latex-specific IgEs: CAP, ALaSTAT and HYTEC. While these tests are highly specific, their sensitivity is rather low (range 75% - 90%). Skin prick testing, on the other hand, has a high specificity (more than 90%),[1,3] however, this type of diagnostic technique may induce anaphylactic reaction in some patients and therefore, should be carried out only by trained healthcare professionals.[15]

3. *Perioperative Precautions*
   A patient with confirmed type I allergy should be advised by his/her healthcare provider to follow immediate precautions, including:
   - Be monitored by an allergist.
   - Wear latex allergy medical alert bracelet.
   - Keep an epinephrine auto-injection kit.

4. *Preparing the Operating Room*
   Facilities that are not latex-safe should prepare the operating room the night before in order to avoid the release of latex particles. Patients should receive scheduling priority in the morning. The anesthesia professionals involved in the case should be informed that the patient has a latex allergy. The patient's latex allergy also needs to be documented in case notes.[3]

5. *Treating Patients in the Operating Room*
   All items containing latex must be removed from the patient care area. Only non-latex medical supplies should be used including, but not limited to:[13]
   - Gloves
   - Catheters
   - IV equipment
   - Surgical tape
   - Tourniquets
   - Ventilation and airway equipment
   - Medication containers without latex stoppers.

   Preoperative prophylaxis of latex allergy patients with antihistamines and corticosteroids has been recommended in the past but many are moving away from this practice.[16] The rationale for not using pretreatment is that it may lessen an early immune response. This may result in anaphylaxis being the first sign of an allergic reaction.[17]
   Other considerations
   - It is unlikely that a type I hypersensitivity reaction will occur in a patient with latex allergy due to exposure to the latex contained in a syringe plunger.[18]
   - Rubber vial stoppers should be punctured once. This is the usual practice of hospital pharmacists to minimize the risk of exposing the patient to latex from this potential source. The use of stopcocks can eliminate the need to inject medications via intravenous tubing latex ports.[19]

Important: Use caution when selecting non-latex gloves. Not all substitutes can equally protect against bloodborne pathogens. Care and investigation should be taken in the selection of substitute gloves.[20]

6. *Recognizing Anaphylaxis during the Perioperative Period*
Some patients may develop anaphylaxis 30 to 60 minutes after being exposed to latex (via absorption of airborne allergens or with mucous membrane exposure) during surgery. This is a serious allergic reaction involving severe difficulty in breathing and/or a sudden drop in blood pressure.[5] Anaphylaxis often presents a diagnostic challenge during anesthesia and surgery because the symptoms may resemble other medical conditions, such as extensive sympathetic blockade. Also, anaphylaxis may be missed in patients who are draped during surgery. Incorrect diagnosis and delayed treatment of anaphylaxis can cause severe health consequences and even death.[8] Bronchospasm and cardiovascular collapse are often the first signs of an anaphylactic reaction.[5] Other symptoms are summarized in Table 1 below.[1]

Once anaphylaxis is recognized, aggressive treatment should follow immediately. Treatment usually involves the following steps:[5,21]

- Discontinue all latex-containing products suspected of causing reaction.
- Maintain airway and administer 100% oxygen.
- Discontinue anesthetic drugs if the event occurs during induction.
- Start treatment with epinephrine as soon as possible.
- Maintain fluid balance.
- Administer where appropriate H1- and H2-receptor blockers, which can help alleviate some symptoms.
- Use a corticosteroid to help prevent or control the late-phase reaction (which can occur up to 36 hours later).

MANAGING HEALTHCARE WORKERS

Healthcare workers with latex allergies may acquire a long-term disability resulting in significant individual and social costs related to health care, insurance and workers'

compensation claims.[11,22] Some healthcare workers may not want to disclose their symptoms/condition to their employer, which may worsen their reaction to latex-containing products over time.[22] Given these consequences, it is important to have preventive measures in place to protect all healthcare workers against latex allergies.

1. *Reasonable Accommodations for Employees who are Diagnosed with Latex Allergy*
Healthcare facilities should take precautions to reduce latex exposure among their employees:[15]
   - Encourage employees to report any symptoms to their immediate supervisor.
   - Advise healthcare workers with latex allergy on treatment options.

   Healthcare workers with confirmed latex allergy should follow these steps to help reduce symptoms and future exposure:[13,15,23,24]
   - Use non-latex gloves only.
   - Avoid areas where powdered latex gloves or other latex products are used and dispensed.
   - Avoid contact with latex products.
   - Wear a latex alert medical bracelet.
   - Seek treatment for allergy.
   - If possible, request to be transferred to a latex safe environment or 'safe zones' defined as areas in which non-latex products are used and latex proteins have been removed from the environment.

2. *General Recommendations Regarding Glove Use Among Healthcare Workers*
In general, healthcare workers should follow precautions to protect themselves at work. If latex gloves need to be worn for barrier protection when handling hazardous materials, healthcare workers should opt for low-protein, powder-free gloves.[20,24] In their study Korniewicz and colleagues were able to demonstrate that although the initial cost of conversion to powder-free, low-protein latex surgical gloves may be high, it can help reduce long-term healthcare costs.[11] Healthcare workers should also take special care of their hands by reducing the amount of time gloves are worn, washing hands with PH balanced soap, and avoiding oil-based hand creams and lotions that can disintegrate gloves. Special care should be exercised when putting on or removing gloves (especially avoiding letting the gloves snap), as latex proteins can be diffused into the air. Using glove liners and wearing double and triple gloves can also help reduce exposure to latex.[15,20]

CONTINUING EDUCATION

Continuing education of patients, their families, healthcare workers, and employers is an important part of management of latex allergy. Patients who are diagnosed with latex allergy and their family members should be educated about how to manage this condition and follow preventive measures to avoid future exposure.[3]

Healthcare workers should receive education and training on how to recognize the signs and symptoms of an allergic

TABLE 1 **Symptoms of anaphylaxis.**	
Awake Patients	**Anesthetized Patients**
• Itchy eyes	• Facial edema
• Generalized pruritus	• Hives (urticaria)
• Shortness of breath	• Rash
• Sneezing	• Skin flushing
• Wheezing	• Bronchospasm
• Nausea and/or vomiting	• Laryngeal edema
• Faintness	• Edema
• Abdominal cramping	• Hypotension
• Diarrhea	• Tachycardia
• Feeling of impending doom	• Cardiac arrest

reaction in patients, prevent latex exposure, and treat allergic and anaphylactic response. Healthcare workers should also be encouraged to seek guidance from their employer if they experience latex allergy symptoms.[3]

Finally, facilities need to establish policies and procedures to ensure that the setting is safe for patients and health care workers.[4]

REFERENCES

1. Demaegd J, Soetens F, Herregods L. Latex allergy: a challenge for anaesthetists. *Acta Anaesthesiol Belg.* 2006; 57(2):127–135.

2. Kumar RP. Latex allergy in clinical practice. *Indian J Dermatol.* Jan 2012; 57(1):66–70.

3. Bernardini R, Catania P, Caffarelli C, et al. Perioperative latex allergy. *Int J Immunopathol Pharmacol.* Jul-Sep 2011; 24(3 Suppl):S55–S60.

4. Elliott BA. Latex allergy: the perspective from the surgical suite. *J Allergy Clin Immunol.* Aug 2002; 110(2 Suppl):S117–S120.

5. Hollnberger H, Gruber E, Frank B. Severe anaphylactic shock without exanthema in a case of unknown latex allergy and review of the literature. *Paediatr Anaesth.* Jul 2002; 12 (6):544–551.

6. Baker L, Hourihane JO. Latex allergy: two educational cases. *Pediatr Allergy Immunol.* Sep 2008; 19(6):477–481.

7. Hudson ME. Dental surgery in pediatric patients with spina bifida and latex allergy. *AORN J.* Jul 2001; 74(1):57–63, 65–56, 69–70 passim; quiz 73–58.

8. Turillazzi E, Greco P, Neri M, Pomara C, Riezzo I, Fineschi V. Anaphylactic latex reaction during anaesthesia: the silent culprit in a fatal case. *Forensic Sci Int.* Jul 18 2008; 179(1):e5–e8.

9. Korniewicz DM, Chookaew N, Brown J, Bookhamer N, Mudd K, Bollinger ME. Impact of converting to powder-free gloves. Decreasing the symptoms of latex exposure in operating room personnel. *AAOHN J.* Mar 2005; 53(3):111–116.

10. Rose D. Latex sensitivity awareness in preoperative assessment. *Br J Perioper Nurs.* Jan 2005; 15(1):27–33.

11. Korniewicz DM, Chookaew N, El-Masri M, Mudd K, Bollinger ME. Conversion to low-protein, powder-free surgical gloves: is it worth the cost? *AAOHN J.* Sep 2005; 53(9):388–393.

12. Brown RH, McAllister MA, Gundlach AM, Hamilton RG. The final steps in converting a health care organization to a latex-safe environment. *Jt Comm J Qual Patient Saf.* Apr 2009; 35(4): 224–228.

13. Sussman G, Milton G. Guidelines for the management of latex allergies and safe latex use in health care facilities. (2010). http://www.acaai.org/allergist/allergies/Types/latex-allergy/Pages/default.aspx. Accessed April 22, 2014.

14. Floyd PT. Latex allergy update. *J Perianesth Nurs.* Feb 2000; 15 (1):26–30.

15. American Association of Nurse A. Health hazards posed by exposure to latex. *Dent Assist.* Nov-Dec 2002; 71(6):36–37.

16. Holzman RS. Clinical management of latex-allergic children. *Anesth Analg.* Sep 1997; 85(3):529–533.

17. Weiss ME, Hirshman CA. Latex allergy. *Can J Anaesth.* Jul 1992; 39(6):528–532.

18. Jones JM, Sussman GL, Beezhold DH. Latex allergen levels of injectable collagen stored in syringes with rubber plungers. *Urology.* Jun 1996; 47(6):898–902.

19. Heitz JW, Bader SO. An evidence-based approach to medication preparation for the surgical patient at risk for latex allergy: is it time to stop being stopper poppers? *J Clin Anesth.* Sep 2010; 22 (6):477–483.

20. Tanner J. Choosing the right surgical glove: an overview and update. *Br J Nurs.* Jun 26- Jul 9 2008;17(12):740-744.

21. Machado JA, da Cunha RC, de Oliveira BH, da Silva J. [Latex-induced anaphylactic reaction in a patient undergoing open appendectomy. Case report]. *Rev Bras Anestesiol.* May-Jun 2011; 61(3):360–366.

22. Bernstein DI. Management of natural rubber latex allergy. *J Allergy Clin Immunol.* Aug 2002; 110(2 Suppl):S111–S116.

23. Monduzzi G, Franco G. Practising evidence-based occupational health in individual workers: how to deal with a latex allergy problem in a health care setting. *Occup Med (Lond).* Jan 2005; 55 (1):3–6.

24. Potential for sensitization and possible allergic reaction to natural rubber latex gloves and other natural rubber products. (2008). http://www.osha.gov/dts/shib/shib012808.html. Accessed April 20, 2014.

INDEX

Note: Page numbers followed by *f* indicate figures, *t* indicate tables, and *b* indicate boxes.